EMQs and MCQs for Medical Finals

EMQs and MCQs for Medical Finals

Jonathan Bath MBBS BSc (Hons)
Resident in General Surgery
John Hopkins Hospital

Rebecca Morgan MBBS BSc (Hons)
Foundation 2 doctor
St. Thomas' Hospital

Mehool Patel MBBS MD MRCP
Consultant Physician in Stroke and Elderly Medicine
University Hospital Lewisham

Blackwell
Publishing

© 2007 Jonathan Bath, Rebecca Morgan & Mehool Patel
Published by Blackwell Publishing

Blackwell Publishing, Inc., 350 Main Street, Malden, MA 02148-5020, USA
Blackwell Publishing Ltd, 9600 Garsington Road, Oxford OX4 2DQ, UK
Blackwell Publishing Asia Pty Ltd, 550 Swanston Street, Carlton, Victoria 3053,
Australia

The right of the Author to be identified as the Author of this Work has been asserted in
accordance with the Copyright, Designs and Patents Act 1988.

First published 2007
1   2007

Library of Congress Cataloging-in-Publication Data

Bath, Jonathan.
     EMQs and MCQs for medical finals / Jonathan Bath, Rebecca Morgan, Mehool Patel.
       p. ; cm.
     ISBN 978-1-4051-5707-0 (alk. paper)
     1. Medicine—Examinations, questions, etc. I. Morgan, Rebecca. II. Patel, Mehool.
III. Title. [DNLM: 1. Medicine—Examination Questions. W 18.2 B331e 2007]

R834.5.B37 2007
610.76—dc22
                                                                              2007000350
ISBN: 978-1-4051-5707-0

A catalogue record for this title is available from the British Library

Set in 9.25/12 Meridien by Charon Tec Ltd (A Macmillan Company), Chennai, India
www.charontec.com

Printed and bound in Singapore by COS Printers Pte Ltd

Commissioning Editor: Martin Sugden
Editorial Assistant: Robin Harries
Development Editor: Hayley Salter
Production Controller: Debbie Wyer

For further information on Blackwell Publishing, visit our website:
http://www.blackwellpublishing.com

The publisher's policy is to use permanent paper from mills that operate a sustainable
forestry policy, and which has been manufactured from pulp processed using acid-free
and elementary chlorine-free practices. Furthermore, the publisher ensures that the text
paper and cover board used have met acceptable environmental accreditation standards.

Contents

Preface

Whilst studying for Finals it was hardly believable the number of textbooks, notes, lectures and other resources that were available to satiate even the most demanding of student. An unhealthy culture of panic buying was almost encouraged, such was the vast amount of information that was expected and required.

However, with such an impressive armament at our fingertips it seemed illogical that there were few avenues for those diligent (or just plain lucky) enough to have accrued sufficient knowledge to want to put it to the test. Question books often provided coverage of topics likely to be encountered in examinations but often left frustration when incorrect choices were not explained.

This question book containing detailed answers was designed to address this need for explanation of not only the correct choice, but also why the other choices were incorrect, thereby providing the reader with positive feedback based on current medical practice. With 450 questions, based across 24 commonly tested areas of medicine, surgery and subspecialities and divided into five practice examination papers covering a mixture of subjects, *EMQs and MCQs for Medical Finals* provides a comprehensive review of these topics as well as providing exposure to frequently encountered question formats to help engender familiarity with examination styles.

All questions are original and written with the memories of Finals still very much fresh in our minds. We hope this book will help alleviate some of the anxiety regarding examinations by helping to prepare students for what is undoubtedly the most challenging test of knowledge faced during one's medical career.

Jonathan Bath
Baltimore

Rebecca Morgan
London

PART **I**

Practice Papers

PAPER 1
Questions

Multiple choice questions (single best answer)

1 A 75-year-old gentleman is referred by his GP to a consultant cardiologist for management of his newly diagnosed atrial fibrillation (AF). Palpitations and occasional shortness of breath are the only symptoms he has noticed and he has no past history of cardiovascular disease, but has suffered a transient ischaemic event in the past. On examination he is found to have an irregular heart rate ranging between 70 and 90 beats per minute and ECG confirms AF. Which of the following is the most appropriate next stage in his management?

- ☐ **a.** Start digoxin for rate control.
- ☐ **b.** Warfarinise the patient to reduce the risk of thromboembolism formation.
- ☐ **c.** Start a beta blocker for associated hypertension.
- ☐ **d.** Organise an echocardiogram.
- ☐ **e.** Refer back to GP as his case can easily be managed in the community.

2 A 38-year-old gentleman attends A&E at 9 p.m. during a busy medical take. He complains of chest pain which has intermittently been present since the morning. On further questioning his pain is central in location with no radiation and some associated nausea. His father suffered with an MI at the age of 65 and his grandfather suffered from peripheral vascular disease. His troponin I is 0.05 (significant >0.1) and ECG shows no ischaemic changes. This gentleman asks you what happens next, what should you tell him?

- ☐ **a.** He needs to be admitted for further bloods tests.
- ☐ **b.** He requires an exercise tolerance test before he is discharged.
- ☐ **c.** An echo will be useful in his further management.
- ☐ **d.** He can be safely discharged without further follow-up.
- ☐ **e.** He should be started on aspirin.

3 An 84-year-old nun presented to A&E 2 weeks after discharge from hospital under the care of the cardiologists. Her presenting complaint is one of feeling faint and dizzy and intermittently short of breath. She mentions that during her last admission she was started on digoxin because she had an irregular heart rate that was racing away. On discharge she claims that she had no problems and only developed this dizziness in the past couple of days. Her drug history includes atenolol 100 mg once daily. Her ECG today shows a rate of approximately 40 beats per minute with no association between P waves and QRS complexes. What is the next step in her management?

- ☐ **a.** Insert a temporary pacing wire.
- ☐ **b.** Give regular atropine.
- ☐ **c.** Start amiodarone 200 mg tds.
- ☐ **d.** Stop atenolol.
- ☐ **e.** Take bloods including drug levels.

4 A 69-year-old man was admitted from A&E 3 days after suffering a myocardial infarction. He was complaining of increasing shortness of breath and on observation was tachypnoeic at rest whilst sitting up. On examination he had no peripheral signs of disease, his jugular venous pressure was raised, he was breathing at 30 breaths per minute and his heart rate was 120/minute. On auscultation there was evidence of a systolic murmur but no other findings. An erect chest X-ray was normal. Which of the following complications of MI is most likely to be the cause of this gentleman's shortness of breath?

- ☐ **a.** Ventricular septal defect.
- ☐ **b.** Recurrent infarction.
- ☐ **c.** Aortic regurgitation.
- ☐ **d.** Heart failure.
- ☐ **e.** Dressler's syndrome.

5 A 45-year-old teacher was referred to the cardiologists after having been admitted with shortness of breath. Her past medical history consists of inflammatory bowel disease but no cardiac problems. On examination her apex was located in the anterior axillary line in the sixth intercostal space. There were no peripheral signs of cardiovascular disease but on auscultation a fourth heart sound was audible. There were no murmurs. Bedside 2D echo showed a dilated heart with an ejection fraction of 20–25%. The likely cause of her dilated cardiomyopathy is:
- [ ] **a.** Viral.
- [ ] **b.** Alcohol.
- [ ] **c.** Outflow obstruction.
- [ ] **d.** Congenital.
- [ ] **e.** Autoimmune.

6 The most appropriate diagnostic investigation in a patient presenting with chest pain and a widened mediastinum is:
- [ ] **a.** 4 limb blood pressure measurements.
- [ ] **b.** LFT's.
- [ ] **c.** Lateral chest x-ray.
- [ ] **d.** CT chest.
- [ ] **e.** ECG.

7 A 16-year-old man presents to hospital complaining of abdominal pain, nausea and vomiting. He has been feeling unwell for the last 3 days since he 'caught a cold' from his younger sister. His past medical history is remarkable only for childhood eczema and type I diabetes mellitus. He is in pain and unable to eat or drink anything because of pain in his stomach. Urine dipstick was taken that showed protein +, ketones ++, glucose +++. Which of the following insulin regimens should this man be started on?
- [ ] **a.** Normal subcutaneous insulin with hourly blood glucose monitoring.
- [ ] **b.** Sliding scale of insulin with hourly blood glucose monitoring.
- [ ] **c.** Constant insulin infusion with hourly blood glucose monitoring.
- [ ] **d.** Change of normal insulin regimen to once daily long-acting insulin.
- [ ] **e.** Increase of normal insulin regimen to double requirements.

8 A 78-year-old woman is brought to accident and emergency from the warden-controlled accommodation where she resides. She was found in her apartment by the warden sitting on the floor and very confused. Past medical history is remarkable for pernicious anaemia, type II diabetes and vitiligo. On examination she is disorientated and scores 3/10 on the abbreviated mental test (AMT). Her abdomen feels lumpy and she is bradycardic at 50 beats a minute with a blood pressure of 152/92 and hypothermic at 34.9°C. Blood glucose was 4.1 mmol/L. Which of the following investigations is most likely to reveal the diagnosis?

☐ **a.** Thyroid function tests.
☐ **b.** Electrocardiography (ECG).
☐ **c.** CT scan of the head.
☐ **d.** Echocardiography.
☐ **e.** Short synacthen test.

9 Which of the following associations is correct?

☐ **a.** Acute glaucoma – low intraocular pressure.
☐ **b.** Conjunctivitis – conjunctival vessels do not blanch on pressure.
☐ **c.** Iritis – dilated pupil.
☐ **d.** Subconjunctival haemorrhage – hazy cornea.
☐ **e.** Acute glaucoma – fixed, dilated pupil.

10 A 53-year-old man presents to his GP with a 2-week history of headache and recent blurred vision. He has been having the headaches at more frequent intervals in the past week and describes them as a 'tight band' around his head. Fundoscopy is performed, which reveals arteriolar narrowing and cotton-wool spots. Some oedema of the optic disc is also reported. Which of the following conditions is this fundoscopic appearance consistent with?

☐ **a.** Diabetic retinopathy.
☐ **b.** Hypertensive retinopathy.
☐ **c.** Age-related macular degeneration.
☐ **d.** CMV retinitis.
☐ **e.** Ankylosing spondylitis.

11 Which area of the breast is most commonly affected by breast cancer?

☐ **a.** Upper outer quadrant.
☐ **b.** Upper inner quadrant.
☐ **c.** Lower outer quadrant.
☐ **d.** Lower inner quadrant.
☐ **e.** Retro-areolar.

12 Risk factors for breast cancer include all of the following EXCEPT:
- ☐ **a.** Nulliparity.
- ☐ **b.** Late pregnancy >30 years.
- ☐ **c.** Early menarche.
- ☐ **d.** Late menopause.
- ☐ **e.** High dietary dairy intake.

13 A 43-year-old man presents to his GP with a 1-week history of a painful swollen left knee. On examination the left knee is painful in all ranges of movement and is warm to touch. There is evidence of a boggy diffuse swelling and routine blood tests reveal a neutrophilia, raised white cell count and pyrexia. Which of the following investigations is the most important to perform?
- ☐ **a.** Blood cultures.
- ☐ **b.** Joint aspiration.
- ☐ **c.** Serum urate levels.
- ☐ **d.** MRI knee.
- ☐ **e.** Skyline views of the knee.

14 A 23-year-old man presents to hospital with back pain and trouble performing at his basketball practices. On examination the only positive findings are of a reduced range of movement in back flexion and tenderness over the left Achilles tendon. Which of the following diagnoses is correct?
- ☐ **a.** Early-onset rheumatoid arthritis.
- ☐ **b.** Left-sided prolapsed lumbar disc.
- ☐ **c.** Right-sided prolapsed lumbar disc.
- ☐ **d.** Ankylosing spondylitis.
- ☐ **e.** Facet-joint arthritis.

15 A 35-year-old man is admitted to the intensive care unit with respiratory failure secondary to a fungal chest infection. His past medical history reveals acute myelogenous leukaemia, splenomegaly and a recent bone marrow transplant. His blood results reveal neutropenia and anaemia. Which of the following should be avoided unless absolutely necessary?
- ☐ **a.** Respiratory system examination.
- ☐ **b.** Abdominal and rectal examination.
- ☐ **c.** Regular suction of nasopharyngeal secretions.
- ☐ **d.** Daily bloods taken via a central venous catheter.
- ☐ **e.** Regular turning to avoid pressure sores.

16 A 31-year-old vegan attends her GP practice complaining of fatigue. The GP is concerned about her dietary content and requests blood tests. She complains of no other symptoms and denies having heavy menses or any bleeds rectally. The GP is concerned about iron deficiency anaemia. Which of the following is not a recognised sign of iron deficiency anaemia?

- ☐ **a.** Koilonychia.
- ☐ **b.** Angular stomatitis.
- ☐ **c.** Dysphagia.
- ☐ **d.** Peripheral neuropathy.
- ☐ **e.** Tongue atrophy.

17 A 10-year-old boy presents to A&E with abdominal pain and fatigue. The onset of the pain has been acute over the past 6 hours and is generalised. On further questioning he has no previous abdominal pathology and no clinical findings on examination. A family history reveals a cousin who suffers from sickle cell disease. Which of the following clinical features is NOT consistent with a diagnosis of sickle cell disease?

- ☐ **a.** Pallor.
- ☐ **b.** Splenomegaly.
- ☐ **c.** Bone pain.
- ☐ **d.** Leg ulcers.
- ☐ **e.** Gallstones.

18 A 54-year-old man is brought to hospital by a concerned neighbour after finding him collapsed at home having taken an overdose of medication. He is assessed by the admitting house officer who elicits a history of suicidal ideation, a recent loss of appetite and lack of enjoyment of usual hobbies. The case is discussed with the duty psychiatrist who advises on further management. Which of the following statements regarding depression is NOT true?

- ☐ **a.** Endogenous depression is more easily treated than exogenous (reactive depression).
- ☐ **b.** Females are more likely to take a medication overdose as mode of suicide than males.
- ☐ **c.** Lack of a confiding relationship is associated with depression.
- ☐ **d.** Antidepressant medication takes action after approximately 2 weeks.
- ☐ **e.** Thyroid disease should always be considered in the differential diagnosis of depression.

19 A 24-year-old man is brought in to hospital by a concerned neighbour after he is found trying to break into an electronics shop as he believed the government was using the television sets to control him. He is agitated on arrival to hospital and is demands to be released saying that it is all part of the government conspiracy keeping him hostage in hospital. He is persuaded to be admitted under the on-call team, however, you are called later than night by the nurse to assess him as he was found by the hospital security trying to escape. Which of the following is the correct course of action?

- ☐ **a.** Admission to hospital under Section 3 of the Mental Health Act.
- ☐ **b.** Cuff and restraint under common law.
- ☐ **c.** Admission to hospital under Section 5(2) of the Mental Health Act.
- ☐ **d.** Documentation of discharge from hospital against medical advice.
- ☐ **e.** Discharge with community psychiatric follow-up.

20 Whilst carrying out an abdominal examination for a patient admitted with chest pain you notice a pulsatile and expansile mass in the abdomen. Upon mentioning it to the patient he confirms that he has been told in the past that he has an abdominal aortic aneurysm (AAA). He adds that he is under yearly surveillance and that it doesn't cause him any problems at present. Which of the following statements about abdominal aortic aneurysms is INCORRECT?

- ☐ **a.** More common in males than females.
- ☐ **b.** 10% have associated popliteal aneurysm.
- ☐ **c.** A diameter >4cm requires operative intervention.
- ☐ **d.** Renal failure is a known postoperative complication of AAA repair.
- ☐ **e.** There is a 5% risk of rupture when aneurysm reaches 6cm diameter.

21 A 64-year-old man presents with a urinary tract infection that has been unresponsive to a 5-day course of antibiotics started by his GP. Further questioning reveals he has suffered with problems with his chest for the last 10 years that he attributes to smoking since he was in his 20s. On examination he has a barrel-shaped chest, there is evidence of use of the accessory muscles of respiration and pursed lip breathing. Which of the following routine blood results is most likely to be found in this patient?

☐ **a.** Lymphopaenia.
☐ **b.** Anaemia.
☐ **c.** Raised MCV.
☐ **d.** Polycythaemia.
☐ **e.** Thrombocytopenia.

22 A 69-year-old man was admitted from A&E 7 days after suffering a myocardial infarction (MI). He was complaining of increasing shortness of breath and on observation was tachypnoeic at rest sitting up. On examination, he had no peripheral signs of disease, his jugular venous pressure was raised, he was breathing at 30 breaths per minute and his heart rate was 120/minute. On auscultation there was evidence of a systolic murmur but no other findings on examination. An erect chest X-ray was normal. Which of the following complications of MI is most likely to be the cause of this gentleman's shortness of breath?

☐ **a.** Ventricular septal defect.
☐ **b.** Recurrent infarction.
☐ **c.** Aortic regurgitation.
☐ **d.** Heart failure.
☐ **e.** Dressler's syndrome.

23 A 7-year-old boy is referred by his GP to the on-call surgeons. He has attended the practice complaining of lower central abdominal pain and vomiting. The pain was acute in onset almost 2 hours prior to presentation but is gradually worsening. He notes that there have been similar episodes of pain in the past which spontaneously resolved themselves. He has no recent history of foreign travel or unusual diet. His temperature is 38.0°C and denies any diarrhoea. Examination of his ears, nose, throat and chest is normal. In this case which of the following must you be sure to check?

- ☐ **a.** Rovsing's sign.
- ☐ **b.** Scrotal examination.
- ☐ **c.** Rectal examination.
- ☐ **d.** Full blood count.
- ☐ **e.** Abdominal X-ray.

24 Two hours after a football game in which a 34-year-old man was struck with the ball in the groin, he is brought to hospital with a swelling in the scrotum that has not resolved with application of an ice-pack. On examination there is a small scar in the right groin, the left testis is lying slightly higher than the right and there is a small, hard lump in the right testis. The testicular adnexae are firm but non-tender. These findings are suggestive of:

- ☐ **a.** Torsion of the hydatid of Morgagni.
- ☐ **b.** Epididymo-orchitis.
- ☐ **c.** Seminoma.
- ☐ **d.** Teratoma.
- ☐ **e.** Scrotal haematoma.

25 A 31-year-old man presents to his GP complaining of an itchy rash on his hands. On questioning he reveals that he works for a Chinese restaurant in the back of kitchen as a dishwasher. On examination of his hands there are multiple excoriated sites on the dorsum and over the fingers of both hands with cracking of the skin over an erythematous base. The most likely diagnosis is:

- ☐ **a.** Dermatitis.
- ☐ **b.** Lichen planus.
- ☐ **c.** Chemical burn.
- ☐ **d.** Porphyria cutanea tarda.
- ☐ **e.** Psoriasis.

26 A 38-year-old man presents to the dermatology clinic with intensely itchy elbows and knees. He states that this has been going on for the past 2 weeks and is interfering with his life to the point that he cannot take it any longer. Systemic enquiry reveals past episodes of malabsorption relieved by a wheat-free diet. He is not allergic to any medication and maintains a gluten-free diet. The most likely cause of his itch is:

☐ **a.** Atypical eczema.
☐ **b.** Psoriasis.
☐ **c.** Dermatitis herpetiformis.
☐ **d.** Scabies.
☐ **e.** Polycythaemia rubra vera.

27 A 14-year-old girl presents to her GP distressed and upset. She tells you that she was in a relationship with an older boy and that they had been engaging in sexual intercourse. She had recently become worried that she was pregnant as they had been having unprotected sex and an over the counter pregnancy test confirmed this. She begs you not to tell her mother and to refer her to a family planning clinic for an abortion. Which of the following is NOT the correct course of action?

☐ **a.** Referral to a family planning clinic.
☐ **b.** Counselling her about contraceptive options.
☐ **c.** Offering her a sexually transmitted infection screen.
☐ **d.** Informing her parents as she is a legal minor.
☐ **e.** Advocating her discussing the pregnancy with her parents.

28 A 33-year-old lady presents to hospital on return from a skiing holiday. She is normally fit and well and describes an incident where her ski got caught in the snow causing her to fall over during which the ski did not release from her foot. She described immediate pain in her right calf which was then alleviated by simple analgesia. Examination and X-ray at the ski resort provide very limited help in a diagnosis. You are asked to see her and make a diagnosis of a ruptured tendo Achilles. What would be your management plan?

☐ **a.** Surgical tendo Achilles repair.
☐ **b.** Above knee backslab.
☐ **c.** Below knee cast with foot in neutral position.
☐ **d.** Below knee cast with foot in equinus position.
☐ **e.** Discharge with GP follow-up.

29 In patients with tibial plateau fractures which of the following nerves is most likely to damaged as a result of the injury?
- ☐ **a.** Common peroneal nerve.
- ☐ **b.** Tibial nerve.
- ☐ **c.** Sciatic nerve.
- ☐ **d.** Femoral nerve.
- ☐ **e.** Lateral cutaneous nerve of thigh.

30 A new non-invasive test for the influenza virus is produced by a pharmaceutical company based on a study of 1340 individuals. The data is published in an infectious disease journal that you are reading in your spare time and is given in table format below:

Test	Disease	
	Positive	Negative
Positive	580	150
Negative	140	450

Which of the following statements regarding statistical aspects of the new test is correct?
- ☐ **a.** The sensitivity of the test is $(580/(580 + 140)) = 80.1\%$.
- ☐ **b.** The positive predictive value of the test is $580/(580 + 140) = 80.1\%$.
- ☐ **c.** There were 150 false negatives in the test.
- ☐ **d.** A high specificity will predict a low false negative rate.
- ☐ **e.** This test should be used as a screening test for influenza?

31 A 36-year-old multiparous woman presents to the emergency gynaecology unit after an episode of vaginal bleeding that was discovered after she was trying on some clothes in the maternity section of a department store. Further questioning reveals she is at 31 weeks' gestation, as confirmed by ultrasound scan. Her vital signs are BP 142/78, temperature 36.7°C, pulse 96/minute. Which of the following is the most likely diagnosis?
- ☐ **a.** Cervical cancer.
- ☐ **b.** Placenta praevia.
- ☐ **c.** Abruptio placentae.
- ☐ **d.** Placenta accrete.
- ☐ **e.** Chorio-amnionitis.

32 A 30-year-old primigravida who is 20 weeks pregnant contacts her midwife for advice about a painful right leg. She tells the midwife that the leg began to swell 2 days earlier and is now acutely painful to walk on. Clinically there is a discrepancy of 7 cm between the diameter of both calves. She has had no other problems during her pregnancy and there is no family history of gestational problems. What is the likely diagnosis in her case?

- ☐ **a.** Cellulitis.
- ☐ **b.** Fat embolus.
- ☐ **c.** Deep vein thrombosis.
- ☐ **d.** Ischaemic limb.
- ☐ **e.** Varicose veins.

33 A 4-year-old child is brought to his GP by his mother who is concerned about poor weight gain. He is at the 15th centile for height and weight and his past medical history includes admissions to hospital for recurrent chest infections and an episode of gastroenteritis. Developmental parameters are normal except for slightly reduced hearing in the right ear, which is slightly erythematous. Which one of the following pathologies is likely in this child?

- ☐ **a.** PAS positive macrophages on intestinal film.
- ☐ **b.** Cobblestoned appearance on barium enema.
- ☐ **c.** Single amino acid defect in a chloride channel transporter.
- ☐ **d.** Double bubble on abdominal X-ray.
- ☐ **e.** Abnormal bone marrow cytology.

34 An adolescent presents to his school doctor with bilateral tender and swollen breasts. He has become increasingly self-conscious of late and has been avoiding physical education classes. On examination there are tender soft masses in the lower quadrants of both breasts. Which of the following is the most appropriate next step in managing this patient?

- ☐ **a.** Urgent referral to social services.
- ☐ **b.** Reassure the patient that this is normal.
- ☐ **c.** Needle aspiration and send fluid for culture and cytology.
- ☐ **d.** Referral to a breast surgeon for excision and biopsy.
- ☐ **e.** Short course of oral prednisolone and 2-week review.

35 A 33-year-old gentleman presents with upper abdominal pain and vomiting. Blood tests demonstrate a raised white cell count and an amylase of 300 IU/L. Of the following differentials, which is the LEAST likely to be correct?

- ☐ **a.** Pancreatitis.
- ☐ **b.** Perforated duodenal ulcer.
- ☐ **c.** Ruptured abdominal aortic aneurysm.
- ☐ **d.** Transverse colon diverticulitis.
- ☐ **e.** Diabetic ketoacidosis.

36 Regarding clinical signs of abdominal disease, which of the following is associated with bowel perforation?

- ☐ **a.** Rovsing's sign.
- ☐ **b.** Murphy's sign.
- ☐ **c.** Rigler's sign.
- ☐ **d.** Kerr's sign.
- ☐ **e.** Trousseau's sign.

37 A 55-year-old woman is 2 days post-fenestration of liver cysts. She is complaining of pain in the abdomen, nausea and malaise. Routine blood tests taken post-operatively show a bilirubin of 135 μmol/L, γ-GT of 210 IU/L, AST of 150 IU/L with a slightly elevated WCC. Which of the following is the most likely explanation?

- ☐ **a.** Biliary sepsis.
- ☐ **b.** Propofol hepatotoxicity.
- ☐ **c.** Common bile duct ligation.
- ☐ **d.** Bile leak.
- ☐ **e.** Cholecystitis.

38 A 65-year-old obese woman underwent an open cholecystectomy for complicated gallstone disease 5 days ago. You are called to see her on the wards as she has become dyspnoeic, irritable and complaining of pain. Observations record a blood pressure of 110/60, pulse 66 and regular and saturations of 94% on 2 L of oxygen. Her past medical history is of ischaemic heart disease and hypertension treated with daily aspirin, atenolol, simvastatin and frusemide. Which of the following post-operative complications is the most likely diagnosis?

- ☐ **a.** Pulmonary embolus.
- ☐ **b.** Post-operative atelectasis.
- ☐ **c.** Myocardial infarction.
- ☐ **d.** Left ventricular failure.
- ☐ **e.** Diaphragmatic injury.

39 Which of the following is LEAST useful in investigating the above complication?

  ☐ **a.** Computed tomography with pulmonary angiography (CT-PA).

  ☐ **b.** Fibrin degradation product (D-dimer).

  ☐ **c.** Arterial blood gas.

  ☐ **d.** Electrocardiogram.

  ☐ **e.** Chest radiograph.

40 A 53-year-old man presents to accident and emergency complaining of a warm, tender swelling in the right groin associated with nausea, vomiting and constipation. On examination there is a tender, 2 cm swelling that is irreducible. The decision for theatre is made and examination intra-operatively the relations of the mass are defined as medial to the inferior epigastric artery and above the inguinal ligament. Which of the following correctly describes this mass?

  ☐ **a.** Spigelian hernia.

  ☐ **b.** Indirect inguinal hernia.

  ☐ **c.** Direct inguinal hernia.

  ☐ **d.** Femoral hernia.

  ☐ **e.** Ventral hernia.

41 A 37-year-old lady is admitted to hospital with what the A&E doctors suspect is a SEVERE asthma attack. Which of the following signs or symptoms is consistent with that diagnosis?

  ☐ **a.** Silent chest, peak expiratory flow rate (PEFR) <33% of predicted.

  ☐ **b.** Tachycardia >110/minute, PEFR <50% of predicted.

  ☐ **c.** Exhaustion, hypotension.

  ☐ **d.** PCO_2 normal or high on arterial sampling.

  ☐ **e.** Completing sentences, respiratory rate 15/minute.

42 A 57-year-old lady is seen complaining of acute onset shortness of breath. She is known to suffer from asthma, which is normally well controlled. Regularly she takes inhalers, both bronchodilators and inhaled steroids. She hasn't suffered an exacerbation of her asthma for a number of years and has never had any ITU admissions. Which of the following is NOT a reasonable differential diagnosis of an acute asthma attack?

  ☐ **a.** Anaphylaxis.

  ☐ **b.** Pneumothorax.

  ☐ **c.** Upper respiratory tract obstruction.

  ☐ **d.** Massive pulmonary embolus.

  ☐ **e.** Upper respiratory tract infection.

43 A 25-year-old woman presents to accident and emergency after a sudden onset of shortness of breath. She has a past medical history of asthma and dysmenorrhoea. She denies any current medication apart from the oral contraceptive pill since her menarche. On examination she is a tall thin woman who is tachypnoeic with a pulse of 122. BP is 94/56 with a raised JVP. ECG demonstrates sinus tachycardia. Which of the following treatments is the most appropriate?

- ☐ **a.** Carotid massage with cardiac monitoring.
- ☐ **b.** Needle aspiration in the second intercostal space anterior chest.
- ☐ **c.** Slow i.v. frusemide infusion.
- ☐ **d.** Nebulised bronchodilators.
- ☐ **e.** Low molecular weight heparin.

44 A 34-year-old man is brought in by his colleagues with acute dyspnoea following an office summer party. Regular medications include salbutamol inhaler and over the counter antihistamines for allergic rhinitis. On examination there is evidence of stridor and some peri-oral swelling. What is the most important next step in managing this patient?

- ☐ **a.** Nebulised salbutamol.
- ☐ **b.** Intramuscular adrenaline.
- ☐ **c.** Intravenous hydrocortisone.
- ☐ **d.** Insertion of a laryngeal mask airway.
- ☐ **e.** Endotracheal intubation.

45 A 22-year-old man is brought in to hospital following a high-speed road traffic accident where he was the driver. On initial assessment he is found to be drowsy with marked facial injury, chest injury consistent with steering wheel impact and multiple areas of subcutaneous emphysema. He is tachycardic with respiratory distress and further respiratory examination reveals a displaced trachea to the left side of the chest. Which of the following is the first step in management?

- ☐ **a.** Endotracheal intubation.
- ☐ **b.** Needle thoracocentesis of the right chest.
- ☐ **c.** Insert a nasopharyngeal airway.
- ☐ **d.** Insert a chest drain with underwater seal.
- ☐ **e.** Perform an emergency tracheostomy.

46 A 63-year-old gentleman presented to casualty with chest pain and shortness of breath. He described the chest pain as right sided and intermittent. The pain and shortness of breath were exacerbated by deep respiratory effort but ameliorated by shallow breathing. He has no risk factors for coronary artery disease. He has a past medical history of severe Parkinson's disease and is cared for by his wife. He takes levodopa and carbidopa but no other medications. On examination he has inspiratory crepitations at the right base but no other findings. Which of the following is the most likely cause for his symptoms?

- ☐ **a.** Atypical pneumonia.
- ☐ **b.** Aspiration pneumonia.
- ☐ **c.** Reflux disease.
- ☐ **d.** Levodopa toxicity.
- ☐ **e.** Parkinson's disease associated heart failure.

47 A 16-year-old girl presents to accident and emergency having taken 35 paracetamol tablets that morning. She is tearful and upset and history taking is difficult as she does not answer questions easily. Her past medical history is of depression and self-harm and childhood eczema. Examination is unremarkable and blood tests reveal an Hb of 10.8, slightly low albumin with normal urea and electrolytes. AST, bilirubin, γ-GT, alkaline phosphatase and ALT are normal. INR is 1.12 with a fibrinogen less than 6 and a normal APTT. Which of the following investigations is the most sensitive indicator of hepatic damage?

- ☐ **a.** AST and ALT.
- ☐ **b.** Alkaline phosphatase.
- ☐ **c.** INR.
- ☐ **d.** Fibrinogen.
- ☐ **e.** Albumin.

48 A 68-year-old woman is admitted to the ward after an elective hip replacement for osteoarthritis. On post-operative day 3 her respiratory function starts to deteriorate and she starts to complain of profuse diarrhoea. A sputum sample is obtained and sent off to the laboratory and appropriate antibiotic therapy commenced. Four days later she is dehydrated with reduced skin turgor. Recent blood results show moderately low potassium, high urea and a stool culture result pending. Which of the following steps is appropriate in managing this patient?
- [ ] **a.** Administration of i.v. potassium at a rate of 20mmol/hour.
- [ ] **b.** Administration of oral metronidazole.
- [ ] **c.** Administration of oral amoxicillin.
- [ ] **d.** Administration of 2 units of blood.
- [ ] **e.** Administration of a potassium sparing diuretic.

49 A 23-year-old woman presents to hospital feeling nauseated, unwell, with loss of appetite. She tells you that this occurred over a month and she was very worried she was pregnant as she had missed her last period. Further questioning reveals no recent history of travel, she drinks two or three glasses of wine a week and has been married for 2 years. Systemic review reveals a 2-week history of a painful right knee that happened after falling whilst ice skating. On examination she is comfortable at rest but has a mild yellow tinge to the sclera and an itchy rash over her forearm. The abdomen is very tender over the right upper quadrant but Murphy's sign is negative. Which of the following diagnoses is most likely?
- [ ] **a.** Viral hepatitis.
- [ ] **b.** Budd–Chiari syndrome.
- [ ] **c.** Cholecystitis.
- [ ] **d.** Autoimmune hepatitis.
- [ ] **e.** McArdle's disease.

50 A 63-year-old man presents to his GP with a month's history of regurgitating food, foul-smelling breath and a sensation of gurgling in her neck when he eats. He describes the regurgitated food as slightly changed but denies any blood or pain when he eats. He has not lost any weight recently and says that apart from the symptoms described he is otherwise fit and well. Which of the following diagnoses is most likely?
- [ ] **a.** Pharyngeal pouch.
- [ ] **b.** Plummer–Vinson syndrome.
- [ ] **c.** Chagas' disease.
- [ ] **d.** Oesophageal carcinoma.
- [ ] **e.** Mallory–Weiss tear.

51 A 34-year-old man with ulcerative colitis presents in the gastro-enterology outpatient clinic with abdominal pain and fatigue. He states the pain has been intermittent for the past 2 weeks and has not settled with simple analgesia. Focussed questioning reveals that the pain is distinct from that of his ulcerative coli-tis flare-ups and he has not experienced any change in bowel habit recently. Routine blood tests taken prior to clinic show a markedly raised alkaline phosphatase with mild hyperbilirubi-naemia. Haemoglobin is slightly reduced but the rest of the blood tests are normal. Which of the following would be the most appropriate next investigation?

☐ **a.** CT scan of the abdomen.
☐ **b.** Endoscopic retrograde cholangiopancreatogram (ERCP).
☐ **c.** Colonoscopy.
☐ **d.** Plain abdominal radiograph.
☐ **e.** Liver biopsy.

52 A 52-year-old man presents to hospital complaining of abdomi-nal pain and diarrhoea. He has had 10 bouts of diarrhoea since the morning and states that the pain is severe. He has noticed that his bowels have become much more watery over the past 2 months and that he has been increasingly breathless. Recently he has stopped taking alcohol as he has noticed that on occasion his face and neck become violently red and he feels hot and nau-seated and attributes this to drinking red wine. On examination he is slightly anxious and breathless whilst lying flat. There is peripheral pitting oedema of the ankles and abdominal examina-tion reveals a 3 cm smooth but tender hepatomegaly. Cardiac sounds are abnormal with a pansystolic murmur and a raised jugular venous pressure. Which of the following investigations is likely to be most useful diagnostically?

☐ **a.** 24-hour urine protein collection.
☐ **b.** Plasma osmolality.
☐ **c.** 24-hour urine 5-hydroxyindoleacetic acid (5-HIAA).
☐ **d.** Urinary osmolality.
☐ **e.** 24-hour urine for 4-hydroxymethoxymandelate (VMA).

53 A 26-year-old man was admitted by ambulance suffering with severe headaches. He described the headaches as the worst pain he had ever experienced and mentioned that concurrently he felt unsteady and drunk. He described the pain as being occipital in location and of rapid onset, being continuous with a duration of up to a minute. He has no relevant past medical or family history of note and works as a truck driver. On examination; he is apyrexial, GCS 15/15 there are no focal neurological signs. What is the next step in investigation of this gentleman's headache?

- ☐ **a.** MRI brain.
- ☐ **b.** CT scan of head.
- ☐ **c.** Lumbar puncture.
- ☐ **d.** Blood cultures.
- ☐ **e.** Admit for neurological observations and regular analgesia.

54 Relatives of a 70-year-old lady were concerned that she appeared to be increasingly confused. On examination she was orientated in time, place and person but did have slurred speech. Further neurological examination revealed bilateral past pointing and trunkal ataxia with no evidence of nystagmus. Routine blood tests revealed no cause for these symptoms. Where is this lady's lesion most likely to be located?

- ☐ **a.** Bilateral basal ganglia.
- ☐ **b.** Left temporo-parietal lobe.
- ☐ **c.** Cerebellar vermis.
- ☐ **d.** Left lateral cerebellar lobe.
- ☐ **e.** Left-sided frontal lobe.

55 A 70-year-old gentleman who is known to be taking warfarin is admitted to hospital with left-sided weakness. He has a history of coronary artery disease for which he is taking the warfarin but examination reveals no other findings of note. Which of the following investigations is the most important to obtain?

- ☐ **a.** Carotid duplex scan.
- ☐ **b.** Echocardiogram.
- ☐ **c.** CT scan of the brain.
- ☐ **d.** INR.
- ☐ **e.** ECG.

56 A 24-year-old lady presents with progressive seizure-like jerking movements of all extremities. She has three siblings all of whom are normal; although a cousin was thought to have suffered with a similar illness and died prematurely at the age of 37 years. No diagnosis was made for her cousin. On admission her GCS was 15/15, although she was slightly confused. A CT scan of her brain was normal but a follow-up MRI scan revealed areas of reduced density bilaterally at the basal ganglia. Routine blood tests revealed deranged liver function tests but nothing else of note. Which of the following is the most likely diagnosis?

- ☐ **a.** Early-onset Parkinson's disease.
- ☐ **b.** Wilson's disease.
- ☐ **c.** Glycogen storage disorder.
- ☐ **d.** Porphyria.
- ☐ **e.** Lead poisoning.

57 A 50-year-old man presents to his GP with headache, tenderness over the scalp and a general feeling of being tired all the time. Focused questioning reveals he also suffers with muscular aches and feels he has been a bit slow of late. Routine bloods were sent off and a 2-week appointment is made to review the results. Which of the following diagnoses is LEAST likely in this man?

- ☐ **a.** Superficial temporal arteritis.
- ☐ **b.** Migraine.
- ☐ **c.** Tension headache.
- ☐ **d.** Viral meningitis.
- ☐ **e.** Cluster headache.

58 A 30-year-old woman was admitted to casualty with a 24-hour history of worsening headaches. She described the headaches as constant with no relieving factors and associated nausea but on direct questioning she confirms that the pain is exacerbated by strong light. On examination there are no peripheral neurological signs but you note papilloedema on fundoscopy. Which of the following options is not a cause of this sign?

- ☐ **a.** Meningitis.
- ☐ **b.** Benign intracranial hypertension.
- ☐ **c.** Cerebellar haemangioblastoma.
- ☐ **d.** Hyperparathyroidism.
- ☐ **e.** Malignant hypertension.

59 A 54-year-old man presents feeling unwell with a failure to pass urine for 24 hours. Blood results taken on admission show a raised urea and creatinine and his blood pressure lying is 165/92. Abdominal palpation reveals a suprapubic dome-shaped mass that is dull to percussion. CT scan of the abdomen reveals a poorly defined peri-aortic mass and a bladder volume estimated to be 1.5 L. Which of the following drugs are most likely responsible for this presentation?

- ☐ **a.** Gold.
- ☐ **b.** Paracetamol.
- ☐ **c.** Acyclovir.
- ☐ **d.** Rosiglitazone.
- ☐ **e.** Methysergide.

60 A 46-year-old woman recently returned from visiting her relatives in Bangladesh. Shortly after her return she developed a fever, became unwell and complained of an ache in her left flank. Detailed questioning reveals a 7k weight loss since her return 3 weeks ago and diarrhoea that has been manifest on and off over the same period. On examination she is tender in the renal angle and a mid-stream urine result demonstrates a sterile pyuria. What is the next step in management for this woman?

- ☐ **a.** Treat for a fungal pyelonephritis.
- ☐ **b.** Treat empirically with a 7-day course of antibiotics.
- ☐ **c.** Intravenous urogram.
- ☐ **d.** Chest X-ray.
- ☐ **e.** Cystoscopy.

Extended matching questions

Chest pain

a. Acute MI.
b. Pneumonia.
c. Pulmonary embolus.
d. Pericarditis.
e. Bornholme's disease.
f. Pneumothorax.
g. Gastro-oesophageal reflux disease.
h. Aortic dissection.

Select the most suitable option for each of the scenarios below:

61 An 87-year-old female nursing home resident has started to complain of chest pain. There are no exacerbating or relieving factors for the pain. The nurses note that she is also short of breath. She suffers with chronic obstructive pulmonary disease which is usually well controlled on inhaled medications.

62 A 30-year-old secretary who has recently recovered from viral chest infection presents to A&E with intermittent chest pain. The chest pain is central in origin with no radiation or any associated symptoms. On examination the chest pain is recreated by exerting gentle pressure on the sternum.

63 A 68-year-old gentleman has complained of retrosternal chest pain. He notes that it is at its worse in the early afternoon and evening. The pain does not wake him from sleep but is recreated when he lies flat. He complains of associated nausea but no vomiting. He takes regular aspirin for coronary artery disease and has recently had a short course of diclofenac for joint pains.

64 A 58-year-old gentleman is brought in to A&E by ambulance following an episode of chest pain at work. His colleague that accompanied him to the hospital mentioned that he described central chest pain which felt like it as tearing through to his back.

65 One week following a total knee replacement a 63-year-old woman starts to complain of chest pain. It is right sided in location and exacerbated by inspiration. It has no radiation or associated symptoms. She had previously complained of a swelling in her right calf which was thought to be related to her joint replacement.

Manifestations of endocrine disease

a. Cushing's syndrome.
b. Acromegaly.
c. Diabetes mellitus.
d. Diabetes insipidus.
e. Phaeochromocytoma.
f. Syndrome of inappropriate ADH secretion (SIADH).
g. Hypothyroidism.
h. Hyperthyroidism.

The following patients have all presented with endocrine disease. Please choose the most likely diagnosis from the list above. Each option can be used once, more than once or not at all.

66 A 54-year-old man presents to the renal clinic for regular follow-up post-live-related kidney transplant. He complains of a feeling of lethargy, weight gain and has been complaining of swelling of his ankles recently. There is no tenderness at the site of renal transplant and ultrasound demonstrates no abnormality. Blood pressure reading is 176/98 with a fasting blood glucose level of 10.2 g/dL. Blood results show a sodium of 148 mmol/L with a potassium of 3.5 mmol/L.

67 A 78-year-old woman is brought to hospital by her neighbour who is concerned that she has become confused recently. On examination she is alert but not orientated in time or place and is noted to be tired and uncooperative during physical examination. Abdominal examination reveals a lumpy quality to the abdomen and areas of erythema *ab igne* on both shins. A keen medical student notes some unusual hair loss over her eyebrows and scalp.

68 A 52-year-old man presents to hospital with shortness of breath and cough productive of green sputum. He complains that he has been feeling weak, thirsty and thinks his high blood pressure medication may be at too high a dose as he has been urinating frequently for the past week and has lost a significant amount of weight over the last month. Past medical history is remarkable for hypertension. Chest radiography confirms a lower respiratory tract infection. Blood results reveal a sodium of 147 mmol/L, potassium of 4.9 mmol/L, urea of 11 mmol/L with a plasma osmolality of 330 mOsm/L. Urine osmolality is verbally reported as being 'high'.

69 A 42-year-old man presents to his GP for a yearly check-up offered in his area. His past medical history is unremarkable and he states that aside from some recent changes in his vision and headaches, both of which he attributes from some new glasses he bought a few weeks ago he feels well. On examination he is a tall and heavy set man who is very tanned from a recent holiday. Cardiovascular, respiratory and abdominal examination is unremarkable but you notice an area of untanned skin around his left ring finger and he tells you regretfully that recently his wedding band has become too tight and is being resized.

70 A 38-year-old man presents to his GP complaining of recurrent anxiety attacks. He describes three or four episodes whilst he has been out in public of feeling light-headed with palpitations and a mild tremor that causes him to want to sit down until the feeling subsides. Focussed questioning reveals he has become constipated recently and he is very anxious that this may be cancer as his family have a history of 'renal and pancreatic growths'.

Rheumatological conditions

a. Gout.
b. Rheumatoid arthritis.
c. Osteoarthritis.
d. Pseudogout.
e. Septic arthritis.
f. Ankylosing spondylitis.
g. Polymyalgia rheumatica.
h. Psoriatic arthropathy.

The following patients have all presented with rheumatological problems. Please choose the most correct diagnosis from the above list. Each option may be used once, more than once or not at all.

71 A 27-year-old girl presents to her GP with pain and swelling in her joints, particularly the small joints of the hands. She has noticed this discomfort for the past month but has no other symptoms other than a bit of malaise and non-specific feeling of 'not being herself'. She had put these symptoms down to having a young child. She takes the combined oral contraceptive pill but no other medications and suffers with no other illnesses.

72 A 47-year-old builder complains of pain in his foot. On examination there is evidence of redness and discomfort in the right hallux although there is no evidence of ulceration or skin changes. Social history reveals an intake of alcohol in the region of 40 units/week, often in binges, and a diet rich in red meat.

73 A 63-year-old lady returns to the rheumatology clinic with pain in the joints of the hands and some loss of function. The ring finger on her right hand has become shortened in length, all other fingers are normal although there is a degree of ulnar deviation. Current medications include topical steroids, tar and regular light therapy.

74 A 23-year-old man presents to his GP with an increasing pain in his lower back and stiffness that is worse in the mornings. He has noticed some intermittent pain in his knees and increasing pain in the soles of his feet towards the end of the day. Spine X-ray reveals squaring of the vertebrae.

75 A 74-year-old lady has suffered with increasing pain in her hip for a number of years, which she tolerates with NSAIDs. Recently she has noticed squaring of the thumb joint on her left hand and the pain in her hip is becoming more problematic and more troublesome towards the end of the day.

Opportunistic infections in HIV/AIDS

a. Pneumocystis jerovici pneumonia.
b. Candidiasis.
c. Toxoplasmosis.
d. *Cryptosporidium* infection.
e. Cryptococcal infection.
f. Varicella zoster pneumonitis.
g. Cytomegaly virus infection.
h. Mycobacterium avium intracellulare.

The following HIV positive patients have all presented with opportunistic infections. Please choose the most correct diagnosis from the above list. Each option may be used once, more than once or not at all.

76 A 34-year-old man presents to hospital with abdominal pain, ☐ crampy in nature and associated with loose watery stools. On examination he is pale, tachycardic and sweaty. He denies eating any seafood recently but had been staying at a friend's farm for the past 2 weeks.

77 A 40-year-old woman presents to hospital with a 3-day history ☐ of headache, nausea, lack of appetite. She has been otherwise fit and healthy and describes the headache as not related to any particular time of day but associated with pain on looking at bright lights.

78 A 28-year-old woman presents to her GP with pain on swallow- ☐ ing solid food and a strange taste in her mouth. She describes the pain as retrosternal in nature and associated only with swallowing; worse with dry and solid food and less with liquids. She denies any significant weight loss.

79 A 45-year-old man is brought to hospital by his friends who ☐ are worried that he has been acting 'out of character' recently. Collateral history reveals a gradual change in his behaviour, becoming more confused and agitated over a 2-month period with an episode of shaking of the limbs and arms that was attributed to medication side-effects. On arrival to accident and emergency he is aggressive, disruptive and would not allow any of the nursing staff to take blood from him.

80 A 32-year-old man was found collapsed at home by his partner and brought by ambulance to accident and emergency. On arrival he is struggling to breathe and is on an oxygen mask. History from the partner reveals a gradual onset over the past 2 weeks of increasing shortness of breath and feeling of tiredness after the simplest of tasks. On examination he is tachypnoeic with a respiratory rate of 34 breaths a minute and on auscultation fine crepitations are heard in the lower and midzones of the lungs.

Treatment of psychiatric disorders

    a. Olanzipine.
    b. Sertraline.
    c. Cognitive behavioural therapy.
    d. Electroconvulsive therapy.
    e. Eye movement desensitisation and reprocessing.
    f. Temazepam.
    g. Reduction in caffeine intake.
    h. Lithium.

The following patients have all presented with a psychiatric disorder. Please choose the most appropriate treatment modality from the above list. Each option may be used once, more than once or not at all.

81 A 34-year-old woman is brought to hospital by a friend who is concerned that recently she has been acting bizarrely; going on shopping trips every other day and spending money in the local betting shop, which she never used to do. She has also been socialising more often than usual and had been throwing house parties every weekend.

82 A 42-year-old aid worker presents to his GP with 5-week history of inability to sleep, a feeling of being on edge and easily startled and nightmares of persecution and violence. He had previously returned from an aid mission overseas where he had to be evacuated due to unsafe conditions.

83 A 24-year-old man who has recently arrived in the United Kingdom is referred to the acute psychiatric clinic by his GP who is concerned that he has been experiencing auditory hallucinations telling him that the immigration officials have been monitoring his activities and are planning to use him as a spy. He become agitated when confronted about these thoughts and claims that people are stealing ideas from his head.

84 A 43-year-old woman presents to her GP complaining of feeling a sense of overwhelming fear associated with shortness of breath and a racing heart beat when she is asked to give a presentation or speak in front of lots of people. She says that the thought of having to do any kind of social activity makes her feel nauseated.

85 A 67-year-old woman is brought to accident and emergency by her neighbour who has been increasingly worried about her behaviour. She is unkempt and was found by her neighbour at home in her chair where she had not moved for 3 days. She has been on antidepressant medication in the past started by her GP. Psychiatric assessment in hospital revealed a low mood with deep suicidal ideation and morbid delusions.

Diseases of the hand

    a. Dupuytren's contracture.
    b. Glomus tumour.
    c. Paronychia.
    d. Nailbed haematoma.
    e. Radial nerve injury.
    f. Lower brachial plexus root injury.
    g. Carpal tunnel syndrome.
    h. Scaphoid fracture.

The following patients have all presented with diseases of the hand. Please choose the most likely diagnosis from the above list. Each option may be used once, more than once, or not at all.

86 A 35-year-old keen gardener presents to her GP with a swollen left index finger. She states that it has caused her throbbing pain for the past 2 weeks and came on after she cut her finger on some rose thorns. There is swelling, redness and tenderness surrounding the nail itself on the left index finger only.

87 A 43-year-old man presents with an extremely painful mass under one of the nails of his right hand. He states that he has become more aware of the mass over the past month. There is a bluish hue to the mass with lifting of the nailbed.

88 A 31-year-old woman is brought in to accident and emergency after cutting herself with a knife following a break-up with her partner. On examination of her hand there are multiple lacerations on the wrist by the base of the thumb. She complains of an inability to extend her wrist.

89 A 13-year-old boy falls onto concrete whilst roller-skating. He is seen by the out of hours GP and is found to have a tender swollen base of the thumb with tenderness in the anatomical snuffbox. He has weakness on making a pincer grip but has normal abductor pollicis brevis function.

90 A 54-year old man who is seen regularly in the endocrinology clinic presents with the complaint that during the night he wakes up with tingling and numbness in his hands that is only relieved by shaking them out. On further questioning he has otherwise been fit and well but states that in recent years he has gone up many shoe sizes and cannot now fit into his favourite hat.

PAPER 2

Questions

Multiple choice questions (single best answer)

1 A 27-year-old man is referred from accident and emergency on a Friday night. He is complaining of pain in his left hand and describes injuring it by punching a wall following a fight with his girlfriend. He notes that the hand is swollen and he is not quite able to form a fist due to the pain and swelling. Neurovascular supply is intact. On X-ray you note a mid-shaft fifth metacarpal fracture that appears to be rotated on the true lateral view. How would you manage this case?

☐ **a.** Below elbow backslab and fracture clinic follow-up.
☐ **b.** Sling for support and outpatient physiotherapy.
☐ **c.** Admit for open reduction and internal fixation of fracture.
☐ **d.** Admit for analgesia and physiotherapy.
☐ **e.** GP review in 1 week.

2 A 58-year-old gentleman was admitted complaining of lower back pain. He noted that the back pain had gradually worsened and had now stopped responding to analgesia. He described some radiation of the pain into his right thigh but denied any sciatica-like symptoms. He was afebrile and had a limited straight leg raise to 30 degrees. Hip movements were good bilaterally. X-rays of his lumbar spine revealed no cause for his symptoms. His past medical history includes angina and a pneumonectomy 9 months earlier for a malignant mesothelioma. Which of the following investigations will provide the best diagnostic information?

☐ **a.** Blood cultures.
☐ **b.** Bone scan.
☐ **c.** MRI spine.
☐ **d.** Lumbar puncture.
☐ **e.** CT spine.

3 A 14-year-old boy is brought to hospital by ambulance having been involved in a road traffic accident. He was in the front seat and was wearing a seatbelt but had been incorrectly belted. He arrives intubated by the ambulance crew and is hypotensive. A FAST scan demonstrates free fluid in the abdomen from a ruptured spleen. He is scheduled for emergency surgery for exploratory laparotomy and splenectomy. As he is being taken to theatre his parents arrive from home and demand that he not be given any blood transfusions as he is a Jehovah's Witness and show you their cards stating so. Which of the following actions is the correct course of action?

- ☐ **a.** Refuse to proceed to surgery without blood.
- ☐ **b.** Proceed to surgery using crystalloid replacement only.
- ☐ **c.** Proceed to surgery as an emergency using blood as necessary.
- ☐ **d.** Reschedule surgery to allow for auto-transfusion.
- ☐ **e.** Apply for a court order to allow surgery to proceed.

4 A young child is brought to her GP by her mother who has noticed she has developed a rash over her face and neck. The child is otherwise well and the mother describes no other symptoms apart from a mild itch that occurs now and again around the lesions. On examination there are multiple small pearly papules with a central umbilicated area of keratin plug distributed randomly over the face and neck. Which of the following is most likely to be the cause of this rash?

- ☐ **a.** Varicella zoster virus (VZV).
- ☐ **b.** Herpes simplex virus (HSV).
- ☐ **c.** Molluscum contagiosum.
- ☐ **d.** Eczema.
- ☐ **e.** Pityriasis versicolor.

5 A 34-year-old man is referred from the surgical team and seen by the dermatologists for an itchy rash in his elbow creases, which he has been scratching for the past week. He is diagnosed with eczema on inspection of the rash. Which of the following patterns is NOT part of the eczema classification?

- ☐ **a.** Atopic eczema.
- ☐ **b.** Asteatotic eczema.
- ☐ **c.** Discoid eczema.
- ☐ **d.** Arthropathic eczema.
- ☐ **e.** Varicose eczema.

6 A 72-year-old Afro-Caribbean man presents to his GP after problems initiating micturition. He has taken to wearing a pad during the day and finds that he has to use the toilet frequently at night, with occasional urinary accidents and post-void dribbling. Abdominal examination is remarkable only for a fullness in the lower abdomen and routine blood tests, urea and electrolytes are normal. The next best step in management is:

- ☐ **a.** Suprapubic catheterisation.
- ☐ **b.** Blood glucose.
- ☐ **c.** Anti-dsDNA antibody.
- ☐ **d.** Prostate-specific antibody.
- ☐ **e.** Ultrasound scan of the renal tract.

7 A 54-year-old man presents feeling unwell with a failure to pass urine for 24 hours. Blood results taken on admission show a raised urea and creatinine and his blood pressure lying is 165/92 mmHg. Abdominal palpation reveals a suprapubic dome-shaped mass that is dull to percussion. CT scan of the abdomen reveals a poorly defined peri-aortic mass and a bladder volume estimated to be 1.5 L. Which of the following drugs are most likely responsible for this presentation?

- ☐ **a.** Gold.
- ☐ **b.** Paracetamol.
- ☐ **c.** Acyclovir.
- ☐ **d.** Rosiglitazone.
- ☐ **e.** Methysergide.

8 A fit 26-year-old lady was admitted to hospital with cellulitis of her left leg later found to be secondary to a spider bite. She was started on intravenous antibiotics – flucloxacillin and benzylpenicillin having no known drug allergies. The on-call house officer was called to see her due to the nurse noticing some facial flushing. On further questioning she admitted to suffering with tingling in her hands and teeth but no shortness of breath or chest tightening. She remained apyrexial throughout. What would be your next course of action?

- ☐ **a.** Consider this to be an anxiety attack and continue treatment with reassurance.
- ☐ **b.** Add in erythromycin as current cover is not adequate.
- ☐ **c.** Change antibiotics due to allergy.
- ☐ **d.** Stop antibiotics, administer steroids and antihistamines.
- ☐ **e.** Continue treatment with topical antibiotics.

9 A 79-year-old lady with known chronic obstructive pulmonary disease has been admitted 6 times in the past 6 months. On this admission she complains of increasing shortness of breath and difficulty in coping at home. On observation from a distance this lady is comfortable at rest with a respiratory rate of 14/minute. At the bedside, observation reveals a tachypnoea and breathing through pursed lips. Arterial blood gas studies for assessing domiciliary oxygen requirements are found to be negative and this has been the case on previous admissions. Physiotherapists have noted that her mobility is good. Your team decides that she is medically fit for discharge, what will be your next step?

☐ **a.** Continue rehabilitation at a local cottage hospital.

☐ **b.** Ask social services for review with nursing home placement in mind.

☐ **c.** Keep patient in hospital until she feels ready to leave.

☐ **d.** Send her home with a GP follow-up immediately.

☐ **e.** Impress on the patient that she is well and that she has no medical problems requiring attention.

10 A 97-year-old lady is referred to the on-call surgical team by her GP. She has been complaining of a cold, painful leg for the past 6 hours. On examination the GP notes that the skin appears to be mottled and notes the absence of pulses below the femoral artery on the affected side. Of note her past medical history includes arrial fibrillation for which she is not anticoagulated. On examination she is noted to have a respiratory rate of 35/minute and evidence of bibasal inspiratory crepitations which chest X-ray confirms as bilateral pneumonia. What diagnosis was the GP concerned about in this lady?

☐ **a.** Buerger's disease.

☐ **b.** Femoral artery embolus.

☐ **c.** Arterial insufficiency.

☐ **d.** Abdominal aortic aneurysm.

☐ **e.** Venous ulceration.

11 A 32-year-old woman presents to her GP complaining of recurrent episodes of intense discomfort associated with shortness of breath, chest pain and palpitations usually whilst she is out in public places. The episodes last between 5 and 10 minutes are usually cease on their own. Her past medical history is unremarkable but she tells you that her family have a history of 'heart attacks' and is worried that her symptoms may be related. Which of the following associations is NOT true?
- ☐ **a.** Irritable bowel syndrome.
- ☐ **b.** Agoraphobia.
- ☐ **c.** Mitral valve prolapse.
- ☐ **d.** Chronic obstructive pulmonary disease (COPD).
- ☐ **e.** Age over 65 years.

12 A 43-year-old man presents to clinic with feelings of a lack of enjoyment of his usual hobbies, a feeling of detachment from his family and friends associated with poor sleep, nightmares and irritability. He describes these changes happening a few months ago and states that he has been easily startled and ill at ease ever since. His past medical history is remarkable only for allergic rhinitis and a recent hospital admission for a head injury following a robbery at his home. Which of the following diagnoses is the most likely?
- ☐ **a.** Acute stress disorder.
- ☐ **b.** Depressive disorder.
- ☐ **c.** Post-traumatic stress disorder (PTSD).
- ☐ **d.** Schizoid personality disorder.
- ☐ **e.** Generalised anxiety disorder (GAD).

13 A 5-year-old girl is brought to her GP by her mother as she is worried about her health. She has always been a well child until recently when she has become increasingly tired and pale. Her mum is concerned that she intermittently suffers with fevers that are not well controlled with paracetamol. She has now gradually developed a rash and the main concern is one of bacterial meningitis. On clinical examination she does not appear to be acutely unwell. She has noticeable pallor of the conjunctiva and has a widespread purpuric rash which blanches on pressure. The GP advises a paediatric review and some blood tests which show low platelet count and a leuko-paenia. What is the likely diagnosis in this case?
- ☐ **a.** Bacterial meningitis.
- ☐ **b.** Acute lymphocytic leukaemia.
- ☐ **c.** Chronic myeloid leukaemia.
- ☐ **d.** Acute myeloid leukaemia.
- ☐ **e.** Viral encephalitis.

14 Which of the following facts about chronic leukaemia is INCORRECT?
- ☐ **a.** CLL is a chronic incurable condition.
- ☐ **b.** Ionising radiation is a known cause of CML.
- ☐ **c.** CLL cells contain the Philadelphia chromosome.
- ☐ **d.** Early disease prognosis for CLL is 8–10 years.
- ☐ **e.** CLL is a malignant disease of B-lymphocytes.

15 A 42-year-old man presents to his GP with a 2-month history of a painless lump in his neck. He has noticed this lump grow slowly bigger and as he had been feeling tired with sweats at night he had thought it was lymph node from a 'head cold'. Recently he has noticed that he cannot enjoy wine or beer anymore because they cause him pain. Which of the following diagnoses is the most likely?
- ☐ **a.** Hodgkin's lymphoma.
- ☐ **b.** Infectious mononucleosis.
- ☐ **c.** Non-Hodgkin's lymphoma.
- ☐ **d.** Polycythaemia rubra vera.
- ☐ **e.** Myelodysplastic syndrome (MDS).

16 A 51-year-old woman presents to accident and emergency with episodes of coughing up blood over a 2-week period. Further questioning reveals a history of weight loss, frequent cough and a feeling of tiredness and malaise. Routine blood tests taken in hospital reveal an erythrocyte sedimentation rate of 70 mm/hour, Sodium of 135 mmol/L, Potassium of 5.3 mmol/L, creatinine of 167 μmol/L, urea of 9.3 mmol/L, with a mild neutrophilia and haemoglobin of 10.2 g/dL. Which of the following investigations is most likely to be positive?

☐ **a.** c-ANCA.
☐ **b.** Anti-glomerular basement membrane.
☐ **c.** Anti-SCL 70.
☐ **d.** Anti-mitochondrial antibodies.
☐ **e.** Rheumatoid factor.

17 A 48-year-old former secretary, known to the rheumatologists, presents to clinic with a 2-week history of tingling over her fingers and hands and numbness over the palms of her fingers and thumbs apart from the little fingers on both hands. On examination there are multiple bilateral joint deformities and tapping over the volar aspect of the wrist exacerbates the symptoms described above. Which of the following treatment options should be considered next?

☐ **a.** Intra-articular steroid injection.
☐ **b.** Carpal tunnel decompression.
☐ **c.** Nerve conduction studies.
☐ **d.** Plain radiographs of both wrists/hands.
☐ **e.** Wrist splinting.

18 Optimal assessment of a breast lump in a 55-year-old lady is best described by which of the following?

☐ **a.** Clinical examination, ultrasound and biopsy.
☐ **b.** Clinical examination and mammogram.
☐ **c.** Ultrasound, mammogram and biopsy.
☐ **d.** Clinical examination, mammogram and biopsy.
☐ **e.** Clinical examination, chest X-ray and biopsy.

19 A 31-year-old lady is referred by her GP as she is complaining of breast pain. She is 1-week post-partum and has been breast feeding but it has now become too painful to continue. The GP notes that on examination there is evidence of a collection in one of the breasts with overlying erythema and associated pain. An ultrasound scan confirms an abscess. What is the most appropriate management?

☐ **a.** Oral flucloxacillin.
☐ **b.** Incision and drainage of abscess.
☐ **c.** Needle aspiration.
☐ **d.** Analgesia and cold compress.
☐ **e.** Admit for i.v. antibiotics.

20 A 34-year-old woman who is under regular review in the rheumatology clinic is seen in accident and emergency with a urinary tract infection. Whilst in hospital she is examined by some medical students who notice that her vision in the right eye is poor with diplopia in the same eye. She has a history of cardiac problems and examination of the cardiac system reveals a soft diastolic murmur heard best in the aortic area. Which of the following diagnoses would this clinical picture be most consistent with?

☐ **a.** William's syndrome.
☐ **b.** Down's syndrome.
☐ **c.** Marfan's syndrome.
☐ **d.** Turner's syndrome.
☐ **e.** Reiter's syndrome.

21 A 64-year-old woman is seen by her GP for a very red, itchy and painful eye. She describes the eye as having the sensation of there being a bit of 'grit stuck in it'. When she is asked about these symptoms she says she has had these symptoms on and off for a long time but never this badly. On further enquiry she suffers from a dry cough and has trouble eating very dry food as she finds it 'sticks to her mouth and is difficult to swallow'. Which of the following diagnoses is the most likely?

☐ **a.** Anterior uveitis.
☐ **b.** Acute glaucoma.
☐ **c.** Subconjunctival haemorrhage.
☐ **d.** Sjögren's syndrome.
☐ **e.** Retinal vein occlusion.

22 A 69-year-old man with type II diabetes mellitus is brought to hospital with confusion, drowsiness and aggressive behaviour. He lives with his daughter who noticed that he had become 'not himself' and had checked his blood sugar, finding it to be 2.3 mmol/L. Which of the following are NOT associated with hypoglycaemic states?

- ☐ **a.** Liver failure.
- ☐ **b.** Gliclazide.
- ☐ **c.** Insulinoma.
- ☐ **d.** Addison's disease.
- ☐ **e.** Cushing's disease.

23 A 58-year-old woman presents to the thyroid clinic to have a check-up for long-term hypothyroidism for which she is taking thyroxine 100μg once daily. She tells you in the clinic that she has read about a novel therapy for thyroid disease that doesn't involve tablets and would like to try this if possible. Her blood results are available in the clinic and demonstrate a high thyroid stimulating hormone and a high T4. Which of the following is most likely to explain these results?

- ☐ **a.** Subclinical hypothyroidism.
- ☐ **b.** Sick euthyroid syndrome.
- ☐ **c.** Non-compliance and overdosing prior to clinic.
- ☐ **d.** Inadequate replacement with thyroxine.
- ☐ **e.** Over-replacement with thyroxine.

24 Mid-ward round a nurse asks you to review one of your well-known patients with acute onset shortness of breath. The nurse is concerned that the patient looks unwell and requests your opinion. You remember that the patient recently suffered an myocardial infarction, on assessment you note that the airway is patent but the patient is acutely short of breath. The first step in your management is:

- ☐ **a.** Contact your senior colleagues for assistance.
- ☐ **b.** Perform an arterial blood gas.
- ☐ **c.** Attach a cardiac monitor.
- ☐ **d.** Request a chest X-ray.
- ☐ **e.** Complete a primary survey.

25 Which of the following is not a clinical finding associated with infective endocarditis?

- ☐ **a.** Osler's nodes.
- ☐ **b.** Retinal haemorrhages.
- ☐ **c.** Splinter haemorrhages.
- ☐ **d.** Clubbing.
- ☐ **e.** Erythema nodosum.

26 An 84-year-old gentleman was given an urgent outpatient cardiology appointment by his GP. He was concerned about the increasing swelling of his legs and his shortness of breath. On examination he was able to walk with sticks but oedema had spread up to his groin. He was notably short of breath and on auscultation he had bibasal inspiratory crepitations up to the midzones. He is currently on digoxin for a history of arterial fibrillation and other medications include furosemide 40 mg once daily. You are asked to admit the patient, what changes will you make to his medications?

- ☐ **a.** Add in bumetanide.
- ☐ **b.** Change furosemide to i.v. and double the daily dose.
- ☐ **c.** Add an ace inhibitor.
- ☐ **d.** Start a beta-blocker.
- ☐ **e.** Add in metolazone.

27 A 35-year-old lady attended accident and emergency with chest pain. She had no history of cardiovascular disease and denied any risk factors. Blood tests showed a positive troponin and ECG showed antero-lateral ischaemic changes. Which of the following illegal drugs are associated with this presentation?

- ☐ **a.** Amphetamines.
- ☐ **b.** Cocaine.
- ☐ **c.** Cannabis.
- ☐ **d.** Heroin.
- ☐ **e.** Rohypnol.

28 A patient on the coronary care unit is a 30-year-old lady. Your consultant suggests that you examine her as she has interesting findings. As you look over you notice that she is a tall slim lady wearing glasses. What would you expect to find on auscultation?

- ☐ **a.** Systolic murmur at the right upper sternal edge.
- ☐ **b.** Diastolic murmur at the right upper sternal edge.
- ☐ **c.** Systolic murmur at lower left sternal edge.
- ☐ **d.** Systolic murmur at the apex.
- ☐ **e.** Diastolic murmur at the apex.

29 In patients newly diagnosed with arterial fibrillation on digoxin therapy, which of the following electrolytes is most important to monitor?

- ☐ **a.** Serum sodium.
- ☐ **b.** Serum potassium.
- ☐ **c.** Serum calcium.
- ☐ **d.** Serum magnesium.
- ☐ **e.** None of the above.

30 A 54-year-old man presents to hospital with lethargy, shortness of breath and complaining of itching all over. His previous notes state he is well known to the renal physicians for chronic renal failure secondary to diabetic nephropathy and is followed up in the joint diabetic/renal clinic regularly. History taking reveals he has been having a lot of trouble recently for arthritic pain in his hip and has been taking some pain medication from the chemists. On examination there is bilateral pitting oedema to the mid-thigh and he is short of breath with a respiratory rate of 30 breaths a minute. Oxygen saturations are at 87% on room air. He provides a list of the current medications he is taking. Which of the following medications has most likely precipitated this admission?

☐ **a.** Erythropoietin.
☐ **b.** Frusemide.
☐ **c.** Ibuprofen.
☐ **d.** Pioglitazone.
☐ **e.** Chlorpheniramine.

31 A 10-year-old boy is brought to hospital by his mother who is worried that he has passing very dark smoky urine. She states that this started this morning and has been intermittent over the course of the days. She is also worried that his face has become more swollen over the last couple of days and he has not been feeling himself. On further questioning the mother tells you that he had been fine up until a nasty bout of 'flu' that he caught from school just over a week ago that required a few days off school. Which of the following diagnoses is the most likely?

☐ **a.** Minimal change glomerulonephritis.
☐ **b.** Post-streptococcal glomerulonephritis.
☐ **c.** Henoch–Schönlein purpura.
☐ **d.** Berger's disease (IgA nephropathy).
☐ **e.** Rapidly progressive glomerulonephritis.

32 A 54-year-old man with chronic renal failure is seen at his regular follow-up with his GP. Blood pressure is taken showing a reading of 145/78 mmHg with a normocytic anaemia, Hb 9.5 g/dl, urea of 11.4 mmol/L and a creatinine of 145 μmol/L. Which of the following is NOT associated with chronic renal failure (CRF)?

☐ **a.** Anorexia.
☐ **b.** Nausea.
☐ **c.** Restless legs.
☐ **d.** Hypokalaemia.
☐ **e.** Hyperphosphataemia.

33 A 43-year-old woman presents to hospital with shortness of breath, malaise and bilateral pitting oedema to the knees. She is treated for acute renal failure and started on a diuretic that acts at the thick ascending limb of the loop of Henlé. Which of the following diuretics acts at this particular site?

- ☐ **a.** Acetazolamide.
- ☐ **b.** Mannitol.
- ☐ **c.** Frusemide.
- ☐ **d.** Bendrofluazide.
- ☐ **e.** Spironolactone.

34 Which of the following states is NOT an indication for renal replacement therapy (dialysis)?

- ☐ **a.** Refractory metabolic acidosis.
- ☐ **b.** Oliguria.
- ☐ **c.** Severe hyperkalaemia.
- ☐ **d.** Uraemic symptoms.
- ☐ **e.** Drug ingestion.

35 Whilst on your general practice attachment you are asked to pay a visit to an 81-year-old gentleman. His wife died 3 years earlier following a large myocardial infarction and since he has been managing at home independently. His daughter is concerned that he doesn't seem to be himself. She notes that he is becoming increasingly forgetful and on occasion doing strange things like leaving the taps running or the oven on when it is not in use. In the case of Alzheimer's disease, which of the following is incorrect?

- ☐ **a.** A CT brain will be normal.
- ☐ **b.** Dysphasia may be the presenting feature.
- ☐ **c.** Brisk reflexes and upgoing plantars are often seen.
- ☐ **d.** There may be relevant family history.
- ☐ **e.** Depression is commonly seen.

36 A 31-year-old bank clerk presents to her GP complaining of the worst headache that she has ever experienced. On taking a history the GP elicits that this headache was acute in onset, sharp in nature and had no exacerbating or alleviating features. She denies any history of trauma. The patient notes that she is stressed at work and mentions a family history of migraines. She denies any nausea, vomiting, hallucinations or visual disturbances but notes that that headache is still present and showing no signs of improvement. Examination is unremarkable and observations are stable. Her past medical history includes dysmenorrhoea for which she takes the oral contraceptive pill but nil else of note. The GP refers her to the on-call medical team for review. Which diagnosis is he particularly concerned about?

☐ **a.** Bacterial meningitis.
☐ **b.** Tension headache.
☐ **c.** Subarachnoid haemorrhage.
☐ **d.** Subdural haemorrhage.
☐ **e.** Benign raised intracranial pressure.

37 A 48-year-old woman presents to hospital complaining of vomiting and diarrhoea. The symptoms started in the early hours of the morning after a staff conference. She denied eating any seafood or drinking any alcohol but states that she did eat the buffet food, which was chicken fried rice and vegetable spring rolls. On examination there are no physical signs apart from a previous lower segment Caesarean section in the abdomen. Which of the following organisms is the most likely infectious agent?

☐ **a.** Rotavirus.
☐ **b.** *Clostridium botulinum*.
☐ **c.** *Cryptosporidium parvum*.
☐ **d.** *Bacillus cereus*.
☐ **e.** *Escherichia coli*.

38 A 68-year-old woman with renal cell cancer presents to hospital with abdominal pain and abdominal distension. She states that her abdomen has been becoming more distended over a 3-week period with pain throughout this time. She also states that she was afraid to come into hospital as she thought this was further spread of the cancer. On examination she has a tender distended abdomen with 4-cm smooth hepatomegaly and evidence of fluid shift. The abdominal veins are dilated and there is evidence of caput medusae at the umbilicus. Which of the following diagnoses is the most likely?

☐ **a.** Viral hepatitis.

☐ **b.** Epstein–Barr virus infection.

☐ **c.** α1-antitrypsin deficiency.

☐ **d.** Wilson's disease.

☐ **e.** Budd–Chiari syndrome.

39 A 26-year-old man presents to his GP with recent change in bowel habit, diarrhoea with mucous and blood-streaks and abdominal pain over a month period. He has also noticed that it has become very painful to pass stool to the extent that he sometimes resists the urge to defaecate until he can hold it no longer. Colonoscopy is arranged that shows multiple areas of cobblestone appearance and aphthous ulceration. Which of the following statements regarding this disease is correct?

☐ **a.** Surgical therapy is likely to be curative.

☐ **b.** Disease is limited to the terminal ileum and distally.

☐ **c.** Transmural involvement is seen on histology.

☐ **d.** Continuous inflammatory change is seen on colonoscopy.

☐ **e.** Barium follow-through is of no use diagnostically.

40 A 23-year-old man presents to accident and emergency feeling lethargic, passing large amounts of urine and complaining of abdominal pain. He states that for the past 2 weeks he has had a cough and has been finding himself more breathless when walking to work. Past medical history is remarkable for type I diabetes mellitus and he is a smoker of 20 cigarettes a day. Urine dipstick done on admission show glucose $++$, ketones $+++$ and trace protein. Venous blood gases results show a pH of 7.29, bicarbonate of 18 mmol/L with a base excess of -3.4 mmol/L. Which of the following treatment regimens should be instituted?

- ☐ **a.** Double the usual basal bolus insulin regimen with strict blood glucose monitoring hourly.
- ☐ **b.** Start short-acting insulin infusion with 5-L fluid replacement of 0.9% sodium chloride with potassium as required over a 24-hour period.
- ☐ **c.** Add a long-acting insulin to the usual basal bolus regimen with 5-L fluid replacement with 0.9% sodium chloride.
- ☐ **d.** Start short-acting insulin infusion to reduce blood glucose to less than 15 mmol/L then restart high-dose oral hypoglycaemic with strict blood glucose measurement.
- ☐ **e.** Start a sliding scale of intermediate-acting insulin with 5-L fluid replacement of 0.9% sodium chloride with basal bolus short-acting insulin as required.

41 A 68-year-old woman presents with pain in her abdomen causing her to vomit. She states she has lost her appetite for food and can't hold anything down. Examination of the abdomen reveals localised tenderness over the left iliac fossa. Digital rectal examination reveals flecks of blood mixed with the stool. Routine blood tests show a white cell count of 17.3×10^9/L, C-reactive protein of 110 mg/l, urea of 6.9 mmol/L and creatinine of 118 μmol/L. Which of the following is NOT an indication for surgery?

- ☐ **a.** Faecal peritonitis.
- ☐ **b.** Colovesical fistula.
- ☐ **c.** Large bowel obstruction.
- ☐ **d.** Tender palpable mass.
- ☐ **e.** Failure to exclude cancer.

42 A 43-year-old man with known alcoholic liver disease presents to hospital with a distended abdomen, pain and yellow discolouration to his skin and sclera. On examination of the chest there are multiple blanching red raised lesions over the upper torso and arms, and loss of chest and axillary hair distribution. Abdominal examination reveals a 5-cm tender hepatomegaly with dilated tortuous veins around the umbilicus. Regarding portal-systemic venous anastomoses in portal hypertension, which of the following associations is NOT correct?

- ☐ **a.** Left gastric with azygous leading to oesophageal varices.
- ☐ **b.** Paraumbilical with inferior epigastric leading to caput medusae.
- ☐ **c.** Superior to middle/inferior rectal leading to rectal varices.
- ☐ **d.** Splenic with left gastric leading to splenic varices.
- ☐ **e.** Retroperitoneal and phrenic leading to diaphragmatic varices.

43 A 77-year-old man with known bibasal lung fibrosis is admitted to hospital for assessment of the need of long-term oxygen at home. He is already on home oxygen as required but his GP is concerned that he may need more regular therapy. Results of an arterial blood gas (ABG) taken on 35% oxygen via facemask are: pH 7.41, PO_2 11.1 kPa, PCO_2 5.4 kPa, bicarbonate 26 mmol/L. Which of the following is most appropriate in this case?

- ☐ **a.** Reduce oxygen to 28% and repeat ABG.
- ☐ **b.** Increase oxygen to 40% and repeat ABG.
- ☐ **c.** 35% is adequate oxygen for this patient.
- ☐ **d.** Increase oxygen to 60% and reassess.
- ☐ **e.** Repeat ABG measurement on air.

44 Whilst working on a busy medical firm at a teaching hospital you are asked to take some medical students to see interesting cases in order to improve their examination skills. You take them to see a 76-year-old gentleman who has the following clinical signs: unilateral ↓ chest expansion, ↓ breath sounds and ↓ percussion note. Which of the following clinical conditions would provide these clinical signs?

- ☐ **a.** Pneumothorax.
- ☐ **b.** Fibrosis.
- ☐ **c.** Consolidation.
- ☐ **d.** Pleural effusion.
- ☐ **e.** Extensive collapse/lobectomy/pneumonectomy.

45 Whilst in surgical pre-assessment clinic you note that a 68-year-old lady who is coming in electively for a knee replacement operation is complaining of shortness of breath. On further questioning you note that this is a chronic problem which the GP has not investigated. Since she is undergoing a general anaesthetic you decide to ask the anaesthetist for advice regarding her pre-operative management. He suggests a chest X-ray and lung function tests. Which of the following flow volume loops would represent a normal appearance?

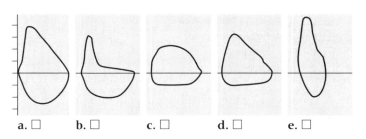

a. ☐   **b.** ☐   **c.** ☐   **d.** ☐   **e.** ☐

46 Whilst on placement at your local GP practice you are asked to see a 78-year-old man who is complaining of shortness of breath. He has no history of respiratory disease and denies use of inhalers. On examination you note that he has a temperature of 38°C and auscultation findings are consistent with a right lower zone pneumonia. Which of the following is the commonest cause of a community acquired pneumonia?

☐ **a.** *Haemophilus influenzae.*
☐ **b.** *Mycoplasma.*
☐ **c.** *Moraxella catarallis.*
☐ **d.** *Streptococcus pneumoniae.*
☐ **e.** *Staphylococcus aureus.*

47 Following making an accurate diagnosis of a community acquired pneumonia, which of the following antibiotics would you start as first-line treatment, bearing in mind that the patient has normal renal function and no known drug allergies?

☐ **a.** Erythromycin.
☐ **b.** Cefalexin.
☐ **c.** Amoxicillin.
☐ **d.** Augmentin.
☐ **e.** Metronidazole.

48 Mr Roberts is a 70-year-old man who has recently returned from a Mediterranean holiday. Over the past few days he has felt like he has the flu. He has been suffering with muscle aches, fever tiredness and has now developed a dry cough. He is becoming increasingly short of breath and his chest X-ray shows a bibasal consolidation. His past medical history includes a myocardial infarction and type II diabetes which is diet controlled. He smokes 10 cigarettes a day. Which of the following organisms is most likely to be the cause of his problem?

☐ **a.** *Legionella.*
☐ **b.** *Mycoplasma pneumoniae.*
☐ **c.** *Chlamydia pneumoniae.*
☐ **d.** *Pneumococcus.*
☐ **e.** *Staphylococcus aureus.*

49 A young child presents with regurgitation of food and vomiting noticed by the mother to occur frequently after meals. She is worried that the child has failed to progress along the normal centile chart and finds that the vomiting is worse when the child lies horizontal after mealtimes. Further investigation reveals a moderate congenital diaphragmatic hernia. Which of the following statements regarding diaphragmatic hernias is correct?

☐ **a.** Traumatic right-sided defects are more common than left-sided defects.
☐ **b.** Large central hernias may present as respiratory distress in neonates.
☐ **c.** Hernias through the foramen of Morgagni are usually significant.
☐ **d.** Congenital hiatal hernias almost always require surgical treatment.
☐ **e.** Traumatic diaphragmatic hernias are usually treated conservatively.

50 Regarding factors associated with peptic ulcer disease, which of the following is NOT considered to be a risk factor for ulceration?

☐ **a.** Pregnancy.
☐ **b.** Male sex.
☐ **c.** Head injury.
☐ **d.** Severe burns.
☐ **e.** Steroids.

51 A 15-year-old boy is admitted for pain in the right iliac fossa associated with nausea and vomiting for 3 days with signs of peritonism. The diagnosis is made and the child taken to the operating theatre. Twelve hours post-operatively the nursing staff are worried as the child is vomiting. Blood pressure and temperature measurements are normal and urine output is good. On examination the abdomen is soft but tender. According to the last entry in the notes he has been allowed to eat and drink but has not managed to keep anything down. Which of the following post-operative complications is most likely to have occurred?

☐ **a.** Small bowel obstruction.
☐ **b.** Anastomotic leak.
☐ **c.** Adverse reaction to anaesthetic agent.
☐ **d.** Acute stress ulceration.
☐ **e.** Post-operative ileus.

52 On seeing the patient you arrive at a diagnosis and decide on further management of the vomiting. Which of the following options should be considered in the first instance?

☐ **a.** Nasogastric tube insertion for oral intake.
☐ **b.** Erect chest radiograph.
☐ **c.** Abdominal radiograph.
☐ **d.** Anti-emetic medication.
☐ **e.** Proton pump inhibitor.

53 A 76-year-old man is referred from his GP to hospital due to recent weight loss, high blood glucose readings of 18 mmol/L and yellow discolouration of the skin and sclera. Routine blood tests reveal markedly deranged liver enzymes, normal urea and electrolytes, and normal full blood count. Examination reveals an obese habitus, yellow discolouration of the skin and sclera, and 5-cm non-tender hepatomegaly. Which of the following diagnoses is the most likely?

☐ **a.** Pancreatic adenocarcinoma.
☐ **b.** Cholangiocarcinoma.
☐ **c.** Choledocholithiasis.
☐ **d.** Hepatitis.
☐ **e.** New-onset diabetes mellitus.

54 A 82-year-old man presents with progressive shortness of breath, paroxysmal nocturnal dyspnoea and orthopnoea over the past 3 weeks. Further questioning reveals a past medical history that is remarkable for osteoarthritis and right knee replacement. He is a heavy smoker and drinks moderate alcohol. Clinical examination reveals tachypnoea, tachycardia and bilateral ankle swelling. Dullness of the percussion note of the right hemithorax is elicited with reduced vocal resonance as well as asymmetrical chest wall movement on inspiration. Auscultation reveals reduced breath sounds to the right midzone and bibasal crepitations. Which of the following should be carried out next?

- ☐ **a.** Echocardiography.
- ☐ **b.** Chest radiography.
- ☐ **c.** Pleural tap and drainage.
- ☐ **d.** Intravenous clarithromycin and amoxicillin.
- ☐ **e.** Electrocardiogram.

55 A 13-year-old boy falls onto concrete whilst roller-skating. He is seen by the out of hours GP and is found to have a tender swollen base of the thumb with tenderness in the anatomical snuffbox. He has weakness on making a pincer grip but has normal abductor pollicis brevis function: Which of the following is the MOST LIKELY diagnosis?

- ☐ **a.** Paronychia.
- ☐ **b.** Nailbed haematoma.
- ☐ **c.** Radial nerve injury.
- ☐ **d.** Lower brachial plexus root injury.
- ☐ **e.** Scaphoid fracture.

56 A 14-year-old girl presents to her GP with severe cramping abdominal pain and diarrhoea for the past 2 weeks. She had a similar episode 8 weeks earlier, which resolved without medical attention. At present the diarrhoea is bloody and bowel motions are associated with crampy abdominal pains. In addition the GP notes oral ulcers, which are painful and according to the patient have been present for the past 3 days. Her family history includes a grandfather who had a colostomy for a gastro intestinal (GI) problem. What is the most likely cause for her symptoms and signs?

- ☐ **a.** Crohn's disease.
- ☐ **b.** Ulcerative colitis.
- ☐ **c.** Henoch–Schönlein purpura.
- ☐ **d.** *Shigella* infection.
- ☐ **e.** *Giardia* infection.

57 A 23-year-old lady has attended the accident and emergency department complaining of a high fever, diarrhoea and vomiting. She has noticed a headache and occasional muscle aches. She has no past medical history of note and has had no recent illnesses. Her menstrual cycle is regular lasting for 5 days a month and her most recent period finished 5 days ago. On examination she appears dehydrated and is hypotensive. What is the most likely diagnosis in her case?
- ☐ **a.** Viral gastroenteritis.
- ☐ **b.** Bowel ischaemia.
- ☐ **c.** Dysmenorrhoea.
- ☐ **d.** Pregnancy.
- ☐ **e.** Toxic shock syndrome.

58 Which of the following associations is incorrect?
- ☐ **a.** *Trichomonas* – yellow discharge.
- ☐ **b.** *Chlamydia* – chronic cervicitis.
- ☐ **c.** Gonorrhoea – urethritis.
- ☐ **d.** *Gardnerella vaginalis* – white discharge.
- ☐ **e.** Atrophic vaginitis – yellow discharge.

59 In estimating the prevalence of disease in a small town, the public health statistician gathers population data including epidemiological data regarding the number of cases and deaths over the past year. There are currently 20,000 people who suffer from the disease. There were 250 deaths over the past year attributed to the disease and 500 new cases were diagnosed in the same period. Information regarding deaths was further broken down into those occurring due to natural causes and those due to violent crime or homicide of which there were 135 and 28, respectively. The population of the town is estimated from voting records to be 140,000. Which of the following correctly describes the prevalence of the disease?
- ☐ **a.** 250/20,000.
- ☐ **b.** 500/140,000.
- ☐ **c.** 500/20,000.
- ☐ **d.** 20,000/140,000.
- ☐ **e.** 250/140,000.

60 Which of the following is NOT a lower motor neurone cause of a facial nerve palsy?
- ☐ **a.** Bell's palsy.
- ☐ **b.** Acoustic neuroma.
- ☐ **c.** Ramsay Hunt Syndrome.
- ☐ **d.** HIV.
- ☐ **e.** Cerebrovascular accident.

Extended matching questions

Hip pain

a. Irritable hip.
b. Fractured neck of femur.
c. Slipped upper femoral epiphysis.
d. Hip dislocation.
e. Peri-prosthetic fracture.
f. Congenital dislocation of the hip.
g. Perthes' disease.
h. Septic arthritis.

61 A 78-year-old overweight lady with a history of osteoarthritis
of the right hip and a total hip replacement presents to accident and emergency. She tried to contact her GP but was unable to get an appointment. She is complaining of pain on the
lateral aspect of her right leg and in her right groin, and has
been unable to weight bear since the morning when she fell
over and landed on her right hip. On examination you note
that her leg is shortened and internally rotated whilst being
held in an adducted position. The neurovascular supply to the
leg is intact.

62 A 7-year-old boy is referred by the GP to the orthopaedic
team for hip pain which has gradually developed over the
past 4 hours. His mother notes that over the same time period
he has developed a limp and is not keen on moving his leg
and is insisting on being carried everywhere. Plain X-rays
show no obvious problem and an ultrasound of the affected
hip shows a collection of fluid. He is afebrile and otherwise well and his hip does not feel hot.

63 An 87-year-old gentleman was referred by the on-call general
☐ practitioner for review. He noted that the patient was a nursing home resident and had suffered a fall a week ago but was still complaining of right hip pain. During the past week he has been treated with regular analgesia and despite this has experienced difficulty in weight bearing due to pain. The on-call GP was asked to review the patient today due to worsening of his hip pain at rest and was reluctant to weight bear or mobilise on that leg. On examination the GP noted that his leg was found to be shortened and externally rotated with tenderness on palpation of the groin and greater trochanter. Straight leg raise was limited due to pain and internal rotation caused severe pain, all other hip movements were satisfactory.

64 A 49-year-old lady presents to accident and emergency 6 weeks
☐ after insertion of a hip resurfacing prosthesis. Since the operation she describes the hip as, 'not ever being quite right'. In the 2 days prior to presentation she noticed increasingly bad pain in her right hip (same side as prosthesis) which radiates into her groin. The pain is preventing her from weight bearing although whilst lying supine all hip movements are possible passively to some degree although they are limited by pain.

65 A 78-year-old man complains of left-sided hip pain. It has been
☐ present for the past 6 hours and is becoming increasingly painful to the point that he is unable to weight bear. His GP is called out to see him and notes a fever of 38°C with pain on palpation of the hip joint and virtually no movement in any direction in the hip. He has a history of having a right total hip replacement 3 years ago. He is referred to the on-call orthopaedic team and blood results show WBC $17.1 * 10^9$/L, CRP 56 mg/L, ESR 24 mm/hr. What is the likely diagnosis?

Substance abuse

    a. Cocaine.
    b. Amphetamines.
    c. LSD.
    d. Phencyclidine (PCP).
    e. Benzodiazepines.
    f. Opioids.
    g. Alcohol.
    h. Barbiturates.
    i. Marijuana.

The following patients have all presented with signs and symptoms of substance abuse. Please choose the most likely substance of abuse from the above list. Each option may be used once, more than once or not at all.

66 A 43-year-old businessman presents to hospital after going for some drinks with colleagues from work. He is restless, stating that he doesn't need to be in hospital and asking when he can go home. On examination he is tachycardic at 120 beats per minute with dilated pupils. Whilst you are examining him he starts to have episodic chest pain.

67 A 52-year-old man is admitted to hospital as he was found wandering the streets confused and 'talking to himself'. He is well known to the local hospitals attending frequently with malnutrition and chest infections. On examination he has heavily injected conjunctiva, appears to be hearing voices and does not readily make eye contact. He is somnolent and exhibits a lack of interest in food or drink when brought to him.

68 A 62-year-old woman is brought to hospital having suffered a fall in the street. On arrival she is disorientated and complaining of chest pain. An ECG performed demonstrates a prolonged QT interval and U waves. On examination she exhibits a lateral gaze palsy and is very unsteady on her feet.

69 A 32-year-old woman is brought to accident and emergency
☐ found collapsed in a nearby residential estate. She is unconscious on arrival and paramedics are securing an endotracheal
tube with 100% oxygen on arrival to hospital. Her blood pressure reading is 90/55 mmHg on her left arm and her temperature is 34.7°C. An arterial blood gas reading taken in hospital
demonstrates a pH of 7.31 with a PO_2 of 15 kPa and a PCO_2 of
6.3 kPa.

70 A 17-year-old high-school student is brought to hospital by his
☐ parents who were concerned about his recent strange behaviour. He was found in his room unable to move his legs and
complaining that his room was all blurry. On arrival to hospital
he is sweating, agitated and violent with a blood pressure of
195/89 mmHg. Neurological examination reveals no pyramidal
abnormality but is remarkable for a florid vertical nystagmus.

Genitourinary discharge

a. Candidiasis.

b. *Trichomonas vaginalis* (TU).

c. *Chlamydia trachomatis*.

d. Lymphogranuloma venereum.

e. *Haemophilus ducreyi*.

f. Bacterial vaginosis.

g. Gonorrhoea.

h. Donovanosis.

The following patients have all presented with genitourinary discharge. Please choose the most correct diagnosis from the above list. Each option may be used once, more than once or not at all.

71 A 33-year-old secretary presents to her GP with an offensive discharge that she noticed 2 days ago. She initially thought it might have been related to her menstrual cycle, however she denies any previous episodes of discharge. A vaginal swab is taken when it is noticed that the discharge smells fishy, however, with a normal appearance to the vagina on speculum examination. Slide microscopy reveals the presence of epithelial clue cells.

72 A 23-year-old man presents to the sexual health clinic with discharge from the penis and a burning sensation on passing urine. He has never had an episode like this before and when questioned he admits to casual sex with multiple partners since breaking up with his girlfriend a month ago. On examination there is a yellowish discharge from the urethra and microscopy shows Gram-negative intracellular diplococci.

73 A 42-year-old man presents to his GP with on itchy rash on his penis. He denies any recent sexual intercourse and has not travelled out of the country for many years. He states he has had the rash for some time with no ill effect. On examination the head of the penis has multiple red lesions with cracked and raw skin. His past medical history is remarkable only for osteoarthritis and type II diabetes mellitus treated with diclofenac and metformin.

74 A 34-year-old woman presents to her GP as she and her husband have been trying for their first child for the past year and a half. She is embarrassed and upset to talk about their sexual habits and is frustrated because all her sisters have borne children already. On further questioning she reveals that she used to work as a prostitute but has 'given that all up now'. An endocervical swab is taken and the organism grown from cell culture is reported as being an obligate intracellular bacterium.

75 A 45-year-old woman presents to her local general practice nurse appointment for a routine smear test. She has not been for regular appointments with the nurse before. Whilst performing the smear test the nurse notices that the surface of the cervix is dotted with small haemorrhages and that there is an offensive, frothy, yellow-green discharge in the vagina with multiple erythematous areas on the vaginal walls.

Seronegative arthritides

a. Reiter's syndrome.
b. Enteropathic arthropathy.
c. Rheumatoid arthritis.
d. Ankylosing spondylitis (AS).
e. Reactive arthritis.
f. Scleroderma.
g. Psoriatic arthropathy.
h. Enthesopathy.

The following patients have all presented with rheumatological problems. Please choose the most correct diagnosis from the above list. Each option may be used once, more than once or not at all.

76 A 31-year-old businessman presents to his GP complaining of an ache in his right knee with an inability to weight bear for the past week. He denies any history of trauma and recent travel history is remarkable only for a 12-hour flight to Thailand a few weeks previously. He denies any previous episodes of joint problems. On examination he is reluctant to remove his trousers when examining the knee and you notice he has a very tender, sore left eye.

77 A 53-year-old man presents to the rheumatology clinic for regular follow-up. He undergoes regular light therapy and his only medications are topical tar and ibuprofen for chronic back pain. On examination he has pitting of his nails on two of the digits on one hand with an asymmetrical oligoarthritis affecting the small joints of both hands.

78 A 20-year-old man presents with a pain in his left foot associated with walking and standing. He works in an office as a sales clerk and denies any particularly strenuous exercise recently. On examination when asked to demonstrate the site of pain he has particular difficulty bending over to touch his foot. Further questioning reveals a similar episode of pain affecting the 'tendon at the back of his right ankle' last year.

79 A 22-year-old man presents to his GP with a 2-month history of pain and stiffness in his back, associated with a reduced range of movement. He noticed this whilst stretching before a football game. He is anxious during the consultation and tells you that he is worried as he has been experiencing a tight sensation around his chest associated with pain that sometimes happens in the morning. Schoeber's test is markedly reduced.

80 A 34-year-old woman presents to hospital with multiple episodes of loose stools associated with some mucous and blood. History taking reveals a history of weight loss, fluctuating diarrhoea and previous hospital admission for a severely painful red eye. She has been investigated previously at her GP for back pain and swollen joints.

Abdominal pain

a. Intussusception.
b. Pyloric stenosis.
c. Hirschsprung's disease.
d. Volvulus.
e. Appendicitis.
f. Nephroblastoma.
g. Inguinal hernia.
h. Constipation.

81 A 9-year-old girl is brought to see the GP by her mother.
☐ She has been complaining of passing heavily bloodstained
urine, which her mother believes represents early menarche.
On further questioning the girl also complains of left-sided
abdominal pain that is constant but has gradually been worsening over the past few weeks. She denies any constitutional
symptoms and generally feels well. On examination she has a
mass in her left loin.

82 A 4-year-old boy is brought to the accident and emergency
☐ department by his worried father. He has noticed that his son
appears to be generally unwell and seems to be adopting a ball-
like position for comfort. He is denying abdominal pain. He has
passed one stool that appeared to be quite abnormal, his father
likens it to red currant jelly. He feels nauseated but has not
vomited. On examination he has a palpable mass in his right
lower quadrant but is not guarding and does not appear to be
clinically peritonitic.

83 A 7-year-old boy presents to his GP with a new-onset
☐ abdominal pain in the past 24 hours. In addition he notes
abdominal distension and constipation for the preceding 2
days. There is evidence of a right-sided abdominal mass which
is resonant to percussion and he is afebrile with no other
abdominal findings.

84 A 6-week-old infant is brought to see his GP as he is suffering
☐ from more frequent episodes of projectile vomiting. His
mother is nervous as she has not had any other children and
he appears to be hungry immediately after vomiting unaltered
milk.

85 A 14-year-old girl is sent home from school after complaining of abdominal pain. She describes the pain as being increasingly constant in the right iliac fossa and has some associated diarrhoea and nausea. On examination she is found to be febrile and have tenderness in the right iliac fossa with some guarding.

Peri-arrest drugs

    a. Atropine.
    b. Adrenaline.
    c. Amiodarone.
    d. Lignocaine.
    e. Magnesium sulphate.
    f. Adenosine.
    g. Verapamil.
    h. Flecainide.

86 This is the drug of choice in sinus, artrial or nodal bradycardias.
☐ It can also be used in pulseless electrical activity with a rate less than 60 beats per minute.

87 This drug is used in the management of torsades de pointes,
☐ ventricular tachyarrhythmias and occasionally in acute asthma.

88 Used in refractory ventricular fibrillation (VF) or pulseless
☐ ventricular tachycardia (VT).

89 Used in paroxysmal supraventricular tachycardia and narrow
☐ complex tachycardia.

90 Used in artrial fibrillation or supraventricular tachycardias with
☐ an accessory pathway.

PAPER 3

Questions

Multiple choice questions (single best answer)

1 A 15-year-old boy is referred to the renal clinic by his GP with a history of worsening haematuria. His mother has been worried recently that he has been taking illicit drugs as he has been finding it more difficult to cope at school and has been falling behind in his schoolwork. He also seems to be less attentive of late and has become more withdrawn, watching television on his own with the volume up loud. Which of the following conditions fits most closely with the clinical history?

☐ **a.** Alport's syndrome.
☐ **b.** Anderson–Fabry disease.
☐ **c.** Goodpasture's syndrome.
☐ **d.** Wegener's granulomatosis.
☐ **e.** Von Hippel–Lindau syndrome.

2 An 80-year-old woman presents to hospital with confusion and pain in her back. She was found by a neighbour wandering near her flat in the early hours of the evening stating that she was going to go to church. Routine blood tests in accident and emergency demonstrate a calcium of 3.1 mmol/L, alkaline phosphatase of 249 IU/L, urea of 12 mmol/L with creatinine of 317 mmol/L and a haemoglobin level of 10.7 g/dL. Plain lumbosacral radiographs were done after eliciting point tenderness over the lower vertebrae that demonstrate punched-out lytic lesions. Which of the following is the most likely diagnosis?

☐ **a.** Paget's disease.
☐ **b.** Sarcoidosis.
☐ **c.** Hyperparathyroidism.
☐ **d.** Myeloma.
☐ **e.** Osteosarcoma.

3 Which of the following is NOT routinely considered as part of a renal screen in the investigation of new-onset renal failure?

☐ **a.** Complement.
☐ **b.** Renal ultrasound.
☐ **c.** Caeruloplasmin and serum copper.
☐ **d.** Anti-neutrophil cytoplasmic antibodies.
☐ **e.** Bence–Jones protein.

4 A 58-year-old woman presents to hospital with headache, blurred vision and palpitations. She states that she has been feeling unwell for about a week prior to coming to hospital and has been having more frequent headaches that are 'all over' her head and associated with blurring of her vision. Her past medical history is unremarkable. She tells you that she is worried that this might be a stroke as her two of her family members suffered from strokes at a young age. Routine observations record a blood pressure reading of 194/110mmHg with a pulse of 115 beats per minute, temperature of 36.4°C with respiratory rate of 22 breaths per minute and oxygen saturations of 99% on room air. Examination findings are unremarkable. Routine blood tests show a sodium level of 136mmol/L, a potassium of 4.8mmol/L with a urea of 10.2mmol/L, creatinine of 172μmol/L and haemoglobin of 9.8g/dL. White cell count and C-reactive protein (CRP) are within normal limits. Which of the following investigations in indicated in the first line?

☐ **a.** Renal ultrasound.
☐ **b.** CT scan of the head.
☐ **c.** Renal biopsy.
☐ **d.** 24-hour urinary metanephrines (VMA).
☐ **e.** Carotid and vertebral artery Dopplers.

5 A 5-year-old boy is referred to the paediatric nephrology clinic by his GP. His father states that his son has been passing dark urine that resembles blackcurrant juice and has noticed that his abdomen has become more swollen on one side than the other. His father is worried that this might be cancer as his own mother died of breast cancer when he was 17 years old. On examination there is a painless mass that moves with respiration in the right flank and a urine sample performed at the clinic shows frank haematuria. Which of the following investigations is most important to obtain with respect to future management?

☐ **a.** CT scan of the abdomen.
☐ **b.** Renal ultrasonography.
☐ **c.** Bilateral surgical biopsies.
☐ **d.** Albumin/creatinine ratio.
☐ **e.** Chest radiography.

6 A 34-year-old man is brought to hospital short of breath and diagnosed with a chest infection. He is treated on amoxicillin and clarithromycin. Shortly after commencement of antibiotic therapy he is found on the ward to be passing only 10mL/h via his urinary catheter although he is well hydrated. Observations reveal a temperature of 38.4°C, blood pressure of 165/96mmHg with a regular pulse of 92 beats per minute (bpm). Examination reveals a diffuse rash over his body. Urinalysis reveals proteinuria and eosinophils and blood tests reveal a markedly raised eosinophil count. Which of the following diagnoses is the most likely?

☐ **a.** Ascending urinary tract infection.
☐ **b.** Haemolytic uraemic syndrome.
☐ **c.** Drug-induced interstitial nephritis.
☐ **d.** Cholesterol embolus.
☐ **e.** Acute tubular necrosis.

7 Whilst on ward cover one evening you are asked to review a 78-year-old lady who is known to have a history of ischaemic heart disease and atrial fibrillation. She was admitted to hospital on this occasion after developing a severe community acquired pneumonia requiring intravenous treatment. The nursing staff are concerned that she seems to have developed a facial asymmetry which was not mentioned in her initial clerking. On your review she notes that this has been there for some time and her GP was investigating the cause prior to her admission into hospital. Which of the following is not known to cause a lower motor neurone facial weakness?

☐ **a.** Head injury.
☐ **b.** Sarcoidosis.
☐ **c.** Guillain–Barré syndrome.
☐ **d.** Lyme disease.
☐ **e.** Medullary infarction.

8 On your emergency medicine rotation you are clerking a 25-year-old patient who has presented with headaches. On the basis of the history you decide that these sound like tension headaches and neurological examination is perfectly normal apart from small pupils that you have noticed. They are equal and reactive to light and accommodation. In which of the following conditions are small pupils characteristic?

☐ **a.** Holmes–Adie syndrome.
☐ **b.** Acute retrobulbar neuritis.
☐ **c.** Amitriptyline overdose.
☐ **d.** Pontine haemorrhage.
☐ **e.** Syphilis.

9 During a busy medical take your Senior House Officer asks you to see a patient who has been referred by accident and emergency with a spastic paraparesis. The patient is a 65-year-old gentleman who denies any past medical problems other than hypertension and an appendicectomy as a child. The family are concerned that this is due to the effect of a stroke and are concerned since he is a non-smoker and has no past cardiac problems. On examination you confirm that he does have a spastic paraparesis. Which of the following conditions would NOT be consistent with that clinical finding?

- ☐ **a.** Demyelating myelopathy.
- ☐ **b.** Spondylosis of the lumbosacral spine.
- ☐ **c.** Motor neurone disease.
- ☐ **d.** Syringomyelia.
- ☐ **e.** Meningioma.

10 Which of the following associations is incorrect?

- ☐ **a.** Hyponatraemia and central pontine myelinolysis.
- ☐ **b.** Hyperthyroidism and tremor.
- ☐ **c.** Hypernatraemia and seizures.
- ☐ **d.** Hypoglycaemia and hemiparesis.
- ☐ **e.** Hypercalcaemia and muscle cramps.

11 A 57-year-old gentleman presents to his GP having noticed that the power in his hand has reduced. He works as a carpenter and has noticed that he is finding it increasingly difficult to carry out tasks that he once considered effortless. He denies any weakness elsewhere and neurological examination is normal other than wasting and weakness in the hypothenar and small muscles of his right hand. Which of the following would NOT account for these signs?

- ☐ **a.** Peripheral motor neuropathies.
- ☐ **b.** Syringomyclia.
- ☐ **c.** Ulnar nerve lesion at the elbow.
- ☐ **d.** Amyotropic lateral sclerosis (ALS).
- ☐ **e.** Osteoarthritis of cervical and thoracic spine.

12 Whilst on your general practice rotation there is concern about a possible local outbreak of bovine spongiform encephalopathy. During the following week you get a number of visits from patients concerned that this will develop into the human form of the disease and are concerned about the risks. Which of the following facts about Creutzfeld–Jakob disease are INCORRECT?

- ☐ **a.** It is caused by a slowly mutating virus.
- ☐ **b.** A typical presentation would involve a progressive dementia.
- ☐ **c.** It has been shown to be transmissible by surgery.
- ☐ **d.** Arises from a conformational change in a prion protein.
- ☐ **e.** Can be tested for with tonsil biopsies.

13 A 78-year-old man presents to hospital after not passing stool for 3 days. He is confused and is accompanied by his carer from the nursing home in which he is resident. A careful history from his daughter reveals he has lost 8 kg in weight over the past 2 months and has been acting unusually over the past month or so. Which of the following tumour markers would be expected to be raised in this disease?

- ☐ **a.** Carcino-embryonic antigen (CEA).
- ☐ **b.** CA 153.
- ☐ **c.** Alpha-fetoprotein (AFP).
- ☐ **d.** Neurone specific enolase (NSE).
- ☐ **e.** Human chorionic gonadotrophin (HCG).

14 A 45-year-old woman is admitted electively to hospital for hepatic cyst fenestration. She makes a good post-operative recovery, however, on the 4th day post-surgery she starts to complain of abdominal pain with fever, nausea and a tender, tense abdomen. Routine blood tests show a high white cell count, a bilirubin of 32 μmol/L, alanine aminotransferase (ALT) of 50 μmol/L and an aspartate transaminase (AST) of 32 μmol/L. Which of the following is the most sensitive diagnostic investigation to perform?

- ☐ **a.** Ultra Sound liver and gallbladder.
- ☐ **b.** HIDA scan.
- ☐ **c.** Plain abdominal radiograph.
- ☐ **d.** CT scan of the abdomen.
- ☐ **e.** ERCP (endoscopic retrograde cholangiopancreatography).

15 A 67-year-old lady completed a week-long course of antibiotics for a hospital-acquired pneumonia. You are reviewing her and she complains that she feels generally unwell. Her observation chart shows a swinging fever and she notes that she is still suffering with a productive cough with foul-smelling sputum. On further questioning she admits chest pain and occasional haemoptysis. You request a chest X-ray and the results show a walled cavity. Which of the following is the most likely diagnosis?

- ☐ **a.** Pleural effusion.
- ☐ **b.** Pulmonary embolus.
- ☐ **c.** Recurrent infection.
- ☐ **d.** Lung abscess.
- ☐ **e.** Empyema.

16 Mr Davies is a 58-year-old gentleman with a history of recurrent pneumonia. He has been referred to the on-call team for management of this current episode of pneumonia as the GP is concerned that he is not able to get on top of this problem in the community. On further questioning you discover that he has been complaining of a persistent cough for the past 2 weeks with copious sputum that is occasionally bloodstained. He is a non-smoker. On examination you note finger clubbing with coarse inspiratory crepitations and occasional wheeze. An erect chest X-ray shows cystic shadows. Which of the following is the most likely diagnosis?

- ☐ **a.** Lung cancer.
- ☐ **b.** Bronchiectasis.
- ☐ **c.** Pulmonary fibrosis.
- ☐ **d.** Pneumonia.
- ☐ **e.** Pulmonary embolus.

17 You are asked to review a chest X-ray for a colleague. You notice a round opacity which of the following is NOT one of your differential diagnoses?

- ☐ **a.** Tuberculosis.
- ☐ **b.** Aspergilloma.
- ☐ **c.** Lung cancer.
- ☐ **d.** Sarcoidosis.
- ☐ **e.** Carcinoid tumour.

18 An 69-year-old gentleman with a past history of lung cancer presents with general fatigue and worsening shortness of breath. He has been undergoing chemotherapy for his lung cancer and is due to be followed up with his oncologist in a few days time. Which of the following are NOT known to be complications of lung cancer?

- ☐ **a.** Hyponatraemia.
- ☐ **b.** Superior vena cava obstruction.
- ☐ **c.** Hoarse voice.
- ☐ **d.** Horner's syndrome.
- ☐ **e.** Pulmonary oedema.

19 Causes of type I respiratory failure include all of the following except?

- ☐ **a.** Pneumonia.
- ☐ **b.** Pulmonary embolus.
- ☐ **c.** Acute exacerbation of asthma.
- ☐ **d.** Acute respiratory distress syndrome.
- ☐ **e.** Pulmonary fibrosis.

20 According to the British Thoracic Society, which of the following is NOT a major risk factor for a pulmonary embolus?

- ☐ **a.** Abdominal malignancy.
- ☐ **b.** Recent hip replacement.
- ☐ **c.** Oral contraceptive pill.
- ☐ **d.** Previous venous thromboembolism.
- ☐ **e.** Immobility.

21 Chest radiography confirms a pleural effusion and a pleural tap and drainage is performed. Pleural fluid analysis reveals a murky dark brown fluid with a protein content of 45 g/dL and heavy lymphocytic involvement. Which of the following is the LEAST likely diagnosis?

- ☐ **a.** Tuberculosis.
- ☐ **b.** Malignancy.
- ☐ **c.** Rheumatoid arthritis.
- ☐ **d.** Liver failure.
- ☐ **e.** Systemic lupus erythematosus.

22 A 44-year-old man is brought in to accident and emergency by helicopter having fallen out of a third floor building. On arrival he has a Glasgow Coma Scale of 4/15 and is intubated and ventilated. Neurological examination reveals unequal pupils and urgent CT scan of the head is performed, which demonstrates midline shift and a left-sided convex enhancing area. Which of the following is the next most appropriate course of action?

- [ ] **a.** Intravenous mannitol to reduce intracranial pressure.
- [ ] **b.** Conservative management with 30 degree head-up nursing.
- [ ] **c.** Intravenous thiopentone to reduce intracranial pressure.
- [ ] **d.** Urgent neurosurgical evacuation of extradural haematoma.
- [ ] **e.** Urgent coiling of burst aneurysm under neuroradiological guidance.

23 A 47-year-old business man is caught in a fire in his office and suffers severe burns to his arms and upper body. He is assessed to have 35% burns to the upper torso, which are not painful to touch and are white in colour. He is admitted to hospital and placed under observation in the burns unit. Which of the following complications of this type of injury is especially important to recognise?

- [ ] **a.** Respiratory distress.
- [ ] **b.** Bacterial infection.
- [ ] **c.** Loss of peripheral pulses.
- [ ] **d.** Severe dehydration.
- [ ] **e.** Acute stress ulceration.

24 An adolescent presents to his school doctor with bilateral tender and swollen breasts. He has become increasingly self-conscious of late and has been avoiding physical education classes. On examination there are tender soft masses in the lower quadrants of both breasts. Which of the following is the most appropriate next step in managing this patient?

- [ ] **a.** Urgent referral to social services.
- [ ] **b.** Reassure the patient that this is normal.
- [ ] **c.** Needle aspiration and send fluid for culture and cytology.
- [ ] **d.** Referral to a breast surgeon for excision and biopsy.
- [ ] **e.** Short course of oral prednisolone and 2-week review.

25 A 43-year-old man comes to hospital with severe pain and tenderness in the left flank. A provisional diagnosis of ureteric obstruction by a renal calculus is made. Intravenous urogram taken shortly after admission to hospital would be most likely to show:

☐ **a.** Reduced size of left kidney.
☐ **b.** Reduced size of right kidney.
☐ **c.** Perfusion defect in the left pelvicalyxceal region.
☐ **d.** Bladder residual post-micturition.
☐ **e.** Delayed excretion by left kidney.

26 A 31-year-old woman is admitted to the surgical team with nausea, bilious vomiting and generalised abdominal pain. She has had multiple previous admissions for abdominal pain and bloody diarrhoea and takes regular low-dose steroids under review by the gastroenterologists. Abdominal X-ray performed on admission demonstrates dilated loops of small bowel. Which of the following is the most likely cause of the radiological findings?

☐ **a.** Meckel's diverticulum.
☐ **b.** Intussusception.
☐ **c.** Adhesions.
☐ **d.** Stricture due to ulcerative colitis.
☐ **e.** Gastro-colic fistula due to Crohn's disease.

27 A 12-year-old boy presents to his GP with several days of generalised tiredness, painful joints in particular the knees, nodular swelling over his elbows and associated low-grade fever with a mild rash on his chest. He has no other medical problems but a few weeks earlier he had complained of a sore throat, which was managed supportively. Which of the following is the most likely diagnosis?

☐ **a.** Rheumatic fever.
☐ **b.** Rheumatoid arthritis.
☐ **c.** Reiter's syndrome.
☐ **d.** Scarlet fever.
☐ **e.** Systemic lupus erythematosus.

28 A 5-year-old boy is brought to see this GP by his parents. He has never visited the practice before but his parents tell you that he has no past medical history of note. At present, they are concerned that he seems to tire easily and complain of pain in his legs. He prefers to stay indoor and watch television rather than playing outdoors with other children. On physical examination, he looks well. His blood pressure reads 138/94mmHg in his right arm and his legs appear to be atrophic and mottled in colour. Which of the following findings are UNLIKELY to be present in this boy?

- ☐ **a.** Reduced lower extremity pulses.
- ☐ **b.** Cyanosis of the toes.
- ☐ **c.** A bicuspid aortic valve on echocardiography.
- ☐ **d.** Rib notching on chest X-ray.
- ☐ **e.** Left ventricular hypertrophy on ECG.

29 A 17-year-old girl seeks advice from her GP for severe abdominal pain. The pain started in her lower abdomen and is central. She has some associated nausea but no vomiting. On further questioning she denies any disturbance to her bowels but notes some dyspareunia and admits to having had unprotected sexual intercourse. She has a low-grade fever and confirms a small amount of smelly vaginal discharge. Which of the following is the most likely diagnosis in this case?

- ☐ **a.** Endometriosis.
- ☐ **b.** Ruptured ovarian cyst.
- ☐ **c.** Pelvic inflammatory disease.
- ☐ **d.** Uterine fibroids.
- ☐ **e.** Mittelschmerz pain.

30 Which of the following facts about carcinoma of the cervix are INCORRECT?

- ☐ **a.** 90% are adenocarcinoma.
- ☐ **b.** Associated with human papilloma virus.
- ☐ **c.** Common presentation is intermenstrual vaginal bleeding.
- ☐ **d.** Cervical erosions may be seen on speculum examination.
- ☐ **e.** The disease may not present until the advanced stage.

31 A research fellow is assessing the effectiveness of a new surgical therapy for melanoma and recruits newly diagnosed melanoma sufferers to the study. He randomises the total participants to either the existing treatment or the novel treatment arm and performs the standard operation for melanoma excision on the first group ($n = 420$). He also performs the newly proposed therapy on the second group ($n = 390$). The treatment arms are double-blinded (both to him and the patients); 6 months after the surgery the patients are seen in clinic to assess for recurrence rates. The following data are obtained:

	Disease present	Disease absent
Standard treatment	80	340
Novel treatment	60	330

Which of the following investigations would be the most suitable for investigating the effect of the novel treatment?
- ☐ **a.** Mann–Whitney U test
- ☐ **b.** Paired *t*-test
- ☐ **c.** Positive-predictive value
- ☐ **d.** Odds ratio
- ☐ **e.** Chi-squared test

32 A 37-year-old lady was admitted to hospital at 2 a.m. following a fall out of her first floor bedroom window. The incidents surrounding the accident were unclear but on arrival to hospital she was immobilised in a hard collar and sandbags and had a GCS of 15 with an obvious left-sided distal radial fracture. On further examination she was found to have left-sided bony pelvic pain which on X-ray was found to be a fracture of the iliac wing. She denied any pain in her thoracic and lumbar spine during a log roll examination and the rectal examination was found to be unremarkable. Examination of her cervical spine elicited no bony tenderness and good flexion and extension without development of any paraesthesiae or pain. Antero-posterior, lateral and peg views of her cervical spine showed no evidence of any fractures, subluxations or dislocations. How should we proceed from here?
- ☐ **a.** Remove hard collar and three-way immobilisation.
- ☐ **b.** Keep just hard collar on.
- ☐ **c.** Keep hard collar and three-way immobilisation *in situ* and organise CT of the cervical spine to confirm the X-ray findings.
- ☐ **d.** Remove hard collar but organise CT of cervical spine urgently
- ☐ **e.** Get flexion and extension cervical spine views.

33 Which of the following signs is NOT an early sign of compartment syndrome?

☐ **a.** Pain in the affected limb on passive movements.
☐ **b.** Pallor.
☐ **c.** Tension of the muscle group.
☐ **d.** Loss of pulse.
☐ **e.** Paraesthesiae.

34 An 87-year-old man is admitted to hospital for shortness of breath and coughing up bloodstained sputum. A chest radiograph demonstrates a ring-shadow in the right upper lobe and CT scan of the chest is suspicious for malignancy. Bronchoscopy and histology confirms the diagnosis. The family are involved daily in the care of the patient and one day the daughters approach you and urge you that if the diagnosis is cancer then for the sake of their father's state of mind can you tell him the results are inconclusive. The family tell you they have just buried their mother having died of breast cancer and they fear their father will not be able to take the news. Which of the following is the correct course of action?

☐ **a.** Comply with their wishes to not let their father know the diagnosis on grounds of compassion.
☐ **b.** Only disclose the diagnosis to the father if he asks directly.
☐ **c.** Allow the grieving period to come to a close and let his GP break the diagnosis once out of hospital.
☐ **d.** State that you understand the delicate situation but inform the patient of his diagnosis as it is his right to know.
☐ **e.** Ask the family to break the diagnosis to their father at an appropriate time.

35 A 54-year-old man presents with pain in his left knee and a rash on his forearm that he has noticed developing over some weeks. He describes the rash as red underneath with a white scale that can be rubbed off to leave little spots of bleeding. The rash is confined to the forearm and involves the elbow and there is a little area of similar looking rash over an old appendix scar. He has also noticed some differences in two of the nails of his right hand with little roughened depressions in the nails themselves. He is seen by his GP who diagnoses the condition and prescribes some medication. Which of the following is NOT used in the treatment of the above skin disorder?

☐ **a.** Topical steroids.
☐ **b.** Tar.
☐ **c.** Aqueous cream.
☐ **d.** PUVA.
☐ **e.** Dapsone.

36 A 6-year-old girl is brought to her GP by her mother who has noticed that she has been scratching incessantly and has become extremely irritable over the past week. The mother can identify no precipitants, however, states that the girl has recently started at a new school and asks if it could be something to do with this. On examination there is a widespread rash over the abdomen with tiny papules over the webspaces and fingers of both hands that are intensely itchy. Associated with the papules are linear tracts that are surrounded by erythema. Which of the following treatments should be instituted?

☐ **a.** Malathion 0.5% cream.
☐ **b.** Flucloxacillin 500mg.
☐ **c.** Conservative management.
☐ **d.** Topical aqueous cream.
☐ **e.** Cold tar.

37 A 73-year-old lady presents to the on-call surgical team complaining of right-sided abdominal pain. On further questioning the pain is mainly in the right flank but does radiate down to the groin. She has noticed dysuria and associated nausea, fever and rigors. On examination there are no palpable masses but she has tenderness on palpation of the renal angle. Urine dipstick is positive for leucocytes, nitrites, glucose and blood. Observations include a temperature of 38.0°C, RR 24/min, Sats 87%, HR 92/min and BP 109/64 mmHg. Which of the following is the most appropriate management for this patient?

☐ **a.** Oral antibiotics and community follow-up.
☐ **b.** i.v. antibiotics and i.v. fluids.
☐ **c.** Catheterise.
☐ **d.** Analgesia.
☐ **e.** Diuretics and i.v. fluids.

38 A 71-year-old man is admitted semi-electively for an anterior resection for a sigmoid cancer. Initial appearances on colonoscopy and CT scanning suggest that the cancer is confined to the bowel. He has been admitted a couple of days early since he is now obstipated and suffering colicky central abdominal pains. The colicky pain is now becoming more constant and there is some concern that he is becoming obstructed. In addition, he notes some dysuria and difficulty in passing urine. What is the likely cause for his urinary symptoms?

☐ **a.** Prostatic metastases.
☐ **b.** Pyelonephritis.
☐ **c.** Bladder cancer.
☐ **d.** External pressure on urinary system.
☐ **e.** Urinary tract infection.

39 A 67-year-old woman presents to accident and emergency with right-sided chest pain and some shortness of breath. Examination reveals a pleural effusion which is confirmed on chest X-ray. Aspiration of the fluid identifies less than 30 g of protein. Which of the following would not be consistent with the above picture?

☐ **a.** Hypothyroidism.
☐ **b.** Liver cirrhosis.
☐ **c.** Nephrotic syndrome.
☐ **d.** Pneumonia.
☐ **e.** Cardiac failure.

40 A university health care centre doctor is called to see a student who has been unwell by worried friends. He has not been attending lectures of late and has been feeling feverish and hot for the last 24 hours. There is an empty packet of ibuprofen 400 mg by his bedside and it is decided to start benzylpenicillin empirically to cover for meningitis. As he is transferred to hospital the ambulance crew notice a non-blanching rash over his right thigh. In hospital his temperature is recorded at 39.1°C and he has started to vomit. Blood cultures are sent off on admission to hospital. What is the most likely cause of vomiting in this man?

☐ **a.** Idiosyncratic reaction to ibuprofen.

☐ **b.** Allergic reaction to benzylpenicillin.

☐ **c.** Neurogenic (central) reaction.

☐ **d.** Systemic inflammatory response to infection.

☐ **e.** NSAID irritation to gastric mucosa.

41 A 63-year-old gentleman was admitted to hospital after suffering with a transient ischaemic attack (TIA). He noticed weakness in his right arm and some changes in his speech, both of which were completely resolved in the 24 hours after onset. On examination, he had no residual neurological findings and no cardiovascular findings of note. Which investigations would be useful to determine the cause for this event and likelihood of future episodes?

☐ **a.** MRI brain.

☐ **b.** Chest X-ray.

☐ **c.** Abdominal ultrasound scan.

☐ **d.** Carotid Doppler scanning.

☐ **e.** ECG.

42 A 63-year-old man is brought to hospital by ambulance following a fall at home. He lives alone and is unaccompanied to hospital. On arrival he is assessed by the emergency staff and appears confused and disorientated but moving all four limbs and communicating, albeit inappropriately. His urine dipstick is positive for leucocytes, nitrites and protein. He scores 3/10 on the abbreviated mental test (AMT) and is uncooperative with physical examination, pulling out his intravenous lines and trying to leave the hospital. Which of the following medications would be of most benefit in managing this patient?

☐ **a.** Haloperidol.

☐ **b.** Lorazepam.

☐ **c.** Memantine.

☐ **d.** Olanzipine.

☐ **e.** Sertraline.

43 A 43-year-old woman is brought to hospital by her husband after he found she had taken an overdose of her medication in her bathroom. Her past medical history is remarkable for hypertension and depression. She denies taking any medication overdose, stating that her husband is simply worrying unnecessarily. On examination she is drowsy with dilated pupils and sluggish reflexes. A tachycardia is clinically evident and electrocardiography is performed that demonstrates a prolonged PR and QT interval. Which of the following medications is most likely responsible for her symptoms?

- ☐ **a.** Tranylcypromine.
- ☐ **b.** Amitriptyline.
- ☐ **c.** Digoxin.
- ☐ **d.** Atenolol.
- ☐ **e.** Sertraline.

44 A 25-year-old man presents to his GP complaining of difficulty sleeping. He complains that he feels very hot at night and finds that his work is suffering during the day. Otherwise he complains of no problems, but on questioning he admits to slight weight loss and examination reveals a unilateral cervical mass. The mass is in the anterior compartment of the neck; it is not tethered to the skin and does not move on swallowing or protrusion of the tongue. What is the most likely diagnosis in this case?

- ☐ **a.** Hodgkin's lymphoma.
- ☐ **b.** Sarcoidosis.
- ☐ **c.** Tuberculosis.
- ☐ **d.** Anxiety.
- ☐ **e.** Acute lymphocytic leukaemia.

45 A 70-year-old lady presents to her GP with vague aches and pains particularly in her back. Other symptoms include polyuria and constipation. She has noticed that she is more prone to picking chest infections over the past few months. An X-ray shows two crush fractures of her lumbar vertebrae. Blood tests taken show a calcium level of 2.96 with a normal albumin level and Phosphate level 0.9. What is the likely diagnosis?

- ☐ **a.** Myeloma.
- ☐ **b.** Myelofibrosis.
- ☐ **c.** Myelodysplasia.
- ☐ **d.** Adrenal tumour.
- ☐ **e.** Prolapsed lumbar disc.

46 A 45-year-old woman presents to accident and emergency with abdominal pain. She is tested for pregnancy, urinary tract infection and undergoes abdominal examination. She is found to have an enlarged spleen with pain localised to the left upper quadrant. Blood tests reveal a haemoglobin level of 9.8 g/dL with an mean cell volume (MCV) of 92 fL. WBC was 26×10^9 and platelet count was 135×10^9. Which of the following chromosomal translocations is most likely to be found in sufferers of this condition?

- ☐ **a.** t(8;14)
- ☐ **b.** t(9;22)
- ☐ **c.** t(14;21)
- ☐ **d.** t(11;22)
- ☐ **e.** t(4;14)

47 Which of the following modalities represents the most useful indicator of the severity of disease in a rheumatoid arthritis sufferer?

- ☐ **a.** Serial radiographs of hands and wrists.
- ☐ **b.** Commencement of biological agents.
- ☐ **c.** Ability to dress and care for oneself.
- ☐ **d.** Number of visits to hospital.
- ☐ **e.** Length of treatment with steroids.

48 A 32-year-old woman presents to hospital with weakness in her left leg and arm with an obvious facial droop on the left hand side. History taking reveals a sudden onset of loss of function of the left side of her body with no loss of consciousness, tongue-biting or associated incontinence of faeces or urine. Past medical history is remarkable only for four miscarriages and peptic ulcer disease. Which of the following diagnoses is most likely?

- ☐ **a.** Systemic sclerosis.
- ☐ **b.** Marfan's syndrome.
- ☐ **c.** Dermatomyositis.
- ☐ **d.** Antiphospholipid syndrome.
- ☐ **e.** Reiter's syndrome.

49 A 23-year-old girl is referred to the breast clinic by her GP. She first sought advice when she noticed a solitary lump in the upper outer aspect of her left breast. She notes that the lump is not painful and there are no overlying changes to the skin. She has no history of breast problems and has no family history of breast cancer. There has been no change in the size of the lump and no association with her menstrual cycle. She admits that it has been present for more than a month but she was too nervous to have it investigated. She denies using any regular medications. Which of the following is the most likely diagnosis?

- ☐ **a.** Fibroadenoma.
- ☐ **b.** Ductal carcinoma *in situ*.
- ☐ **c.** Invasive ductal carcinoma.
- ☐ **d.** Breast cyst.
- ☐ **e.** Breast abscess.

50 A 69-year-old gentleman is seen by his GP for gradual onset gynaecomastia. The patient has tolerated the development of the condition hoping that it would resolve spontaneously although it continues to gradually worsen. He has a history of alcohol abuse, drinking approximately 70 units per week and has been hospitalised with pancreatitis and acute liver failure in the past. Which of the following is the most likely cause for his gynaecomastia?

- ☐ **a.** Physiological.
- ☐ **b.** Liver failure.
- ☐ **c.** Kleinfelter's syndrome.
- ☐ **d.** Hyperthyroidism.
- ☐ **e.** Drugs including spironolactone.

51 A 74-year-old woman is referred to accident and emergency with a history of pain and redness in her right eye that is associated with blurred vision and distortion of her vision leading her to see 'haloes' around objects. When asked if anything makes the pain better or worse she tells you that it seems to come on in the early evening. Which of the following diagnoses is the most likely?

- ☐ **a.** Endophthalmitis.
- ☐ **b.** Acute glaucoma.
- ☐ **c.** Retinitis pigmentosa.
- ☐ **d.** Retinal detachment.
- ☐ **e.** Retinal artery occlusion.

52 A 59-year-old man presents to hospital with progressive deterioration in visual acuity over as period of weeks such that he had trouble focussing on even the closest of objects and had had to stop driving completely. He found that he was experiencing glare when in bright sunlight and had taken to wearing sunglasses when outside. On examination there was frank opacity of the left pupil with reduced clarity of the right pupil and visual acuity was reduced to hand waving in the left eye. Which of the following has NOT been associated with the development of posterior subcapsular cataract?

☐ **a.** Obesity.
☐ **b.** Steroids.
☐ **c.** Hypertriglyceridaemia.
☐ **d.** Hypertension.
☐ **e.** Hypoglycaemia.

53 A 72-year-old woman presents to hospital with shortness of breath. She is found to have a significant cardiac history of ischaemic heart disease with previous coronary artery bypass grafting and ventricular arrhythmias, which she has had for many years. As part of the work-up for shortness of breath she has blood tests taken that demonstrate a slightly high white cell count and C-reactive protein. Thyroid function test, however, returns abnormal. Which of the following medications is most likely responsible for the deterioration in thyroid function?

☐ **a.** Atenolol.
☐ **b.** Atorvastatin.
☐ **c.** Amlodipine.
☐ **d.** Amiodarone.
☐ **e.** Acarbose.

54 Regarding hyperthyroidism, which of the following statements is correct?

☐ **a.** T3 is more abundantly produced than T4.
☐ **b.** Lid retraction can be used to monitor therapy.
☐ **c.** Beta-blockade is always required long term for tachycardia.
☐ **d.** T4 is more potent than T3.
☐ **e.** High T4, T3 and TSH levels are seen in thyrotoxicosis.

55 A 75-year-old gentleman is admitted to hospital following intermittent chest pain for the past 24 hours. His chest pain was central in location with no radiation but was relieved by GTN spray in 3 minutes. His troponin level was positive and ECG showed fixed inverted T waves laterally. He has a past history of peripheral vascular disease. The next stage of his management should include:

- ☐ **a.** An exercise tolerance test (ETT).
- ☐ **b.** A thallium cardiac scan.
- ☐ **c.** Serial ECGs.
- ☐ **d.** CT chest.
- ☐ **e.** Coronary angiogram.

56 A 78-year-old lady was referred to the cardiologist during her inpatient stay for increasing attacks of angina. She is currently using PRN GTN spray, verapamil and enalapril. She has noticed that the frequency of her angina attacks is increasing and her symptoms are becoming more severe at rest. What changes in her medications will improve her symptoms?

- ☐ **a.** Change verapamil to diltiazem and start isosorbide mononitrate.
- ☐ **b.** Give regular nitrates.
- ☐ **c.** Change ace inhibitor.
- ☐ **d.** Add in beta-blocker.
- ☐ **e.** Start digoxin.

57 An 81-year-old gentleman is admitted to hospital with chest pain and a diagnosis of a Non-ST Elevation MI (NSTEMI) is made. Which of the following is the most appropriate immediate medical management?

- ☐ **a.** Aspirin, warfarin and beta-blocker.
- ☐ **b.** Aspirin, clopidogrel, clexane and GTN spray.
- ☐ **c.** Clopidogrel, GTN spray and warfarin.
- ☐ **d.** Clopidogrel, clexane and warfarin.
- ☐ **e.** Clexane, warfarin, beta-blocker and statin.

58 A 58-year-old man presents with new-onset chest pain and shortness of breath. ECG shows atrial fibrillation with a rate of 180 beats per minute. He has no past cardiac history. The most appropriate management would be:

☐ **a.** Oxygen, digoxin i.v.
☐ **b.** Oxygen, beta-blockers.
☐ **c.** Oxygen, heparin, warfarin.
☐ **d.** Oxygen, heparin, i.v. amiodarone.
☐ **e.** Oxygen, heparin and synchronized DC shock.

59 A 70-year-old man presents with chest pain. His ECG shows an acute myocardial infraction (MI) with a new left bundle branch block. On admission he is given 100% oxygen, morphine, metoclopramide, GTN spray and aspirin. On further questioning you elicit that he suffered a haemorrhagic stroke a year ago. The next most appropriate step in management is:

☐ **a.** Coronary artery bypass surgery.
☐ **b.** Thrombolytic therapy with streptokinase.
☐ **c.** Percutaneous transluminal coronary angioplasty (PTCA).
☐ **d.** Heparin infusion.
☐ **e.** i.v. glycoprotein Iib/IIIa inhibitor.

60 Which of the following is NOT a contraindication to thrombolysis following a diagnosis of an acute MI?

☐ **a.** Previous allergic reaction.
☐ **b.** Cerebral infarct 2 years ago.
☐ **c.** Suspected aortic dissection.
☐ **d.** Heavy vaginal bleeding.
☐ **e.** Hypotension.

Extended matching questions

Glomerulonephritides

a. Minimal change disease.
b. IgA nephropathy (Berger's disease).
c. Focal segmental glomerulosclerosis.
d. Post-streptococcal glomerulonephritis.
e. Rapidly progressive glomerulonephritis (RPGN).
f. Membranous glomerulonephritis.
g. Wegener's granulomatosis.
h. Henoch–Schönlein purpura (HSP).
i. Systemic-lupus erythematosus.

The following patients have all presented with renal disease. Please choose the most likely option from the list above. Each option can be used once, more than once or not at all.

61 A 10-year-old boy is brought to hospital with a rash over his buttocks associated with abdominal pain and vomiting. In accident and emergency he is accompanied by his mother and stepfather. His mother had left him for the weekend with the stepfather and was called to come back from her holiday as he had started to have some bloody stools associated with the rash. Social services had been notified on arrival to hospital.

62 A 30-year-old man presents to hospital complaining that his urine has been very dark recently, resembling coffee at worst. He has been under the weather recently and has taken a few days off work with a very sore throat and coryzal symptoms. Urine dipstick in hospital returns highly positive for blood and protein. He is admitted for supportive management and is scheduled for a renal biopsy, which shows mesangial proliferation with a positive immunofluorescence pattern.

63 A 5-year-old boy is referred to hospital and seen with his father who is worried that he has been listless. He is not sure why his GP suggested he should come to accident and emergency and is keen to 'get some tablets and go home'. On examination the child is tired and irritable and has some swelling around his eyes. Carefully considered renal biopsy is remarkable only for some podocyte fusion on electron microscopy.

64 A 40-year-old woman is admitted from accident and emergency
☐ with a history of arthralgia, facial rash, chest pain and neuropsychiatric symptoms. She is investigated for the cause of her symptoms and undergoes urine dipstick, simple blood tests, electrocardiology, porphyria and sickle screens and troponin initially. She is found to have renal failure with poor urine output and a decision to perform a renal biopsy is taken, which demonstrates wire-loop lesions on light microscopy.

65 A 28-year-old man presents with shortness of breath, haemoptysis, swollen legs and face, and haematuria. He describes feeling progressively more unwell in the weeks preceding admission but was afraid that this 'might be the end'. Clinically he exhibits signs of renal failure and his blood results show a glomerular filtration rate of 8 mL/min (severe). He is admitted to hospital and rapidly deteriorates over a matter of weeks requiring emergency renal replacement therapy. Autoantibody screen returns positive for anti-glomerular basement membrane and renal biopsy demonstrates a florid necrotising glomerulonephritis with crescent formation.

Dementia

    a. Alzheimer's dementia.
    b. Creutzfeldt–Jakob disease.
    c. Multi-infarct dementia.
    d. Frontotemporal dementia.
    e. HIV dementia.
    f. Alcohol-related dementia.
    g. Lewy-body dementia.
    h. Pseudo-dementia.

The following patients have all presented with dementia. Please choose the most correct diagnosis from the above list. Each option may be used once, more than once or not at all.

66 A 65-year-old man is brought to his GP by his wife. She is worried that recently he has been behaving more and more unusually and out of character for him. He has become more forgetful of late and she often gets the impression that he has trouble focusing on her when she is talking to him. His past medical history details two previous admissions to hospital under the neurologists for transient ischaemic attack and stroke.

67 A 68-year-old man is brought to accident and emergency having fallen and broken his hip. Further questioning reveals he is confused and upon talking to a relative a history of tremors and long-standing hypertension is gained. Mini-mental state examination yields a score of 21 and on examination he exhibits bradykinesia, a shuffling gait and a unilateral tremor of his right hand. The relative states that he often seems to hallucinate and become restless.

68 A 61-year-old woman is brought in by the police to hospital found wandering at night in her dressing gown. Mini-mental state examination reveals a score of 18. Her daughter describes her mother as more aggressive recently and often has trouble remembering who she is when she comes to visit. The daughter also states that she has been told by her mother's neighbour on more than one occasion that he has been called at odd times in the night by her.

69 A 58-year-old woman, recently widowed, is brought to hospital by her relatives. She was found at home to have no food in her cupboard and a neighbour who helps her clean found her lying in bed in a poor state of hygiene. Her mini-mental state examination score was 24 and during the test she became very agitated and tearful.

70 A 31-year-old man from Botswana is brought to accident and emergency by the police. He was found at 2 o'clock in the morning holding a knife and wandering the street outside his house. He maintains that somebody is poisoning him and making him feel terrible and he complains of a 'flu-like illness'. On examination he is a slim man with poor nutrition and vital signs reveal a low-grade pyrexia.

Lower gastrointestinal bleeding

   a. Angiodysplasia.
   b. Osler–Weber–Rendu syndrome.
   c. Colorectal carcinoma.
   d. Haemorrhoids.
   e. Drug-induced bleeding.
   f. Mesenteric embolus.
   g. Inflammatory bowel disease.
   h. Diverticulitis.
   i. Inherited coagulopathy.
   j. Rectal polyp.

The following patients have all suffered from bleeding from the lower gastrointestinal tract. Please choose the more correct diagnosis from the above list. Each option may be used once, more than once or not at all.

71 A 43-year-old man presents with bright red rectal bleeding. He denies any pain and states that it came on suddenly with no warning. He has not had any change in bowel habit and does not take any regular medication. Past medical history is remarkable for a total knee replacement 5 years ago and an inpatient admission under the ENT surgeons for a severe nosebleed as a child.

72 A 62-year-old woman presents with rectal bleeding on passing stool. Bleeding is seen on the toilet paper and in the toilet bowl. She states that she has had a few episodes of small fresh bleeding but denies any weight loss or diarrhoea. She describes a feeling of something descending in the rectum when she strains at stool and often feels the urge to defaecate but without success. In fact she suffers from constipation and is due to see her GP for a repeat prescription for senna and lactulose as she has run out.

73 A 67-year-old man presents with rectal bleeding with no warning or associated change in bowel habit. He has experienced episodes of bleeding like this in the past, which usually settle on their own. Referred by his GP to hospital for the last serious episode of rectal bleeding he underwent colonoscopy, which demonstrated a small vascular abnormality.

74 A 54-year-old man presents to the dermatology clinic with a history of multiple red lesions on his nose and around his mouth. He has been suffering recurrent nosebleeds intermittently since he was a child and has had the lesions as long as he can remember. Past medical history is remarkable only for an aspirin allergy that caused severe rectal bleeding. On examination there are multiple, small red lesions that blanch on pressure over them distributed over the face, lips, nose and mouth.

75 A 67-year-old man complains of abdominal pain and rectal bleeding. He has recently been started on digoxin and atenolol for an episode of shortness of breath and palpitations and was due for an anticoagulation clinic appointment to commence on warfarin. He is brought to hospital collapsed in the street and had passed fresh blood per rectum in accident and emergency. Clinically he exhibits signs of shock and requires fluid resuscitation and blood transfusion.

Shortness of breath

a. Atelectasis.
b. Lung cancer.
c. Aspiration pneumonia.
d. Pneumothorax.
e. Exacerbation of asthma/COPD.
f. Pulmonary embolus.
g. Congestive cardiac failure.

76 A 74-year-old gentleman is 1 day post-operatively from his total
☐ hip replacement for the treatment of arthritis affecting his hip.
Immediately post-operatively he made a good recovery and did
not complain of excessive pain. He has a history of COPD and
hypertension but no other medical problems. The nurses are
concerned about him as they have just done his observations
and he has a temperature of 38.5°C, whilst he is not complaining of any pain he feels short of breath and has noticed a dry
cough. What is the most likely cause for his shortness of breath?

77 You are a member of the cardiac arrest team and you are called
☐ to a medical ward where a patient has arrested. You remember
the patient as you had been asked to see him previously to dose
his warfarin as he was being treated for a pulmonary embolus. The nurses mention that he was complaining of increasing
shortness of breath in the hours up to the arrest which seemed
to be somewhat alleviated by administration of oxygen and his
nebuliser. Upon attaching the cardiac monitor you note that the
rhythm is asystole, despite 3 cycles of cardio-pulmonary resuscitation there is no change in his status and death is confirmed.
What is the likely cause for this man's demise?

78 An 80-year-old gentleman has been admitted for the investiga-
☐ tion of his recurrent falls. A full screen of blood tests including a full blood count and urea and electrolytes has shown no
abnormalities. You come to review him after the weekend on
Monday morning and the nursing staff are concerned that he
is not quite himself. He appears to be slumped over to one side
and you notice some slurred speech. You are told by the nursing staff that he has been eating well over the weekend but
they have noticed that he has developed a cough this morning.
What is the most likely diagnosis in this case?

79 A 49-year-old lady presents with increasing shortness of breath. She was seen by her GP earlier in the day who was concerned that clinically she had a pleural effusion and asked her to attend accident and emergency for an urgent chest X-ray and medical review. She is normally fit and well and works as a banker. Of late she has been complaining of mild shortness of breath but she has attributed it to the fact that she has been smoking more than usual due to the stress of work. On clinical examination there are no peripheral signs of respiratory disease although her respiratory rate is 20/min. There is dullness to percussion at the right base and reduced chest expansion and breath sounds in the same area. A chest X-ray confirms a pleural effusion, what is the likely diagnosis?

80 A 74-year-old lady presents acutely short of breath. She mentions that she has been increasingly dyspnoeic over the past week but her breathing has worsened significantly over the past 24 hours. She denies any associated chest pain but confirms that she has a slightly productive cough. On further questioning she admits that she could not pick up her repeat prescription for her inhalers as she was too short of breath and has been without her salbutamol and spiriva for 5 days. On examination her respiratory rate is 18/min and auscultation reveals widespread wheeze with some crepitations heard in the left upper zone. What is the likely diagnosis?

Acute abdomen

  a. Appendicitis.
  b. Pancreatitis.
  c. Diverticulitis.
  d. Intussusception.
  e. Sigmoid volvulus.
  f. Perforated peptic ulcer.
  g. Ruptured abdominal aortic aneurysm.
  h. Basal pneumonia.
  i. Rectosigmoid carcinoma.
  j. Appendiceal carcinoid.

The following patients have all presented with abdominal complaints. Please choose the most correct diagnosis from the above list. Each option may be used once, more than once, or not at all.

81 A 15-year-old boy presents to his GP with a 2 day history of vomiting, nausea and loss of appetite. On examination he is generally tender but more so over the right side of his abdomen. Blood tests reveal a low-grade pyrexia, high white cell count and raised C-reactive protein.

82 A 65-year-old woman is brought to hospital complaining of bright red blood in her stools. On examination she is tender in the left iliac fossa with a hard non-fluctuant mass palpable in the same region. Blood tests reveal a high white cell count, C-reactive protein of 135 and a temperature of 37.9°C.

83 A 72-year-old man presents to accident and emergency with a history of weight loss, confusion and abdominal pain. He is from a nursing home where the nurses state that he has not opened his bowels for 2 days and has become increasingly unwell over the past few weeks. Blood results reveal a haemoglobin of 7.2 g/dL, MCV of 74.3 fL, urea of 9.4 mmol/L and creatinine of 155 μmol/L.

84 A 45-year-old stockbroker presents to hospital complaining of severe abdominal pain. He states that he has not been eating for the past week due to pain and has felt nauseated and has vomited twice this morning. On examination his abdomen is tense with absent bowel sounds and is very tender over the epigastrium.

85 A 57-year-old woman is brought to hospital by ambulance with
☐ abdominal pain. She has vomited green fluid this morning and
has been very constipated since yesterday. Past medical history
reveals high blood pressure and cholesterol treated with atenolol and simvastatin. On examination she is sitting forward on
the bed and in pain. Clinically the abdomen is exquisitely tender
over the epigastrium. Bowel sounds are present and there are
no masses. Chest examination reveals a respiratory rate of 26
breaths per minute with reduced breath sounds in the left base.

Relevant milestones

    a. 0–3 months.
    b. 3–6 months.
    c. 6–9 months.
    d. 9–12 months.
    e. 12–18 months.
    f. 18–24 months.
    g. 2–5 years.
    h. 5–10 years.

86 This child has a heart rate of 95–140/min, a respiratory rate of
☐ 25 breaths per minute, and a systolic BP of 90mmHg.

87 The child sits unaided.
☐

88 First dose of diphtheria, tetanus, pertussis, polio, *Haemophilus*
☐ *influenza B* and meningitis C vaccination is administered in
accordance with the normal vaccination schedule in the United
Kingdom.

89 Persistent runny nose, mild fever, shortness of breath with asso-
☐ ciated dry cough and wheeze. On examination accessory muscles are being used and there are fine end inspiratory crackles
on the chest.

90 Able to follow movements with eyes.
☐

Questions

Multiple choice questions (single best answer)

1 Which of the following are the physiological changes that are well known to occur during pregnancy?
- ☐ **a.** Increased cardiac output by 30%.
- ☐ **b.** Increase in blood volume by 30%.
- ☐ **c.** Slight drop in haemoglobin.
- ☐ **d.** Decreased oesophageal sphincter pressure resulting in heartburn.
- ☐ **e.** Increased venous pressure in the pelvis.

2 Which of the following is NOT a risk factor for ectopic pregnancy?
- ☐ **a.** Pelvic inflammatory disease.
- ☐ **b.** Pelvic surgery/adhesions.
- ☐ **c.** Intrauterine contraceptive device (IUCD).
- ☐ **d.** Progesterone-only pill.
- ☐ **e.** Previous Caesarean section.

3 An 18-month-old boy has tetralogy of Fallot. His symptoms include irritability, cyanosis and tachypnoea. He has suffered one episode of syncope. Which of the following manoeuvres is the best treatment for these episodes?
- ☐ **a.** Reassure the parents that these episodes will resolve themselves.
- ☐ **b.** Lifting the lower extremities above the level of the heart.
- ☐ **c.** Dropping the legs off the side of the bed.
- ☐ **d.** Bringing his knees up to his chest.
- ☐ **e.** Making the child adopt the Trendelenburg position.

4 A 2-week-old male infant is brought into the accident and emergency department by his parents because of persistent vomiting. They have stated that he forcibly vomits almost immediately after eating and the vomit appears to be partially digested food. There is no bile or blood in the vomit. He opens his bowels 3 times a day. His observations are all stable and on examination there is a small non-tender, palpable mass in the epigastrium. Bowel sounds are present and there are no other findings on examination. Which of the following investigations is the most useful initial investigation to perform?

☐ **a.** CT scan of the abdomen.
☐ **b.** Barium swallow.
☐ **c.** Abdominal ultrasound scan.
☐ **d.** Abdominal X-ray.
☐ **e.** Laparoscopy.

5 A 22-year-old man is brought in to hospital following a high-speed road traffic accident where he was the driver. On initial assessment he is found to be drowsy with marked facial injury, chest injury consistent with steering wheel impact and multiple areas of subcutaneous emphysema. He is tachycardic with respiratory distress and further respiratory examination reveals a displaced trachea to the left side of the chest. Which of the following is the correct step in management?

☐ **a.** Endotracheal intubation.
☐ **b.** Needle thoracocentesis of the right chest.
☐ **c.** Insert a nasopharyngeal airway.
☐ **d.** Insert a chest drain with underwater seal.
☐ **e.** Perform an emergency cricothyroidotomy.

6 Features commonly associated with the clinical presentation of acute pancreatitis are:

☐ **a.** Jaundice.
☐ **b.** Pseudocyst formation.
☐ **c.** Hypercalcaemia.
☐ **d.** Bowel necrosis.
☐ **e.** Raised albumin.

7 A 65-year-old known diabetic recently diagnosed with chronic renal failure presents to his GP with acute onset of pain, paraesthesia and pallor in his right leg. On examination the GP notes an absent dorsalis pedis pulse and notes that the skin on his leg is cool and the pallor is emphasised by raising his leg. These symptoms and signs are characteristic of which of the following conditions?

- ☐ **a.** Arterial occlusion.
- ☐ **b.** Venous insufficiency.
- ☐ **c.** Cellulitis.
- ☐ **d.** Reduced circulating volume.
- ☐ **e.** Vasculitis.

8 A 24-year-old man is brought in by ambulance following a road traffic accident. He is drowsy with a Glasgow Coma Scale (GCS) of 11/15. CT scan of chest, abdomen and pelvis is performed revealing multiple long bone and rib fractures and free fluid in the abdomen and pelvis. Clinically he is globally tender over the abdomen with blood pressure 100/60mmHg, pulse 120beats per minute, urine output 10mL/h and respiratory rate of 35 breaths per minute. Which of the following is the correct next step in management?

- ☐ **a.** Urgent orthopaedic referral to exclude fat embolus.
- ☐ **b.** Intravenous noradrenaline for hypotension.
- ☐ **c.** Rapid sequence intubation and ventilation.
- ☐ **d.** Emergency exploratory laparotomy.
- ☐ **e.** Fluid resuscitation and repeat urgent CT abdomen.

9 Post-operatively the nursing staff call you concerned that the above patient is oozing from the wound site and through all the injury dressings. A set of emergency blood tests for full blood count, biochemistry and coagulation screen taken at the time of admission are normal. Past medical history reveals asthma. On the ward the staff nurse in charge of his care who spoke to you on the phone is at the blood bank collecting more packed red cells for transfusion. Which of the following is the correct course of action?

- ☐ **a.** Administration of 4 units of fresh frozen plasma and 2 pools of platelets.
- ☐ **b.** Exploratory laparotomy to control bleeding.
- ☐ **c.** Urgent blood tests for coagulation screen and full blood count.
- ☐ **d.** Administration of 4 units of packed red cells to replace loss.
- ☐ **e.** Urgent haemophilia A and B screen with 10mg vitamin K injection.

10 A 75-year-old woman presents with abdominal pain and confusion. Her past medical history is remarkable for advanced transitional cell carcinoma of the bladder managed palliatively for symptom control. Urine dipstick is positive for blood, protein and leucocytes. Urea is 32.6 mmol/L, creatinine is 457 μmol/L, sodium 140 mmol/L and potassium 4.7 mmol/L. She is catheterised and has been anuric for the past 12 hours and an urgent ultrasound scan of the kidneys and bladder reveal hydroureter and hydronephrosis bilaterally with an abnormal bladder appearance and volume of 15 mL. Which of the following is the most appropriate next step?

☐ **a.** Insertion of suprapubic catheter.
☐ **b.** 5-day course of intravenous cefuroxime.
☐ **c.** 3L of intravenous fluids over 12 hours.
☐ **d.** Urgent decompressive bilateral nephrostomy.
☐ **e.** Urgent renal referral with dialysis.

11 A pulmonary embolus can be a life-threatening condition. Its recognition is of vital importance as it is a potentially treatable condition. Which of the following is NOT consistent with a diagnosis of a pulmonary embolus?

☐ **a.** Normal chest X-ray.
☐ **b.** Arterial blood gas $\downarrow PaO_2$, $\uparrow PCO_2$.
☐ **c.** ECG – tachycardia $S_I Q_{III} T_{III}$.
☐ **d.** Hypotension.
☐ **e.** Unilateral calf swelling.

12 Following many procedures in respiratory medicine chest X-rays are requested to exclude development of a pneumothorax. Which of the following is not known to be a cause of pneumothorax?

☐ **a.** Asthma.
☐ **b.** Lung abscess.
☐ **c.** Connective tissue disorder.
☐ **d.** Pulmonary embolus.
☐ **e.** Spontaneous.

13 A 62-year-old man is brought to hospital complaining of agonising pain in his abdomen. He was admitted for laparoscopic cholecystectomy a week ago and has only recently returned home. He states that the pain is intermittently sharp but is there in the background all the time and he has been drenched in sweat at night. You elicit he has been experiencing some rigors and many of his friends say that his skin has changed colour. On examination he is sweaty and jaundiced. The abdomen is tender in the right upper quadrant but there is no rebound, guarding or rigidity. Bowel sounds are present. He is pyrexic at 38.2°C with a respiratory rate of 24 breaths per minute. Which of the following most accurately describes the clinical picture?

☐ **a.** Reynolds pentad.

☐ **b.** Fitz–Hugh–Curtis syndrome.

☐ **c.** Leriche's syndrome.

☐ **d.** Wernicke–Korsakoff syndrome.

☐ **e.** Charcot's triad.

14 A 60-year-old man presents to his GP complaining of feeling tired all the time. He is accompanied by his wife who was adamant that he comes as he has not been himself for some weeks. He is otherwise fit and well with no past medical history and attributes his tiredness to age, however, confides that his friends keep on asking him if he has been away on holiday as he looks slightly tanned. On examination there is a faint bronzed appearance to the skin, the sclera are slightly yellow-tinged and there are non-blanching red lesions on the upper body. Cardiac examination reveals a third heart sound and tachycardia with mild pitting oedema to both ankles. The abdomen is soft but tender in the right upper quadrant with a 2 cm palpable liver edge. Routine blood tests demonstrate raised bilirubin, alanine aminotransferase and aspartate transaminase with a random blood glucose level of 14 mmol/L. Haematinics done at a routine check-up a month ago demonstrated a raised serum ferritin with a raised serum iron and decreased total iron binding capacity (TIBC). Which of the following investigations would be LEAST useful in confirming the diagnosis?

☐ **a.** MRI scan.

☐ **b.** Fasting transferrin saturation.

☐ **c.** Liver biopsy.

☐ **d.** Liver ultrasound scan.

☐ **e.** C282Y mutation screen.

15 A 25-year-old woman who works as a waitress presents to accident and emergency after several accidents at work. On further questioning she admits to being rather unsteady in carrying heavy loads and customers have been having trouble understanding her speech. On examination she is an anxious but otherwise healthy woman, noted to have a tremor and dysarthria. Careful examination of the eye reveals an area of pigmentation at the junction between cornea and sclera. Which of the following investigations is the most discriminative in making the diagnosis?

☐ **a.** Four-vessel neck angiography.
☐ **b.** Serum bilirubin and liver enzymes.
☐ **c.** Thyroid function tests.
☐ **d.** Serum copper and ceruloplasmin.
☐ **e.** Peripheral blood film and vitamin B_{12} levels.

16 A 30-year-old man complains of severe lower right-sided abdominal pain. The pain causes difficulty in walking to the examination couch but examination reveals rebound tenderness and blood tests reveal a slightly elevated white cell count. On administration of a bolus dose of normal saline intravenously he states that his pain feels much better. Which of the following options explain this phenomenon?

☐ **a.** He has borderline personality disorder.
☐ **b.** His pain is psychogenic.
☐ **c.** He is responding to a placebo.
☐ **d.** His pain is somatic in origin.
☐ **e.** His electrolyte abnormalities are corrected.

17 A 60-year-old female patient makes an appointment with her GP to discuss her recently depressed mood. She describes early morning waking, a reduced libido and a reduced enjoyment of hobbies. She has a history of diabetes, hypertension and degenerative joint disease, for all of which she is receiving optimal treatment. She has recently been started on a new medication. Which of the following drugs is most likely to be the cause of her depressed mood?

☐ **a.** Non-steroidal anti-inflammatory drugs (NSAIDs).
☐ **b.** Oral hypoglycaemic drugs.
☐ **c.** Antihypertensive drugs.
☐ **d.** Calcium supplements.
☐ **e.** Digoxin.

18 An 80-year-old male returns to his GP for a routine appointment following having some blood tests taken for a general health screen. Which of the following results is abnormal for this patient?

☐ **a.** Mild glucose intolerance.

☐ **b.** Increased autoantibody production.

☐ **c.** Raised alkaline phosphatase.

☐ **d.** Reduced creatinine clearance.

☐ **e.** Increase in haemoglobin concentration.

19 During your final year OSCE examination you are asked to examine the neurology of a patient's upper limb. You suspect a lesion of the median nerve. Which of the following facts about the median nerve is INCORRECT?

☐ **a.** It supplies the muscles of the thenar eminence.

☐ **b.** It contains fibres of C6 and C7.

☐ **c.** Passes around the lateral epicondyle.

☐ **d.** Provides sensory supply to the lateral $3^1/_2$ digits of the hand.

☐ **e.** May become trapped in the carpal tunnel.

20 A 41-year-old man is brought in to accident and emergency by ambulance after suffering a seizure. According to his friend who accompanied him, he has no history of epilepsy and has never suffered a seizure before. His friend denies that he takes any medications on a regular basis but mentions that he is homeless and has been known to be involved with illegal substances in the past. Whilst you are obtaining this history the patient suffers a further generalised tonic–clonic seizure which lasts in the region of 2 minutes and is terminated with administration of rectal diazepam. Which of the following is not a cause of generalised tonic–clonic seizures?

☐ **a.** Alcohol abuse.

☐ **b.** Hypoglycaemia.

☐ **c.** Glioma.

☐ **d.** Antidepressant overdose.

☐ **e.** Benzodiazepine overdose.

21 A 45-year-old lady attends her GP practice because of worsening headaches. She suspects that they are actually migraines as she has a family history of this and they last in excess of 6 hours commonly despite taking adequate analgesia. As she is interested in finding out which stronger analgesia she can have you decide to educate her on the known risk factors for migraines. Which of the following is NOT a known risk factor for migraine?

☐ **a.** Caffeine withdrawal.
☐ **b.** Cheese.
☐ **c.** Oral contraceptives.
☐ **d.** Travel.
☐ **e.** Depression.

22 A 17-year-old girl presents to accident and emergency after suffering a witnessed blackout. Her friend who was with her at the time denied any seizure-like activity and the patient denied any aura or post-blackout symptoms. She has no known past medical history and takes no regular medications. Which of the following investigations would be the LEAST useful in this case?

☐ **a.** ECG.
☐ **b.** Serum glucose.
☐ **c.** ECHO.
☐ **d.** FBC.
☐ **e.** CT brain.

23 A 57-year-old gentleman presents to his GP generally feeling tired and complaining of weakness. He has no relevant past medical history and takes no regular medications. On direct questioning he denies any constitutional symptoms and has no family history of note. On examination the GP notices a waddling gait and bilateral proximal myopathy in his lower limbs. Causes of proximal myopathy include all of the following EXCEPT:

☐ **a.** Hypercalcaemia.
☐ **b.** Steroid use.
☐ **c.** Alcoholism.
☐ **d.** Syphilis infection.
☐ **e.** Myasthenia gravis.

24 A 78-year-old man attends his GP practice complaining that his eyesight has recently been deteriorating. He notes that he has suffered with bilateral cataracts in the past, which were surgically removed but has never had any other problems with his eyesight. His other past medical history includes a transient ischaemic attack (TIA) and peripheral vascular disease. He takes regular bendrofluazide and aspirin. On examination there is no obvious ptosis. Whilst mapping out the visual fields you note that he has a deficit in the lateral aspect of his right eye and the medial aspect of his left visual field. In both the cases his central field of vision remains. Where is the lesion?

- ☐ **a.** Optic chiasm.
- ☐ **b.** Left optic tract.
- ☐ **c.** Lower fibres of optic radiation (temporal lobe).
- ☐ **d.** Right optic nerve.
- ☐ **e.** Optic radiation posterior parietal lobe.

25 A 78-year-old man presents to his GP with a swelling in his scrotum associated with a dragging sensation. His past medical history is remarkable for episodes of haematuria under investigation by the urologists and a recent admission to hospital 2 months ago complaining of flank pain with a course of antibiotics for a suspected pyelonephritis. On examination there is a mass in the left hemiscrotum that transmits a cough impulse and is described in the notes like a 'bag of worms'. Which of the following is the most likely diagnosis?

- ☐ **a.** Testicular carcinoma.
- ☐ **b.** Bladder carcinoma.
- ☐ **c.** Nephroblastoma (Wilm's tumour).
- ☐ **d.** Renal cell carcinoma.
- ☐ **e.** Prostate carcinoma.

26 Which of the following is NOT typically seen in nephrotic syndrome?

- ☐ **a.** Proteinuria.
- ☐ **b.** Hypoalbuminaemia.
- ☐ **c.** Oedema.
- ☐ **d.** Hypercholesterolaemia.
- ☐ **e.** Haematuria.

27 A 45-year-old man with known chronic renal failure secondary
to diabetic nephropathy presents to accident and emergency
with shortness of breath, cough productive of green sputum
and swollen ankles. Routine biochemistry is taken and reveals
worsening of renal failure with a potassium level of 6.8 mmol/L.
Which of the following treatment options of hyperkalaemia is
correct as first-line therapy?

☐ **a.** Calcium resonium 15 g mixed with water.
☐ **b.** Calcium gluconate.
☐ **c.** Calcium gluconate then insulin/dextrose infusion.
☐ **d.** Haemodialysis.
☐ **e.** Fluid restriction and potassium-poor-diet.

28 A 34-year-old man presents to hospital with episodes of
severe nosebleeds and of 'coughing up blood'. He has previously been referred to the ENT surgeons from his GP with episodic epistaxis and underwent nasal packing on an admission
2 months previously. Routine blood tests are taken and the
results of the haematological investigations are available with
biochemistry awaited. Haemoglobin is 9.8 g/dL with an mean
cell volume (MCV) of 87 fL, white cell count is 9.3×10^9/L with
platelets of 270×10^9/L. Whilst taking a history from him you
notice that he has been losing weight over the past months,
feeling nauseated and has been experiencing progressive swelling of the ankles associated with itching. Which of the following
investigations is indicated in the first instance?

☐ **a.** Autoantibody screen.
☐ **b.** Endoscopy.
☐ **c.** Renal biopsy.
☐ **d.** 24-hour urine protein collection.
☐ **e.** CT chest.

29 Regarding renal disease and urinalysis results, which of the following associations is correct?

☐ **a.** Glucose – starvation.
☐ **b.** Bilirubin – haemolytic anaemia.
☐ **c.** Red-cell casts – glomerulonephritis.
☐ **d.** Cystine crystals – gout.
☐ **e.** Nitrites – high-carbohydrate, low-protein diet.

30 A 50-year-old man presents to his GP for an annual medical check-up as offered by the practice and undergoes a physical examination and blood taking including lipid profile and diabetes screening. Blood pressure is found to be high with a raised creatinine and urea. Urine dipstick is suggestive of urinary tract infection. Renal ultrasonography is performed as an outpatient, the results of which demonstrate enlarged kidneys. Which of the following conditions is NOT associated with renal enlargement?

- ☐ **a.** Amyloidosis.
- ☐ **b.** Congenital single kidney.
- ☐ **c.** Chronic renal failure.
- ☐ **d.** Polycystic kidney disease.
- ☐ **e.** Renal cell carcinoma.

31 Following a motorbike accident, the 38-year-old rider complains of shoulder pain. Other injuries include abrasions over his shins and face but luckily no fractures. He is reluctant to move his arm due to pain and it is being held in internal rotation. Antero-posterior X-ray views show no obvious fractures or displacement. What should be the next step in your management or investigation of this man?

- ☐ **a.** Apply a broad arm sling and regular analgesia.
- ☐ **b.** Request a lateral X-ray of the shoulder.
- ☐ **c.** Ultrasound the shoulder to investigate for a soft tissue injury.
- ☐ **d.** Fracture clinic appointment in a couple of days.
- ☐ **e.** Shoulder arthroscopy to investigate for rotator cuff injury.

32 You are on-call as an orthopaedic house officer and are asked to review an X-ray by the accident and emergency staff. The patient is an 8-year-old child who has banged her elbow on a door frame. She has mild bruising and swelling over the affected elbow but a good range of movement. Which of the following growth plates would you expect still to be visible on her elbow X-ray?

- ☐ **a.** Capitalum and lateral epicondyle only.
- ☐ **b.** Medial and lateral epicondyles only.
- ☐ **c.** Trochlear, olecranon and lateral epicondyle.
- ☐ **d.** Capitalum and trochlear.
- ☐ **e.** Olecranon, lateral and medial epicondyles.

33 Regarding descriptive terms used in dermatology, which of the following associations is correct?

- ☐ **a.** Macule – a small raised circumscribed area of skin less than 0.5 cm across.
- ☐ **b.** Vesicle – a small collection of fluid within the skin less than 0.5 cm across.
- ☐ **c.** Bulla – a small flat area of circumscribed skin change.
- ☐ **d.** Nodule – a small visible and/or palpable lump less than 0.5 cm across.
- ☐ **e.** Weal – a localised collection of pus within the epidermis.

34 A 70-year-old man presents to hospital with shortness of breath and pleuritic chest pain. A history is taken of productive green sputum with chest pain worse on inspiration and localised to the right side of the chest. On examination there are reduced breath sounds at the right base and crackles. You notice as you are examining the back and chest that there are multiple flat segmental brown lesions that are well demarcated on the skin. The lesions have the appearance of being stuck onto the skin and the patient states he has had these 'moles' for years ever since he had a check-up with his GP who noticed them. Which of the following is the most likely diagnosis?

- ☐ **a.** Malignant melanoma.
- ☐ **b.** Campbell de Morgan spots.
- ☐ **c.** Keratoacanthoma.
- ☐ **d.** Seborrhoeic keratoses.
- ☐ **e.** Basal cell carcinoma (BCC).

35 Which of the following causes of scrotal swellings is painless?

- ☐ **a.** Torsion of the testis.
- ☐ **b.** Epididymitis.
- ☐ **c.** Testicular cancer.
- ☐ **d.** Orchitis.
- ☐ **e.** Hydrocele.

36 A 56-year-old man is seen by his GP for a singular episode of haematuria. The man is keen to be treated with antibiotics for what he has assumed is a urinary tract infection as he is unable to take time off work. He has no past medical history of note and denies any relevant family history. On examination the abdomen is soft, non-tender and has no palpable masses. The GP decides to refer him onto the urologist for a cystoscopy. What is the most likely cause of this man's haematuria?

- [ ] **a.** Prostate cancer.
- [ ] **b.** Bladder cancer.
- [ ] **c.** Renal cell carcinoma.
- [ ] **d.** Benign prostatic hypertrophy.
- [ ] **e.** Prostatism.

37 A 23-year-old Jewish man presented to the accident and emergency department after the sudden onset of abdominal cramping and complaining of a sudden desire to defaecate. On further questioning he admits to noticing some mucus accompanying the stool and has passed occasional small amounts of fresh blood. Which of the following is the most likely diagnosis?

- [ ] **a.** Pseudomembranous colitis.
- [ ] **b.** Ischaemic colitis.
- [ ] **c.** Ulcerative colitis.
- [ ] **d.** Angiodysplasia.
- [ ] **e.** Haemorrhoids.

38 A 74-year-old man is brought to accident and emergency by ambulance after he complained of shortness of breath and chest pain. He describes feeling progressively more short of breath in the preceding weeks associated with some chest pain and palpitations. On examination there are signs of a left lower lobe pneumonia and an irregular pulse with a rate of 146 beats per minute. Temperature is 37.9°C, blood pressure is 124/86 mmHg and oxygen saturations are 99% on 10 L. Which of the following management options is correct?

- [ ] **a.** Digoxin 500 µg every 12 hours then digoxin maintenance with anticoagulation.
- [ ] **b.** Digoxin one-off stat dose then anticoagulation.
- [ ] **c.** Beta-blocker one-off stat dose then digoxin maintenance.
- [ ] **d.** Beta-blocker one-off stat dose then anticoagulation.
- [ ] **e.** Digoxin 500 µg every 12 hours then beta-blocker maintenance.

39 A 28-year-old man is seen by his GP for a vaccination prior to travel abroad. During the consultation he is preoccupied with the forms that are being filled in, requesting to have copies of all documentation and becoming increasingly worried that the government will find out about his trip abroad. When asked about friends and family contacts he becomes agitated and denies having any close friends saying that they would just spy on him. Which one of the following diagnoses is most likely?

- ☐ **a.** Antisocial personality disorder.
- ☐ **b.** Schizotypal personality disorder.
- ☐ **c.** Schizoid personality disorder.
- ☐ **d.** Dependent personality disorder.
- ☐ **e.** Avoidant personality disorder.

40 Regarding dementia, which of the following is NOT a recognised feature of this condition?

- ☐ **a.** Fluctuating level of consciousness.
- ☐ **b.** Sundowning effect.
- ☐ **c.** Mood changes.
- ☐ **d.** Personality changes.
- ☐ **e.** Potentially reversible.

41 A 79-year-old lady is seen by her GP for her annual blood tests. She notes that she has been increasingly tired of late but attributed it to her age. Her full blood count shows a macrocytic anaemia with a normal B12 and folate level, low platelet count and a neutropaenia. Blood film showed abnormal looking cells. The GP is concerned about a haematological condition and refers to the local haematologist for a diagnostic bone marrow aspiration. The results confirm hypercellularity and dysplasia. What is the likely diagnosis in this case?

- ☐ **a.** Myeloma.
- ☐ **b.** Myelofibrosis.
- ☐ **c.** Acute lymphocytic leukaemia.
- ☐ **d.** Chronic lymphocytic leukaemia.
- ☐ **e.** Myelodysplasia.

42 A 48-year-old gentleman presents to his GP complaining of tiredness, headaches and visual disturbance. Having excluded any hard neurological symptoms the GP organised blood tests that show an Hb of 20g/dL. He smokes 30 cigarettes a day and has done for many years. Which of the following is UNLIKELY to be the cause of his symptoms?

- ☐ **a.** COPD.
- ☐ **b.** Gaisbock's syndrome.
- ☐ **c.** Polycythaemia rubra vera.
- ☐ **d.** Dehydration.
- ☐ **e.** Ischaemic heart disease.

43 A 6-year-old child is brought into see the GP because of ear pain. He is complaining of constant dull pain in his right ear with some associated tinnitus and hearing loss. He has no other medical problems of note and has been fully vaccinated to date. His mother mentions that he is just making a recovery from a recent upper respiratory tract infection. What is the most likely cause of his symptoms?

- ☐ **a.** Mastoiditis.
- ☐ **b.** Otitis externa.
- ☐ **c.** Otitis media.
- ☐ **d.** Tympanic membrane rupture.
- ☐ **e.** Cholesteatoma.

44 A 15-year-old boy presents to accident and emergency complaining of a sore throat. On further questioning, he explains that he has had a sore throat for the previous 2 days with associated discomfort when swallowing food or drinks. Direct questioning reveals an associated headache and objectively his temperature is 38.5°C. Examination reveals bilateral swollen masses at the posterior aspect of the tongue with no associated pus. He has some cervical lymphadenopathy bilaterally but no other lymphadenopathy. Which of the following is the most likely diagnosis?

- ☐ **a.** Tonsillitis.
- ☐ **b.** Quinsy.
- ☐ **c.** Retropharyngeal abscess.
- ☐ **d.** Candida infection.
- ☐ **e.** Infectious mononucleosis.

45 A 36-year-old woman presents to the GP with widespread muscle aches, left-sided chest pain and cough, and a rash on her face that has appeared over the past months. She is a known epileptic and has been taking medication for many years. Which of the following medications is NOT associated with drug-induced lupus?

☐ **a.** Isoniazid.
☐ **b.** Hydralazine.
☐ **c.** Phenytoin.
☐ **d.** Procainamide.
☐ **e.** Prednisolone.

46 Regarding antiphospholipid syndrome, which of the following autoantibodies is most strongly associated with this condition?

☐ **a.** Anticardiolipin antibodies.
☐ **b.** Antinuclear antibodies.
☐ **c.** Antireticulin antibodies.
☐ **d.** Anti-Ro antibodies.
☐ **e.** Antineutrophil cytoplasmic antibodies.

47 Which of the following facts about ductal carcinoma *in situ* is incorrect?

☐ **a.** It is a malignant condition.
☐ **b.** Of breast cancers it is the most common.
☐ **c.** It is not capable of metastasising.
☐ **d.** It may present with an isolated breast lump.
☐ **e.** Does not produce nipple discharge.

48 Mastectomy is usually the treatment of choice for breast cancer in all of the following situations EXCEPT:

☐ **a.** Large tumour greater than 4 cm.
☐ **b.** Multi-focal cancer.
☐ **c.** Centrally located cancer.
☐ **d.** Fibroadenoma.
☐ **e.** Patient choice.

49 A 67-year-old diabetic man is seen by his GP for follow-up of glycaemic control and monitoring. He is overweight and slightly hypertensive and as part of his screening fundoscopy is undertaken, which demonstrates changes documented as being consistent with those seen in proliferative diabetic retinopathy. Which of the following complications is associated with this condition?

☐ **a.** Retinal detachment.

☐ **b.** Aqueous haemorrhage.

☐ **c.** Retinal vein thrombosis.

☐ **d.** Optic neuritis.

☐ **e.** Bitemporal hemianopia.

50 An 18-month-old boy is brought to hospital by his mother who is worried that he looks 'cross-eyed'. She describes a history in her family of eye problems and says that she thinks her father had his right eye taken out at a young age. On clinical examination of the eye there is a white reflective reflex in the left eye with obvious divergent squint. Which of the following is the most likely diagnosis?

☐ **a.** Congenital cataract.

☐ **b.** Endophthalmitis.

☐ **c.** Retinoblastoma.

☐ **d.** Ocular tuberculosis.

☐ **e.** Retinopathy of prematurity (ROP).

51 A 45-year-old man presents to hospital complaining of visual disturbance. He has noticed that over the past months his vision has become progressively worse such that he is unable to see pedestrians on the sides of the road when he is driving and has almost been involved in road traffic accidents because of this. His wife comments that he looks different to photos taken just months before and has gone up shoe and hat sizes. Which of the following is the most common pathology associated with this disease?

☐ **a.** Craniopharyngioma.

☐ **b.** Hypothalamic glioma.

☐ **c.** Pituitary adenoma.

☐ **d.** Parasella meningioma.

☐ **e.** Metastatic lymphoma.

52 An 84-year-old woman is brought to hospital after found collapsed at home by a concerned neighbour. On arrival she is found to have a low blood pressure and significant orthostatic hypotension. Intravenous fluid therapy is instituted, which temporarily stabilises the blood pressure at 110/60 mmHg. She is admitted and you are called to the ward as she is still requiring large amounts of fluids to keep her blood pressure above 90 mmHg systolic. Other vital signs are, however, stable and she is afebrile. Her past medical history is significant for recurrent flares of rheumatoid arthritis requiring steroids, eczema as a child and hypertension. Her neighbour tells you that she has not been taking her medications for the past few days because she had had some vomiting and diarrhoea. Which of the following is the most likely explanation?

- ☐ **a.** Intravascular depletion due to vomiting and diarrhoea.
- ☐ **b.** Septic shock due to gastrointestinal infection.
- ☐ **c.** Haemorrhagic stroke due to hypertension.
- ☐ **d.** Vasovagal syncope due to repeated forceful vomiting.
- ☐ **e.** Medication-induced adrenocorticoid axis depression.

53 Empirical antibiotic therapy for infective endocarditis is:

- ☐ **a.** Flucloxacillin and benzylpenicillin.
- ☐ **b.** Benzylpenicillin and gentamycin.
- ☐ **c.** Gentamycin and flucloxacillin.
- ☐ **d.** Amoxicillin and metronidazole.
- ☐ **e.** Cefuroxime and flucloxacillin.

54 Which one of the following physical signs is not associated with cardiovascular disease?

- ☐ **a.** De Musset's sign.
- ☐ **b.** Quinke's sign.
- ☐ **c.** Kussmaul's sign.
- ☐ **d.** Corrigan's sign.
- ☐ **e.** Cullen's sign.

55 A 40-year-old gentleman presents to his GP practice with a 3-day history of central chest pain relieved by sitting forward but exacerbated by inspiration or lying flat. He has no past cardiac history and is on no relevant medications. He has recently recovered from a viral upper respiratory tract illness and his ECG shows widespread concave upwards ST segment elevation. On examination he is afebrile and has no other signs or clinical findings, what is the most appropriate management of this patient?

☐ **a.** NSAIDs and rest.

☐ **b.** Troponin and CK levels.

☐ **c.** ECHO.

☐ **d.** CXR.

☐ **e.** Referral to accident and emergency department.

56 Which of the following is not a feature of cardiac tamponade?

☐ **a.** Bradycardia.

☐ **b.** Pulsus paradoxus.

☐ **c.** Hypotension.

☐ **d.** Raised jugular venous pressure.

☐ **e.** Diminished heart sounds.

57 Which of the following statements is incorrect?

☐ **a.** A bicuspid aortic valve is more likely to calcify than a tricuspid valve.

☐ **b.** A patent ductus arteriosus (PDA) is not compatible with life.

☐ **c.** A machinery murmur is heard with PDA.

☐ **d.** Coarctation of the aorta is associated with Turner's syndrome.

☐ **e.** Chronic hypothyroidism predisposes to atherosclerosis.

58 Which of the following associations is incorrect?

a. Ehlers–Danlos syndrome – mitral valve prolapse.

b. Turner's syndrome – coarctation of aorta.

c. Cushing's syndrome – hypertension.

d. Hypothyroidism – tachycardia.

e. Noonan's syndrome – pulmonary stenosis.

59 A 29-year-old lady who has recently returned from a holiday to Dubai presents with chest pain and shortness of breath. She has no past history of cardiac or respiratory problems and on further questioning you elicit that she takes the oral contraceptive pill. Her examination is unremarkable although she is tachypnoeic. Chest X-ray shows no evidence of pneumonia or pneumothorax. Her D-dimer test is positive and arterial blood gas confirms that she is hypoxic on room air. You diagnose a pulmonary embolus. Which of the following represents the treatment regime that you would start?

- □ **a.** Aspirin, dalteparin and warfarin.
- □ **b.** Low molecular weight heparin and warfarin.
- □ **c.** Aspirin, clopidogrel and warfarin.
- □ **d.** Aspirin and warfarin.
- □ **e.** Unfractionated heparin and warfarin.

60 A 70-year-old gentleman presents to casualty with clinically what appears to be a large pleural effusion. A sample is aspirated using an aseptic technique and its analysis shows straw-coloured fluid, protein 35g/L and no blood. Which of the following conditions would be consistent with this analysis?

- □ **a.** Constrictive pericarditis.
- □ **b.** Cirrhosis of the liver.
- □ **c.** Hypothyroidism.
- □ **d.** Bronchogenic carcinoma.
- □ **e.** Nephrotic syndrome.

Extended matching questions

Contraceptives

Select one of the following contraceptive solutions for each clinical vignette.

a. Combined oral contraceptive pill.
b. Progesterone-only pill.
c. Intrauterine contraceptive device.
d. Depo-provera intramuscular injection.
e. Abstinence.
f. Low-dose oestrogen combined contraceptive.
g. Emergency contraceptive pill.
h. Contraceptive patch.

61 A 16-year-old girl attends her GP complaining of worsening
☐ dysmenorrhoea. She notes that the pain associatedwith her period has gradually been worsening and she has also noticed worsening bleeding. She denies any risk factors for venous-thrombosis.

62 A 37-year-old lady has recently entered into a new relationship.
☐ She had previously not relied on any hormonal contraception as she had used barrier methods for interactions with casual partners. She is clinically obese and is a heavy smoker, she has no past history of venous thrombosis. She works as an office clerk but is well known to be forgetful.

63 A 21-year-old girl seeks help from her GP. She has a regular
☐ partner and normally uses the combined oral contraceptive pill for protection. More recently she has suffered with a diarrhoeal illness that has resolved. She had sex with her regular partner the night before but has since started to worry that although she has not missed any contraceptive pills that they may not have been absorbed due to her recent illness.

64 A 22-year-old medical student has been advised that she should
☐ change her contraceptive. She is currently using the combined oral contraceptive pill but at her regular follow-up appointment she is told that her blood pressure is too high to be issued with a repeat prescription.

65 A 37-year-old multiparous woman has attended the GP practice
☐ to discuss contraceptive options. She has used combined oral contraceptives in the past but since having her last child has decided that she wants a more reliable option.

Upper gastrointestinal bleeding

a. Mallory–Weiss tear.
b. Oesophageal varices.
c. Barrett's oesophagus.
d. Gastritis.
e. Peptic ulceration.
f. Boerhaave's syndrome.
g. Gastric carcinoma.
h. Aorto-enteric fistula.
i. Cricopharyngeal carcinoma.
j. Oesophageal carcinoma.

The following patients have all presented with haematemesis. Please choose the most correct diagnosis from the above list. Each option may be used once, more than once or not at all.

66 A 64-year-old woman presents to accident and emergency with a month's history of progressive difficulty in swallowing, especially for solid food with associated regurgitation of food. She has noticed when she vomits that there are often bright red streaks of blood mixed with the food. Recently she has been complaining that her dresses seem to be too big for her.

67 A 34-year-old accountant presents to hospital on a Friday night with a history of vomiting, severe retching and haematemesis of two cupfuls of fresh blood. He is intoxicated and is pale, anxious and there is bloodstaining around his mouth. His colleagues tell you that they were at a social event together at a local buffet restaurant and that he usually never gets drunk but had been drinking heavily on this occasion.

68 A 54-year-old man is brought in by ambulance to accident and emergency after collapsing at his home 10 minutes away from the hospital. On arrival he looks pale with a Glasgow Coma Scale (GCS) of 6 and there is bloodstaining down his shirt, trousers and around his mouth. He is breathing heavily and collateral history from his wife reveals a large bright red bleed associated with pain in his chest about 15 minutes ago. His past medical history includes a previous abdominal aortic aneurysm repair, asthma and hypertension.

69 A 43-year-old woman is 3 days post-laparoscopic gastric bypass
☐ for morbid obesity. The nurses call you early in the morning as she started to bring up dark red blood with intermittent bouts of vomiting. A sample of the vomitus has been kept and you notice a characteristic heavily dark brown appearance to the blood consistent with coffee ground vomiting. Her drug prescription chart reveals once daily aspirin for previous myocardial infarction, diclofenac (NSAID) tablets for knee arthritis and paracetamol.

70 A 58-year-old man presents to his GP with a 6-week history
☐ of feeling tired at work and inability to sleep well at night. On further questioning he says that he has been not able to tolerate food well recently with severe vomiting after meals and more recently small flecks of blood mixed in with the food. His wife adds that he has been losing weight and although he has been vomiting a lot he still feels hungry after meals. He asks you whether he will still be able to donate blood on a regular basis as he is blood group A and has been asked regularly for donations.

Respiratory investigations

    a. Lung function tests.
    b. Chest X-ray.
    c. Arterial blood gas.
    d. CT chest.
    e. V/Q scan.
    f. CTPA.
    g. Peak expiratory flow rate (PEFR).
    h. FBC.

Which is the most appropriate investigation for each of the scenarios below?

71 A 17-year-old girl has been admitted with acute onset shortness of breath believed by her GP to be a deterioration in her normally well-controlled asthma. She has suffered with asthma since the age of 5 years and is normally well controlled, she has never had any hospital admissions. She usually takes regular salbutamol and beclomethasone.

72 A 76-year-old gentleman has been admitted under the care of the medics for inpatient management of his pneumonia. You are called to the ward to see him as the nurses are concerned that his saturations have dropped despite him being on oxygen. He is not complaining of worsening shortness of breath. He had a chest X-ray done earlier that day that showed a lobar pneumonia.

73 A 27-year-old patient with a history of Marfan's disease presents to accident and emergency with new onset shortness of breath. He has not had any recent illnesses and has not been exerting himself or playing any sports in the past couple of days. He is not complaining of a cough but has noticed a small amount of right-sided chest pain since the onset of the shortness of breath.

74 A 51-year-old lady has recently returned from holiday in the Caribbean. Since her return she has noticed a minor pleuritic chest pain, which she thought would resolve with time; 2 days on, the pain is worsening and she has developed shortness of breath. On examination her saturations on room air are 89%, her chest is clear with good air entry and she has no swelling of her calves. D-dimer test is positive and chest X-ray is normal.

75 A 41-year-old gentleman is referred by his GP to the respiratory clinic for investigation of his worsening dyspnoea and dry cough. He has no past respiratory history and his GP is concerned about finger clubbing, which he has noticed on routine examination. On auscultation of his chest he has noticed fine end inspiratory crackles and chest X-ray shows a ground-glass appearance.

Causes of hepatomegaly

a. Congestive cardiac failure.
b. Riedel's lobe.
c. Gaucher's disease.
d. Leukaemia.
e. Metastatic disease.
f. Hodgkin's disease.
g. Viral hepatitis.
h. Amyloid.
i. Alcoholic hepatitis.
j. Budd–Chiari syndrome.

The following patients have all presented with hepatomegaly. Please choose the more correct diagnosis from the above list. Each option may be used once, more than once or not at all.

76 A 45-year-old man is due to join a new company as a finance director. Prior to his contract starting he books in to have a medical check-up at his GP. He states he feels in good health although tired recently, which he attributes to the stress of changing firms. As part of the routine examination he has blood tests sent and is examined clinically. On examination of the abdomen there is a 2 cm smooth and non-tender enlarged mass in the right upper quadrant. The rest of the examination is normal.

77 A 54-year-old patient who is seen regularly for many years in the rheumatology clinic for management of rheumatoid arthritis presents to hospital with a 2-week history of lethargy, progressive shortness of breath and facial swelling. She has noticed a vague discomfort under her right ribs and states that she feels her body has become more swollen recently. Additionally she has not been able to use her hands as much recently, although she is convinced that it is not due to her rheumatoid disease flaring up. Abdominal examination reveals mild tenderness in the flanks and a 3 cm smooth non-tender mass in the right upper quadrant.

78 A 73-year-old man presents to hospital complaining of an inability
☐ to open his bowels for the past 2 days. He states that he has
not been feeling bright for the past months and has been feeling
nauseated and anorexic. Further questioning reveals a 10 kg
weight loss over the past 2 months and he puts this down to not
eating like he used to as a young man. On examination of the
abdomen there is a 4 cm craggy non-tender liver edge. Digital
rectal examination reveals an empty rectum and a firm 3 cm
poorly defined mass on palpation.

79 A 65-year-old woman presents to hospital with shortness of
☐ breath, reduced exercise tolerance and gross peripheral oedema.
She is well known to the cardiologists who have been treating her left heart failure over many years since her myocardial
infarction. Echocardiography a year ago confirmed a poorly
functioning left ventricle with an ejection fraction of 35% and
right ventricle hypertrophy. On examination of the cardiovascular system she has a raised jugular venous pressure of 9 cm
of H_2O, a third heart sound, systolic murmur heard best at the
right lower sternal edge and tachycardia with marked bilateral
pitting oedema to the knee. Respiratory system reveals crepitations to the midzone bilaterally. Abdominal examination reveals
a distended abdomen with a 3 cm pulsatile and mildly tender
liver edge.

80 A 45-year-old man presents to accident and emergency with
☐ falls and confusion. He is admitted to the medical ward and
started on pabrinex and vitamin B_{12} by intravenous infusion and is written up for chlordiazepoxide (heminevrin) in a
reducing dose over 4 days. On examination he is malnourished
and there is a faint jaundice detectable in the skin and sclera.
Abdominal examination is difficult as the patient is not co-
operative but you notice there is pain in the right upper quadrant and a very tender 2 cm smoothly enlarged liver edge.

Investigation of renal disease

a. Renal biopsy.
b. Autoantibody screen.
c. Renal tract ultrasound.
d. 24-hour protein collection.
e. Daily urea and creatinine.
f. Bence–Jones protein.
g. Intravenous urogram.
h. Renal artery Dopplers.
i. CT scan of abdomen.

The following patients have all presented with renal disease. Please choose the key diagnostic investigation from the list above. Each option can be used once, more than once or not at all.

81 A 34-year-old man complains of arthralgia, abdominal pain and vomiting, a facial rash that is worse in the summer and haematuria. Urea and creatinine are slightly elevated with urinalysis demonstrating red-cell casts. Past medical history is remarkable for childhood eczema.

82 A 42-year-old woman with a past medical history of left hemispheric stroke presents to hospital with signs and symptoms of renal failure. She has been seen by her GP for hypertension and abdominal pain with outpatient investigations pending.

83 A 78-year-old woman is brought to hospital complaining of abdominal pain and is referred to the surgeons. She has been saying that her mother is due to visit her today and that somebody must have broken her lower back as she is in agony. Her blood results show a creatinine level of 295 μmol/L and a calcium level of 3.03 mmol/L.

84 A 32-year-old man presents with shortness of breath and swollen legs and face. He describes feeling progressively more unwell in the weeks preceding admission. On examination there are signs of renal failure. He is admitted to hospital and rapidly deteriorates over a matter of weeks requiring emergency renal replacement therapy.

85 A 72-year-old man is admitted to the ward with chest pain and managed on the acute coronary syndrome protocol. He is found to be hypertensive and hypercholesterolaemic and started on an HMG-CoA reductase inhibitor (statin) and an angiotensin-converting enzyme inhibitor (ACE-I). You are called to the ward to see him as he suddenly desaturates and become acutely short of breath. Once stabilised with frusemide, morphine and oxygen blood tests show a much increased creatinine and urea. You are asked to investigate the cause of this sudden deterioration in renal function.

Causes of headaches

  a. Tension headache.
  b. Subarachnoid haemorrhage.
  c. Subdural haemorrhage.
  d. Extradural haemorrhage.
  e. Cavernous sinus thrombosis.
  f. Meningitis.
  g. Sinusitis.
  h. Cluster headache.

86 A 37-year-old man presents to his GP com plaining of
☐ headache. He notes that it is mainly behind his left eye and
in his forehead. He has been suffering from sinusitis in the
preceding week and assumes that it is caused by this. He has
become increasingly worried as he has noticed that his eye
seems to bulge more on that side and has restricted movement.

87 A 47-year-old lady with a longstanding history of epilepsy has
☐ been brought in by her family as she is suffering with a fluctuation in her conscious level and seems to have some weakness
on the right hand side of her body. She has been suffering with
an increasing number of fits recently. This has come on quite
suddenly over the past 6 hours.

88 A 48-year-old office worker presents with a 3-month history of
☐ worsening headaches. She mentions that they are worse during
the afternoon and evening and are exacerbated by stress. She
describes that pain as band-like around her head and on examination has no neurological deficit.

89 A 35-year-old lady comes home form her stressful job and sud-
☐ denly notices an almighty headache. It is located at the back
of her head and by the time you see her she describes it as the
worst pain she has ever experienced. She notices associated nausea but no vomiting and starts to complain of neck stiffness.

90 A 17-year-old boy who is normally well presents to his general
☐ practitioner with a headache. He has suffered with a recent flu-
like infection but has recovered. He notes that his eyes feel like
they are bulging and the main bulk of the pain is behind his eyes
bilaterally. On clinical examination there is no neurological deficit but you notice pain on palpation over the maxilla bilaterally.

PAPER 5

Questions

Multiple choice questions (single best answer)

1 A 40-year-old lady collapsed during an aerobics class and was brought to accident and emergency by ambulance in asystole. She has no past cardiac history of note and has been generally fit and well recently. Which of the following is the most likely cause of her arrest?
   ☐ **a.** Pulmonary embolus.
   ☐ **b.** Hypertrophic obstructive cardiomyopathy.
   ☐ **c.** Acute myocardial infarction.
   ☐ **d.** Severe pneumonia.
   ☐ **e.** Pneumothorax.

2 Where in the clotting cascade does warfarin exert its effect?
   ☐ **a.** Factor Xa.
   ☐ **b.** Factor II.
   ☐ **c.** Vitamin K.
   ☐ **d.** Vitamin A.
   ☐ **e.** Factor XII.

3 Statins work by competitive inhibition of:
   ☐ **a.** 3-hydroxymethylglutaryl coenzyme A (HMG Co-A) reductase.
   ☐ **b.** Cytochrome p450.
   ☐ **c.** Succinate Co-A dehydrogenase.
   ☐ **d.** 2-Peroxide dismutase.
   ☐ **e.** 21-hydroxylase.

4 Which of the following drugs has both a treatment and diagnostic role in narrow complex tachycardias?
   ☐ **a.** Atenolol.
   ☐ **b.** Amiodarone.
   ☐ **c.** Adenosine.
   ☐ **d.** Atorvastatin.
   ☐ **e.** Amlodipine.

5 You are based at a GP practice and are reviewing a patient with known coronary artery disease. He is a 60-year-old man who is currently taking aspirin, metformin, diclofenac, diltiazem, simvastatin, omeprazole and enalapril. One week ago he was seen by one of your colleagues with abdominal pains and general muscle aches. Blood tests done at the time show deranged liver function tests and a creatinine kinase of 524μmol/L. Which of his medications is likely to be the cause of his symptoms?

☐ **a.** Diltiazem.
☐ **b.** Simvastatin.
☐ **c.** Metformin.
☐ **d.** Diclofenac.
☐ **e.** Enalapril.

6 Which of the following cardiac rhythms is 'shockable' (unsynchronised DC shock)?

☐ **a.** Atrial fibrillation.
☐ **b.** Ventricular fibrillation.
☐ **c.** Sinus rhythm.
☐ **d.** Pulseless electrical activity.
☐ **e.** Asystole.

7 A 23-year-old man presents to hospital complaining of headaches, palpitations and sweating, and nausea and vomiting. He started to have symptoms a few months back and has been experiencing these intermittently. Whilst carrying out observation of vital signs the nurse records a blood pressure of 198/124mmHg with a heart rate of 116 beats per minute. Routine blood tests are requested along with a 24-hour urine collection for catecholamines. Which of the following options is the next appropriate step?

☐ **a.** CT scan of the abdomen.
☐ **b.** Surgical intervention.
☐ **c.** Lowering of blood pressure with phentolamine.
☐ **d.** Lowering of blood pressure with esmolol.
☐ **e.** Renal artery Doppler study.

8 Regarding motor innervation to ocular structures, which of the following associations is NOT correct?

☐ **a.** Levator palpebrae superioris – sympathetic nervous system.
☐ **b.** Lateral rectus muscle – abducens nerve.
☐ **c.** Superior oblique – trochlear nerve.
☐ **d.** Lacrimal glands – parasympathetic nervous system.
☐ **e.** Medial rectus muscle – abducens nerve.

9 A 76-year-old lady presents to her GP with a breast lump. She has noted that it has been present for the past 11 months and has been growing in size. It causes no pain or discomfort and as a result she hasn't sought help until now. On examination the GP notes that there is a lump approximately 5 cm in diameter, overlying skin ulceration and in-drawing of the nipple on that side. She has no family history of breast problems. What is the most likely diagnosis?

☐ **a.** Breast cyst.
☐ **b.** Breast abscess.
☐ **c.** Locally invasive breast cancer.
☐ **d.** Ductal carcinoma *in situ*.
☐ **e.** Mastitis.

10 Which of the following associations is INCORRECT?

☐ **a.** Crohn's disease and iron deficiency anaemia.
☐ **b.** Myelodysplasia and macrocytic anaemia.·
☐ **c.** Pregnancy and normocytic anaemia.
☐ **d.** Thalassaemia and macrocytic anaemia.
☐ **e.** Hypothyroidism and macrocytic anaemia.

11 A 54-year-old man is brought in by ambulance having collapsed at home. He is breathless on arrival and drowsy with a tachycardia of 130 beats a minute. His wife accompanies him and explains that he had been complaining of stomach pains and passing very dark stool for the past couple of days and had taken some aspirin for the pains. On examination in addition to the above findings he has a drop in his blood pressure of 25 mmHg from lying to sitting and digital rectal examination reveals dark offensive stool. Blood tests reveal a urea of 11.3 mmol/L, a haemoglobin of 8.5 g/dL with normal electrolytes and creatinine. Which of the following is the most appropriate course of action?

☐ **a.** Referral to surgeons for an urgent laparotomy.
☐ **b.** 2-unit blood transfusion and colonoscopy.
☐ **c.** Urgent upper gastrointestinal endoscopy.
☐ **d.** Coeliac arteriography.
☐ **e.** Proton pump inhibition and routine endoscopy.

12 A 37-year-old man presents to accident and emergency complaining of the worst groin pain that he has ever experienced. He feels that he may have strained his groin playing football earlier in the week but notes that the pain seems to begin in the flank. It is unilateral only affecting his left side and is colicky in nature. On questioning he agrees that the pain is worse on urinating. Dipstick reveals microscopic haematuria. He has no past history of abdominal problems and has had no operations in the past. His observations reveal a heart rate of 120 beats/minute, respiratory rate 24 breaths/minute, sats 92%, blood pressure 157/91 mmHg. What is the likely diagnosis?

☐ **a.** Pyelonephritis.
☐ **b.** Renal calculus.
☐ **c.** Ureteric calculus.
☐ **d.** Renal cell carcinoma.
☐ **e.** Prostatism.

13 A 63-year-old man with poorly controlled type II diabetes mellitus is referred to the dermatology clinic with a history of a darkly pigmented rash under both arms with thickened skin and a rough texture to the skin. He also complains of some thickening of the skin over his palms making him embarrassed to shake anyone's hand. Which of the following cutaneous manifestations is NOT associated with diabetes?

☐ **a.** Necrobiosis lipoidica diabeticorum.
☐ **b.** Acanthosis nigricans.
☐ **c.** Lipoatrophy.
☐ **d.** Granuloma annulare.
☐ **e.** Pyoderma gangrenosum.

14 An otherwise fit and well 41-year-old lady is referred by accident and emergency for treatment of her ankle fracture. She sustained the initial injury by falling over at home and she thinks that she may have inverted her ankle. On clinical examination there is mild swelling over the lateral epicondyle of her right leg, which is tender on palpation. She can dorsiflex her foot to 90 degrees and plantarflex to 30 degrees but all movements are painful. The distal neurovascular supply is intact. X-rays show an isolated fracture of the distal fibula above the syndesmosis with no talar shift. Which of the following is the most appropriate management of this injury?

☐ **a.** Apply a backslab to the leg and give regular analgesia.

☐ **b.** Admit for internal fixation.

☐ **c.** Place in a walking cast.

☐ **d.** Apply a cylinder cast and bring back to fracture clinic.

☐ **e.** Apply an elasticated dressing and advise non-weight bearing for 6 weeks.

15 Which of the following facts about primary post-partum haemorrhage is INCORRECT?

☐ **a.** It is 500mL or greater of blood lost per vagina in the first 12 hours after delivery.

☐ **b.** Commonest cause is retained products of conception.

☐ **c.** Other causes include intrauterine infection.

☐ **d.** Bleeding may be treated with i.v. oxytocin.

☐ **e.** Vaginal bleeding 1–6 weeks after delivery is considered post-partum haemorrhage.

16 A 67-year-old Caucasian gentleman complains of abdominal pain after eating. The pain is described as severe and has been associated with abdominal distension and vomiting on occasion. Over the past few months he has lost approximately 7 kg, which he attributes to a reduced appetite due to fear of the ensuing pain after eating. In between incidents of pain abdominal examination is normal although a bruit is heard over the right femoral artery. Further examination of his vascular system reveals reduced distal pulses bilaterally in both legs. Abdominal X-ray and other imaging studies including colonoscopy and barium studies have failed to reveal the cause of his pain. Which of the following is most likely to be the cause of his problem?

☐ **a.** Neoplastic.

☐ **b.** Inflammatory.

☐ **c.** Congenital.

☐ **d.** Psychogenic.

☐ **e.** Ischaemic.

17 Which of the following is not associated with the Glasgow criteria for predicting the severity of acute pancreatitis?

- ☐ **a.** $PO_2 < 8$ kPa.
- ☐ **b.** Glucose > 10 mmol/L.
- ☐ **c.** Urea < 10 mmol/L.
- ☐ **d.** Age > 55 years.
- ☐ **e.** Albumin < 32 g/L.

18 Which of the following relationships is correct?

- ☐ **a.** Femoral hernia – high incidence of strangulation in females.
- ☐ **b.** Ventral hernia – most common in neonates.
- ☐ **c.** Direct hernia – herniates into the scrotal sac.
- ☐ **d.** Pantaloon hernia – hernia protrudes either side of femoral artery.
- ☐ **e.** Indirect hernia – herniates through the superficial ring only.

19 A 75-year-old gentleman undergoes a cholecystectomy for recurrent bouts of gallstones. Ten days after the surgery he develops pain and swelling of the right parotid gland. Which of the following is most likely to be the cause of the parotid swelling?

- ☐ **a.** Haemorrhage into the parotid gland.
- ☐ **b.** *Staphylococcus aureus* infection.
- ☐ **c.** Trauma to the gland during surgery.
- ☐ **d.** Stone formation and obstruction of the parotid duct.
- ☐ **e.** Mumps infection.

20 A 37-year-old man is a driver involved in a road traffic accident. On examination he is found to have point tenderness over the lower left ribs and tachycardia and falling blood pressure among other signs of hypovolaemic shock. Breath sounds are normal bilaterally. These findings are most likely to be due to which of the following?

- ☐ **a.** Rupture of liver capsule.
- ☐ **b.** Rupture of spleen.
- ☐ **c.** Cardiac contusions.
- ☐ **d.** Abdominal aorta transaction.
- ☐ **e.** Haemothorax secondary to pulmonary contusions.

21 A 74-year-old man is 1-day post-transurethral resection of the prostate (TURP) for benign prostatic hyperplasia. The nurse calls a doctor to review this gentleman as he is uncomfortable and in pain on the ward. There is nothing remarkable on general examination; however, on inspecting the catheter for potential blockage it is discovered that there is a tight constricting band just proximal to the glans penis, which is swollen and pale. What abnormality does this gentleman have?

- [ ] **a.** Phimosis.
- [ ] **b.** Paraphimosis.
- [ ] **c.** Epispadias.
- [ ] **d.** Hypospadias.
- [ ] **e.** Peyronie's disease.

22 A 78-year-old non-smoker with a history of chronic obstructive pulmonary disease (COPD) has been admitted to the day assessment unit for home oxygen assessment. She has noticed increasing breathlessness of late both on exertion and intermittently at rest. You perform an arterial blood gas (ABG) on air and the results are as follows: pH 7.40, PO_2 7.3 kPa and PCO_2 4.8 kPa. What would be your next step in the assessment?

- [ ] **a.** Increase her oxygen to 60% and repeat ABG in 1 hour.
- [ ] **b.** Discharge her, she doesn't require domiciliary oxygen.
- [ ] **c.** Try 28% and repeat ABG in 1 hour.
- [ ] **d.** Recheck ABG on air in 1 hour.
- [ ] **e.** Ask patient to mobilise and recheck ABG afterwards.

23 A 25-year-old Afro-Caribbean office worker has been referred to the respiratory clinic for investigation of dry cough, mild chest pain and reduced exercise tolerance. He is complaining of a rash on his shins and occasional joint aches. A chest X-ray performed shows bilateral hilar lymphadenopathy. What is the most likely diagnosis?

- [ ] **a.** Sarcoidosis.
- [ ] **b.** Tuberculosis.
- [ ] **c.** Asthma.
- [ ] **d.** Pulmonary fibrosis.
- [ ] **e.** Malignancy.

24 Which of the following associations is incorrect?

- [ ] **a.** Pulmonary fibrosis – fine end inspiratory crackles.
- [ ] **b.** Extrinsic allergic alveolitis – type I respiratory failure.
- [ ] **c.** Pulmonary embolus – hypoxia.
- [ ] **d.** Cystic fibrosis – fine crepitations.
- [ ] **e.** Pneumonectomy – reduced breath sounds.

25 Whilst looking through the past medical history notes of one of your inpatients (admitted for ENT surgery) you note that she suffers with fibrosing alveolitis. Causes of this include all of the following EXCEPT:

☐ **a.** Cryptogenic.
☐ **b.** Rheumatoid arthritis.
☐ **c.** Sjögren's syndrome.
☐ **d.** Ulcerative colitis.
☐ **e.** *Aspergillus.*

26 A 69-year-old lady is admitted on your medical take. She has had two other admissions earlier this year for recurrent pleural effusions, on both occasions samples of fluid failed to reveal a cause for the effusion. On this occasion she is short of breath, chest X-ray shows a right-sided pleural effusion for which a chest drain is inserted to provide symptomatic relief. A sample of the fluid from this admission shows malignant cells and a repeat X-ray after drainage shows pleural thickening. A pleural biopsy confirms your suspected diagnosis of mesothelioma. Which of the following facts about mesothelioma is not true?

☐ **a.** Can occur in either pleura or peritoneum.
☐ **b.** The period between exposure and development of cancer is approximately 40 years.
☐ **c.** Pleural mesothelioma is more common on the right than the left side.
☐ **d.** Prognosis is approximately 2 years.
☐ **e.** Incidence is more common in females than males.

27 During your pre-operative assessment clinic a patient notes that he feels incredibly tired during the day and his wife mentions that he occasionally stops breathing at night and wakes up gasping for breath. He is being admitted for hip surgery under spinal anaesthesia but you suggest that he sees his GP about his sleep symptoms. Which of the following is not a clinical feature of sleep apnoea?

☐ **a.** Recurrent cough.
☐ **b.** Daytime somnolence.
☐ **c.** Reduced libido.
☐ **d.** Morning headache.
☐ **e.** Reduced cognitive performance.

28 A 65-year-old gentleman sees his GP on his wife's recommendation as she has noticed that he is becoming increasingly short of breath on exertion. At rest he is asymptomatic and he has noticed that everything seems to take his a little bit longer but hasn't noticed that he is having difficulty in breathing. On examination his GP notes bibasal crepitations with a mildly raised jugular venous pressure. There were no peripheral signs of respiratory disease. The GP organises a chest X-ray to confirm the diagnosis but believes that this gentleman is suffering with cor pulmonale. Cause of cor pulmonale includes all of the following EXCEPT:

☐ **a.** Pulmonary fibrosis.
☐ **b.** Primary pulmonary hypertension.
☐ **c.** Sickle cell disease.
☐ **d.** Enlarged adenoids in children.
☐ **e.** Acute asthma.

29 A 65-year-old gentleman presents acutely short of breath. He has no history of respiratory disease and is having further difficulty with every inspiration. On examination you note use of accessory muscles and tracheal deviation to the left-hand side. On the right you note increased resonance on percussion, reduced breath sounds and reduced chest expansion on that side. What is the next step in your management?

☐ **a.** Chest X-ray.
☐ **b.** Arterial blood gas.
☐ **c.** Insert large bore cannula into second intercostal space on right-hand side.
☐ **d.** Insert chest drain.
☐ **e.** Administer bronchodilators.

30 A 56-year-old homeless man presents with abdominal pain and mild shortness of breath. After appropriate questioning and examination chest and abdominal radiology is requested. Chest X-ray demonstrates a right-sided pleural effusion and the abdominal X-ray shows an absent psoas shadow. What is the most useful next investigation to aid in diagnosis?

☐ **a.** Pleural tap.
☐ **b.** Serum glucose.
☐ **c.** Serum amylase.
☐ **d.** Trans-oesophageal echo.
☐ **e.** Endoscopy.

31 A 24-year-old man presents to his GP with a rash on the head of his penis. He is extremely reluctant to talk about the rash and feels that he has done something wrong. Questioning reveals the rash appeared slowly over the course of the past 2 weeks and it itchy and causes him discomfort during the day. He denies any dysuria or urethral discharge but does say that he has noticed he needs to urinate more frequently and has been feeling lethargic and very thirsty. He does not have a sexual partner and has not had sexual intercourse in the last 6 months. On examination there are multiple areas of underlying erythema with a whitish layer to them. Which of the following investigations is likely to confirm the diagnosis?

☐ **a.** Blood glucose level.
☐ **b.** Erythrocyte sedimentation rate.
☐ **c.** Urine analysis.
☐ **d.** HTLV 1 and 2 assays.
☐ **e.** Full blood count.

32 A 45-year-old woman presents to her GP with a sensation of food sticking in her throat when she has a meal associated with some pain. She states that the sensation is worse with solids and dry food and she complains of no problems with drinking liquids. Her past medical history is unremarkable and the only medication she takes is an antacid preparation bought from her local chemist. On examination she is obese and perspiring slightly. The abdomen is distended in line with her body habitus and is soft and non-tender. Cardiac and respiratory systems examination shows no abnormality. Which of the following diagnoses is the most likely cause for her dysphagia?

☐ **a.** Systemic sclerosis.
☐ **b.** Reflux oesophagitis stricture.
☐ **c.** Radiation oesophagitis.
☐ **d.** Oesophageal carcinoma.
☐ **e.** Oesophageal candidiasis.

33 A 52-year-old man presents to his GP with bilateral symmetrically enlarged breasts. He states that he noticed an increase in the size of the breasts over the past few months and initially put it down to lack of exercise. He is worried that now they resemble female breasts and he has become very self-conscious about them. His past medical history is remarkable for gastro-oesophageal reflux disease and angina. Which of the following medications is most likely responsible for gynaecomastia in this man?

- ☐ **a.** Atenolol.
- ☐ **b.** Gaviscon.
- ☐ **c.** Cimetidine.
- ☐ **d.** Enalapril.
- ☐ **e.** Aspirin.

34 A 52-year-old businessman presents to accident and emergency anxious and worried. He has been passing bright red blood with stools that is apparent on the toilet paper and can be seen in the toilet bowel. He denies any pain whilst passing stools but does say that he has to spend long on the toilet and strains most times to pass stool. On examination he is anxious but otherwise healthy. Cardiac examination reveals a mild tachycardia and respiratory examination shows evidence of a mild tremor with a respiratory rate of 24 breaths per minute. Abdominal examination reveals no abnormality, however, on digital rectal examination there are soft fluctuant masses felt at 11, 3 and 7 o'clock with the patient in the lithotomy position and a few spots of fresh red blood on the glove. Which of the following diagnoses is most likely in this man?

- ☐ **a.** Rectosigmoid carcinoma.
- ☐ **b.** Anal fissure.
- ☐ **c.** Angiodysplasia.
- ☐ **d.** Inflammatory bowel disorder.
- ☐ **e.** Haemorrhoids.

35 A 74-year-old woman presents to her GP with a lack of energy and tiredness that continues throughout the day independent of her sleeping habit. She denies any other symptoms but has had to visit the shops more frequently than usual to buy some new dresses as her old ones do not fit her any more. Routine blood tests show a white cell count of 11×10^9/L, haemoglobin of 7.4 g/dL, MCV of 72 fL, urea of 6.9 mmol/L, creatinine of 147 μmol/L, aspartate transaminase of 58 units/L, alanine aminotransferase of 79 units/L with a bilirubin of 30 μmol/L. Which of the following investigations would NOT form part of the investigational work-up?

☐ **a.** Liver biopsy.

☐ **b.** CT scan of abdomen.

☐ **c.** Chest radiography.

☐ **d.** Colonoscopy.

☐ **e.** Oesophagogastroduodenoscopy (OGD).

36 A 35-year-old woman presents to hospital over a 2-month period complaining of abdominal pain in her left lower quadrant with abdominal distension and progressive shortness of breath. In the last discharge notification a transvaginal ultrasound was performed, which demonstrated a cystic mass in the left ovary reported as most likely a benign mass with further investigation recommended. On examination the abdomen is distended with evidence of shifting dullness but soft and non-tender. Which of the following eponymous syndromes describes this clinical picture?

☐ **a.** Jarisch–Herxheimer reaction.

☐ **b.** Meig's syndrome.

☐ **c.** Fitz–Hugh–Curtis syndrome.

☐ **d.** Peyronie's disease.

☐ **e.** Raynaud's syndrome.

37 A 34-year-old woman presents to accident and emergency complaining of severe abdominal pain associated with weakness of both legs. She states that the symptoms started in the morning and have steadily gotten worse. She complains of abdominal pain that is generalised but much worse in the suprapubic region but denies any dysuria. A sample of urine for dipstick was dark in colour but was negative for blood, protein or nitrites on testing. On examination the abdomen is soft but tender over the suprapubic region and neurological examination reveals markedly reduced sensation in the distal lower limbs but normal tone, power and co-ordination. You notice that during the examination she has been frantically looking through her observations and drug charts and stating that no documentation must be taken as the government have been spying on her. Which of the following investigations would be most useful in making the diagnosis?

- ☐ **a.** 24-hour urinary protein collection.
- ☐ **b.** Thyroid function tests.
- ☐ **c.** Urinary porphobilinogen levels.
- ☐ **d.** CT scan of the abdomen.
- ☐ **e.** Urinary metanephrines (HMMA/VMA).

38 An elderly man is admitted to hospital following a fall and fractured neck of femur. He made a slow recovery but for the past 4 days has been more confused and asking when he can see his wife who died 4 years ago. The nursing staff notice that recently he has lost control of his bowels and is incontinent of watery, foul-smelling stools up to 4 times a day. Physical examination reveals a slightly distended abdomen with active bowel sounds and digital rectal examination reveals hard faeces but no blood or masses. An abdominal radiograph shows a patchy ground-glass appearance throughout the distribution of the colon. Which of the following is the most likely cause?

- ☐ **a.** Faecal impaction.
- ☐ **b.** Cholesterol embolus.
- ☐ **c.** Sigmoid volvulus.
- ☐ **d.** Cauda equina syndrome.
- ☐ **e.** *Clostridium difficile* infection.

39 A 45-year-old-man is involved in a fight and is knifed in the abdomen. He is taken to theatre as an emergency by the surgical team and requires 7 unit blood transfusion with colostomy formation. His recovery is complicated by the development of acute respiratory distress syndrome and he spends 2 weeks sedated and ventilated on the intensive care unit. Parenteral nutrition (TPN) is instituted on day 4 of his ICU admission and continued throughout until his transfer to the ward. You are reviewing his blood tests on the surgical ward and notice that the haemoglobin is 11.4 g/dL with normal electrolytes but bilirubin of 23 μmol/L, aspartate transaminase of 113 units/L, alanine aminotransferase of 89 units/L, alkaline phosphatase of 423 units/L and γ-GT of 101 units/L. Which of the following is the most likely explanation for the derangement in liver enzymes?

- ☐ **a.** Blood transfusion reaction.
- ☐ **b.** Parenteral nutrition related.
- ☐ **c.** Biliary leak.
- ☐ **d.** Hepatitis secondary to blood transfusion.
- ☐ **e.** Sedation-related side-effect.

40 Which of the following facts about multiple sclerosis is not true?

- ☐ **a.** It has a relapsing/remitting course.
- ☐ **b.** 97% of MS patients have oligoclonal bands in CSF.
- ☐ **c.** Clinical picture is caused by demyelination in central nervous system (CNS).
- ☐ **d.** Good treatments are available.
- ☐ **e.** Symptoms are worsened by immersion in a hot bath.

41 A 37-year-old school teacher undergoes a lumbar puncture for a history highly suggestive of a bacterial meningitis. A CT scan performed prior to the lumbar puncture showed no evidence of raised intracranial pressure. Which of the following findings on analysis of CSF would rule AGAINST a diagnosis of bacterial meningitis?

- ☐ **a.** Normal CSF pressure.
- ☐ **b.** Moderately/severely raised protein level.
- ☐ **c.** >50 polymorphs.
- ☐ **d.** Glucose – low.
- ☐ **e.** Raised opening CSF pressure.

42 A 51-year-old gentleman is referred by his GP for worsening back pain. He works as an electrician and the GP is concerned that he is unable to continue working due to the pain. On questioning, he has had a 'niggling pain' in his lower back for a few months but this morning, 4 hours prior to presentation he notes that all of a sudden the pain became far worse, very sharp in nature with no radiation. Simple analgesia has not relieved the pain. He notes that he wants to pass urine but feels unable to and is complaining of saddle anaesthesia. Which of the following investigations is most diagnostic?

- ☐ **a.** Thoraco-lumbar spine X-rays.
- ☐ **b.** MRI spine.
- ☐ **c.** Bloods including erythrocyte sedimentation rate and C-reative protein.
- ☐ **d.** CT head.
- ☐ **e.** Nerve conduction studies.

43 An 11-year-old girl is diagnosed as having type I diabetes mellitus. Tests were carried out after she noticed that she was constantly thirsty and passing large volumes of urine. Although the diagnosis has shocked her she is keen to find out more about the long-term problems associated with the condition. Her family are particularly concerned that she may develop neurological complications in later life. Which of the following is NOT known to be associated with diabetes?

- ☐ **a.** Third nerve palsy.
- ☐ **b.** Bilateral pupillary abnormalities.
- ☐ **c.** Transient hemiparesis.
- ☐ **d.** Headaches.
- ☐ **e.** Autonomic neuropathy.

44 A 56-year-old woman presents to her GP complaining of intense stabbing pain over her left cheek and forehead. The pain lasted a few seconds in duration and resolved itself. She notes that she always has the pain on the left side and it is often made worse by touching the skin. She has no relevant past medical history and finds simple analgesia unhelpful. Which of the following conditions is most likely to account for her symptoms?

- ☐ **a.** Trigeminal neuralgia.
- ☐ **b.** Cluster headache.
- ☐ **c.** Parotitis.
- ☐ **d.** Temporal arteritis.
- ☐ **e.** Otitis media.

45 A 73-year-old man is brought to the GP by his wife as she has noticed that he is not quite walking normally. On further questioning the wife notes that his gait has been deteriorating for some time and is now shuffling and slow to initiate. Which of the following is associated with Parkinson's disease?

- [ ] **a.** Waddling.
- [ ] **b.** Wide base.
- [ ] **c.** High stepping.
- [ ] **d.** Difficulty initiating movements.
- [ ] **e.** CNS demyelination.

46 A 15-year-old boy is brought in by ambulance after sustaining a head injury during a football match. His mother was told that another player accidentally kicked the ball at his head and it hit the left side, just between his eye and ear. He did not lose consciousness but was slightly drowsy after the incident. He persuaded friends to take him home as he felt well, he refused to attend hospital. On arrival at home he was fine but over the next few hours became slightly more drowsy and complained of a headache. His symptoms were assumed by his family to be due to tiredness but 6 hours after the incident they noted that he was becoming less responsive and called an ambulance. What is the likely diagnosis?

- [ ] **a.** Subdural haemorrhage.
- [ ] **b.** Extradural haemorrhage.
- [ ] **c.** Subarachnoid haemorrhage.
- [ ] **d.** Intracranial venous thrombosis.
- [ ] **e.** Stroke.

47 A 78-year-old lady that has been a resident on the acute medical ward for the past 10 days following admission for a urinary tract infection has become increasingly confused. Over the past day she has been found to have a fluctuating level of consciousness whilst being disorientated in time and place. She seems to have become withdrawn but intermittently becomes very noisy and agitated. The family have raised their concerns about the cause of her symptoms and note that she seems to be quite depressed in the mood and muddled in her thinking. What is the likely cause for her symptoms?

- [ ] **a.** Dementia.
- [ ] **b.** Delirium.
- [ ] **c.** Schizophrenia.
- [ ] **d.** Depression.
- [ ] **e.** Cerebral mass.

48 You are asked to assess a patient on the ward. He is a 73-year-old man and has been suffering with what you diagnose as a peripheral neuropathy. Which of the following is NOT a cause of a peripheral neuropathy?

☐ **a.** Diabetes.

☐ **b.** B12 deficiency.

☐ **c.** Hereditary.

☐ **d.** Alcohol.

☐ **e.** Paracetamol overdose.

49 Whilst on call you reluctantly agree to clerk a patient whom according to the GP is simply 'off legs'. On examination the patient gives a vague history of noticing weakness in his lower limbs but seems a little confused. The rest of the history is obtained from the helpful neighbour who has accompanied him. She notes that in his medicine box there was atenolol and losartan but is certain that he takes no other medicines. Whilst carrying out a thorough neurological examination you note that he has bilateral pin-point pupils. Which of the following would account for his pupils?

☐ **a.** Pontine haemorrhage.

☐ **b.** Frontal lobe infarct.

☐ **c.** Atenolol overdose.

☐ **d.** Cerebellar mass.

☐ **e.** Multiple sclerosis.

50 A 78-year-old woman is scheduled to have a low colonic resection for colonic carcinoma and is brought in to hospital. Blood tests were performed pre-operatively, which demonstrate normal renal function, slightly deranged liver enzymes and normal blood counts. She undergoes surgery and is sent back to the wards with no immediate post-surgical complications. The following day you are called to see her on the wards as she is feeling nauseated and has been vomiting shortly after being given her analgesic injection. You prescribe anti-emesis in the form of cyclizine and request she is reviewed with her blood tests the following day. Blood results taken at the end of the second post-operative day demonstrate a urea of 12.3 mmol/L, creatinine 172 μmol/L with potassium of 4.4 mmol/L and sodium of 146 mmol/L. Which of the following is the most likely cause of renal failure in this woman?

- ☐ **a.** Analgesic nephropathy.
- ☐ **b.** Dehydration.
- ☐ **c.** Renal metastases.
- ☐ **d.** Post-surgical rhabdomyolysis.
- ☐ **e.** Urinary retention.

51 A 73-year-old woman with end-stage renal failure undergoes haemodialysis 3 times a week at a local satellite dialysis centre. She is known to have diabetic nephropathy and is seen in the joint renal/diabetic clinic on a regular basis. Which of the following complications has NOT been described as associated with long-term dialysis?

- ☐ **a.** Carpal tunnel syndrome.
- ☐ **b.** Bleeding tendency.
- ☐ **c.** Bone fractures.
- ☐ **d.** Aluminium toxicity.
- ☐ **e.** Reversal of renal function.

52 A 42-year-old woman presents to hospital with fever, sweats and loss of appetite. She describes a history of 6-kg weight loss over a 2-month period with pain in her mid-back. Past medical history reveals a wide local excision of a breast cancer 8 years ago and asthma as a child. Blood tests reveal a haemoglobin of 11.8 g/dL, a urea of 10.4 mmol/L with a creatinine of 192 μmol/L. Serum corrected calcium is 3.12 mmol/L. Metastatic malignancy is strongly suspected. Which of the following investigations should NOT be performed immediately?

- ☐ **a.** Staging CT scan.
- ☐ **b.** Liver ultrasound.
- ☐ **c.** Breast examination.
- ☐ **d.** Mammography.
- ☐ **e.** Thoracic spine radiographs.

53 A 67-year-old woman is admitted under the care of the general surgeons with abdominal pain and vomiting. Her current medications are atenolol, metformin, simvastatin, as required paracetamol and regular aspirin. She is diagnosed as having pancreatitis and a CT scan is arranged as an inpatient, which confirms the diagnosis. Clinically her pancreatitis improves. Two days into her hospital admission you are called to see her in the afternoon as she has not been passing urine since midday the day before and has been complaining of shortness of breath. Which of the following medications is likely responsible for this secondary deterioration?

☐ **a.** Atenolol.
☐ **b.** Metformin.
☐ **c.** Simvastatin.
☐ **d.** Paracetamol.
☐ **e.** Aspirin.

54 A 54-year-old man presents to accident and emergency with abdominal pain and is investigated by the surgical on-call team. He describes the pain as in his left flank with radiation to the front and has noticed that his face and legs have become more swollen over the past 3 days. A urine sample sent was noticed by the nursing staff to be bloodstained. Urine dipstick taken on admission showed heavy protcinuria, positive for blood but negative for nitrites and leucocytes. Clinical examination reveals a very tender left flank and abdomen with evidence of a fullness in the same region. He is apyrexic with a blood pressure of 180/78 mmHg and blood tests show moderate renal failure with D-dimer of 7580. On reviewing his medical notes it is noted that he has frequently been admitted to hospital with episodes of nephrotic syndrome and that he suffers from eczema. Which of the following is the most likely diagnosis?

☐ **a.** Pyelonephritis.
☐ **b.** Addisonian crisis.
☐ **c.** Pancreatitis.
☐ **d.** Renal vein thrombosis.
☐ **e.** Pulmonary embolus.

55 A 75-year-old woman presents to hospital with chest pain and mild shortness of breath. She describes a 3-day history of a cough productive of green sputum and is diagnosed with lower respiratory tract infection. Her past medical history includes osteoarthritis, chronic renal failure and hysterectomy. Her prescription chart shows oral amoxicillin and clarithromycin, regular paracetamol and diclofenac for pain, as required sodium docusate for constipation. You are called to see her 2 days later as her urine output has dropped from 35 to 10mL/hour over 24 hours. Which of the medications on her prescription chart is the most precipitant of deterioration in renal function?

☐ **a.** Amoxicillin.
☐ **b.** Clarithromycin.
☐ **c.** Paracetamol.
☐ **d.** Diclofenac.
☐ **e.** Sodium docusate.

56 A 58-year-old man who has been followed up in the renal clinic for chronic renal failure for many years presents to hospital in end-stage renal failure (ESRF). The management options are explained to him and he is listed for cadaveric renal transplantation and managed expectantly with haemodialysis 3 times weekly. Which of the following is an ABSOLUTE contraindication to renal transplantation?

☐ **a.** Severe depression.
☐ **b.** Excised skin cancer.
☐ **c.** Heart failure.
☐ **d.** Recent urinary tract infection.
☐ **e.** Chronic hepatitis C.

57 Which of the following is NOT a true cause of haematuria?

☐ **a.** Glomerulonephritis.
☐ **b.** Ureteric stone.
☐ **c.** Schistosomiasis.
☐ **d.** Rifampicin.
☐ **e.** Malaria.

58 A 37-year-old man is brought in by ambulance to hospital after suffering an industrial accident where he was trapped underneath an iron girder. He has a Glasgow Coma Scale of 10/15 on arrival and has extensive injuries to his lower limbs for which he was given paracetamol in the ambulance. A radiographic screen of his limbs reveals bilateral complex fractures of tibia and fibula and extensive soft tissue swelling. Initial biochemical blood tests show deranged renal function with a creatinine of 196 μmol/L and he is very oliguric. What is the most likely diagnosis?

- ☐ **a.** Renal contusion.
- ☐ **b.** Rhabdomyolysis.
- ☐ **c.** Cholesterol embolus.
- ☐ **d.** Acute interstitial nephritis.
- ☐ **e.** Urethral rupture.

59 Regarding the above case, which of the following investigations would be most useful to perform next?

- ☐ **a.** Creatinine kinase.
- ☐ **b.** Renal ultrasound scan.
- ☐ **c.** 24-hour urine protein collection.
- ☐ **d.** Bence–Jones protein.
- ☐ **e.** Renal artery Dopplers.

60 During a walk-in clinic in general practice you are asked to see a patient who has been complaining of headaches, palpitations and occasional blurred vision. You take the blood pressure whilst listening to the history and find a reading of 185/98 mmHg. Which of the following renal conditions is NOT usually associated with hypertension?

- ☐ **a.** Renal artery stenosis (RAS).
- ☐ **b.** Recurrent urinary tract infections.
- ☐ **c.** Polycystic kidney disease.
- ☐ **d.** Glomerulonephritis.
- ☐ **e.** Severe acute pyelonephritis.

Extended matching questions

Cardiovascular investigations

Which of the following is the most appropriate investigation?

   a. Chest X-ray.
   b. ECG.
   c. Echocardiogram.
   d. Exercise tolerance test (ETT).
   e. Diagnostic coronary angiogram.
   f. 24-hour tape.
   g. Cardiac perfusion scan.
   h. 24-hour blood pressure monitor.

61 A 58-year-old secretary with a past history of hypertension presents with intermittent new-onset chest pain. This was first noticed during a holiday to the United States. Whilst on holiday an ECG was taken which showed lateral T-wave inversions. An ECG repeated on admission showed some associated ST depression. This ECG was identical to one taken by the patient's GP in the interim period. Her troponin level was mildly positive. An exercise test showed no acute changes.

62 A 74-year-old lady complains of periods of dizziness with occasional associated blackouts. She is on no regular medicines.

63 A 69-year-old lady with a recent diagnosis of atrial fibrillation (AF) enquires about the risks associated with the condition. She is concerned that a cerebrovascular accident is associated with AF and asks about anticoagulation. Which of the above investigations would aid your decision about anticoagulation in this lady?

64 A 68-year-old man who was admitted with troponin negative chest pain but T-wave inversion asks about his risks of progressing onto cardiac problems. Which investigation would aid in stratifying his risk?

65 A 72-year-old lady is admitted for shortness of breath. On examination pulmonary oedema is diagnosed. This is medically treated but she complains of intermittent dizziness and periods of her heart racing. On examination you note that her heart rate is 60 beats per minute, the observation chart notes that her heart rate is persistently above 100 beats per minute. Which investigation would provide diagnostic information in this case?

Specific pneumonias

a. Pneumococcal.
b. Staphylococcal.
c. *Klebsiella.*
d. *Pseudomonas.*
e. *Mycoplasma.*
f. *Legionella.*
g. *Chlamydia.*
h. *Streptococcus.*

66 An 80-year-old lady with a history of chronic obstructive
☐ pulmonary disease and heart failure is admitted via her GP with
a 2-day history of cough and fever with a suspicion of a pneumonia. Her chest X-ray shows a right lower lobe pneumonia.
Which is the likeliest pathogen?

67 A 30-year-old man with a history of cystic fibrosis presents to
☐ the GP with a 5-day history of worsening productive cough
and fever. Which of the bacteria is likely to be the cause of his
pneumonia?

68 A 24-year-old man presents to his GP feeling generally under
☐ the weather, complains of myalgia, headaches and malaise.
He has noticed a productive cough and some mild shortness
of breath, although on auscultation there is very little to hear.
The GP refers him to casualty as he is unsure about the clinical
picture. What is the GP concerned about?

69 A 34-year-old street dweller presents to accident and emergency
☐ with a productive cough and fever. He is keen to be treated and
leave but on examination he is an unkempt man with signs of
needle marks on his forearms, although he denies any drug
abuse. On auscultation there are inspiratory crepitations in the
left midzone and chest X-ray confirms a consolidation. What is
the likely cause?

70 A 45-year-old businessman who has recently returned from a
☐ business trip to Europe presents to his GP with a 3-day history of a dry cough and associated chest pain and diarrhoea. He
mentioned that he felt like he had the 'flu for a few days before
the cough came on but persisted with the symptoms as he had
to go to work. On attendance at the GP he has a fever of 40°C
with bibasal inspiratory crepitations.

P5 QUESTIONS

Causes of upper abdominal pain

a. Hepatitis.
b. Cholecystitis.
c. Cystic liver disease.
d. Lower lobe pneumonia.
e. Ruptured spleen.
f. Diabetic ketoacidosis (DKA).
g. Myocardial infarction.
h. Subphrenic abscess.

The following patients have all presented with abdominal complaints. Please choose the most correct diagnosis from the above list. Each option may be used once, more than once or not at all.

71 A 42-year-old haemophiliac presents to hospital with pain in the right upper quadrant and a mild yellow tinge to the skin. He complains of feeling nauseated with poor appetite and feeling very tired at work. Examination reveals a smoothly enlarged tender liver edge 4 cm from the right costal margin.

72 A 63-year-old nursing home resident is brought in by ambulance to hospital as the nursing staff are worried that she has become increasingly confused and unsteady on her feet. The accompanying letter from the nursing home states that she suffered a stroke 3 years ago with persistent dysphagia. She is normally nil by mouth and fed via a PEG tube; however, one of the nursing staff had noticed some regurgitation of feed and stopped the PEG feeding this morning.

73 A 25-year-old man presents to accident and emergency with severe upper abdominal pain. He is sweating and breathing heavily on arrival with a respiratory rate of 34 breaths per minute. Focused history taking reveals he has recently suffered 'a bad cold' and has not been able to take his regular medication recently due to feeling nauseated. From his medical notes he is under regular yearly review in the eye clinic and is seen regularly by the renal physicians. Routine investigations reveal a pH of 7.25, PaO_2 of 14 kPa with a $PaCO_2$ of 3.8 kPa. White cell count is raised as is the C-reactive peptide and serum amylase is 420.

74 A 43-year-old woman is seen in the general surgery clinic and admitted to hospital with abdominal pain associated with vomiting and nausea. On examination she is an obese woman with tenderness over the right upper quadrant. An ultrasound of the abdomen was requested and during the investigation she was noticed to catch her breath when the probe was placed over the right upper quadrant. Blood tests revealed a raised white cell count and C-reactive peptide.

75 A 64-year-old woman is 6 days post-laparoscopic liver cyst fenestration. You are called to assess her on the wards one night as she is complaining of pain over the right upper quadrant and has been spiking fevers throughout the night. At the bedside you examine her and she looks sweaty, in pain and pale. She has a small vacuum-assisted drain placed on the right side but there is no evidence of localised infection around the entry site. Chest radiology, urine, sputum and faeces culture reveal no source of infection. Over the next couple of days she repeatedly develops high swinging fevers and pain in the right shoulder tip.

Management of diarrhoeal illnesses

a. Oral metronidazole.
b. Fluid rehydration and insulin infusion.
c. Phosphate enema.
d. Systemic steroids with or without mesalazine.
e. Carbimazole and beta-blockade.
f. Synthetic pancreatic enzymes (Pancrex).
g. Oral rehydration therapy.
h. Proton pump inhibition with or without endoscopy.
i. Psychiatric counselling.
j. Intravenous cefuroxime and metronidazole.

The following patients have all presented with diarrhoeal illnesses. Please choose the more correct diagnosis from the above list. Each option may be used once, more than once or not at all.

76 A 26-year-old woman presents to accident and emergency with increased frequency of stool, passing up to six motions a day. She feels very weak and states that she has been passing blood mixed with the stool, mucous and loose stools since yesterday evening. She denies any recent foreign travel and has been married for the past 2 years with no extra-marital partners. It is noted by an observant onlooker that she has a very tender red eye and on review of systems she has been complaining of pain in her knee that she has noticed over the past few days.

77 A 64-year-old man has been recently admitted to hospital with a chest infection and treated on intravenous clarithromycin and amoxicillin for suspected community-acquired pneumonia. A week into his course of antibiotics he started complaining to the nursing staff of an inability to hold his stool with faecal incontinence that he has never had before. The nursing staff note that the stools are offensive and slightly green tinged.

78 A 32-year-old known diabetic presents to hospital complaining of polyuria, polydipsia, diarrhoea and fatigue. He had recently come back from a backpacking holiday in Europe and thinks he may have caught something there as he has been exhibiting coryzal features and a productive cough of green sputum for the past 3 days. Blood glucose measurement shows a glucose of 27.6 mmol/L with significant dehydration, ketones ++ in the urine with a venous gas measurement recording a pH of 7.31 and a slightly reduced bicarbonate.

79 A 45-year-old man presents to his GP complaining of recent
☐ changes in his weight, mood and bowel habit. He has noticed
that over the past few months he has become increasingly heat
intolerant such that taking his son sledging in the snow caused
him to sweat profusely and he could wear no more than a pair
of shorts and a t-shirt. Recently he has been feeling more anxious about his career and family although he states there is
no basis to the anxiety. His wife states he has lost about 6 kg
of weight over the past month and he attributes this to regular
bouts of loose stools up to 5 times a day over the same period.

80 A 16-year-old girl is brought to hospital by her mother with
☐ diarrhoea and recent rapid loss of weight. Her mother tells you
that she has noticed that her daughter has become more withdrawn at school and has been spending more time in her room
these days. When enquiring about eating habits the mother
states that she has been eating good healthy amounts but is
always keen to leave the table when she is done and won't
wait for the rest of the family to finish. On examination the
girl is underweight for her height and has noticeable blistering
over the knuckles on both hands. She has some soft swellings
at the base of the jaw and these are non-mobile and diffuse in
character.

Causes of haematuria

a. Prostatic hyperplasia.
b. Renal cell carcinoma.
c. Schistosomiasis.
d. Bladder carcinoma.
e. Tuberculosis.
f. Urinary tract infection (UTI).
g. Glomerulonephritis.
h. Renal contusion.
i. Renal vein thrombosis.

The following patients have all presented with haematuria. Please choose the most likely diagnosis from the list above. Each option can be used once, more than once or not at all.

81 A 63-year-old Afro-Caribbean man presents to his general practitioner with problems passing urine over the past 2 months. He has been noticing that he has to get up to go to the toilet frequently and when he has been he feels that he needs to go again 'less than 5 minutes afterwards'. He is distressed because he has recently discovered blood in his urine and is worried he has cancer.

82 An 82-year-old woman is brought to hospital by her carer who discovered she had been passing frank blood in the urine that was not associated with any pain. The carer was unsure how long this had been going on for. The patient is not taking any anticoagulation and had otherwise been fit and well. An occupational history revealed she worked for many years in the dye industry.

83 A 43-year-old man presents to hospital with abdominal pain, haematuria and symptoms of dysuria. He states that these symptoms have been getting progressively worse over a month's period after a watersports holiday in Egypt. He also describes an itchy papular rash over his lower legs.

84 A 78-year-old woman is brought to hospital by her worried neighbours as she has been acting 'not herself' and has been found wandering around in the evening in just her nightgown and slippers. On examination she has an abbreviated mental test score of 3 out of 10, is found to be pyrexic and has tenderness over her suprapubic region. A urine sample taken is reddish-orange in colour.

85 A 34-year-old man presents to hospital after suffering a fall whilst under the influence of alcohol. He is inebriated on arrival and unable to give a full history apart from that of falling from the standing position onto his right flank. He is in pain and clutching his back and when he rolls to his left side you notice some bruising over his lower right posterior ribs. He is incontinent and the nursing staff notice his urine is very dark red.

Peripheral nerve lesions

   a. Common peroneal nerve.
   b. Median nerve.
   c. Tibial nerve.
   d. Radial nerve.
   e. Obturator nerve.
   f. Lateral cutaneous nerve of the thigh.
   g. Ulnar nerve.
   h. Axillary nerve.

Which nerve is likely to account for the symptoms in each of these cases?

86 A 27-year-old man has been admitted to hospital following a footballing injury. He remembers that during the match, another one of the players went for the ball but hit his leg on the postero-lateral aspect. His leg was immediately painful but he also noticed that he was experiencing difficulty in lifting his foot up towards him and also everting his foot.

87 A 43-year-old man has suffered an anterior dislocation of his humerus following trauma. He describes weakness in shoulder elevation and abduction, with numbness, and altered sensation over the lateral aspect of the arm.

88 A 49-year-old secretary visits her GP as she is becoming increasingly worried about numbness and tingling in both of her hands. She mentions that it affects the lateral three and a half fingers and it often wakes her at night.

89 A 76-year-old lady suffered a fall, which resulted in a fracture of her proximal ulna bone. Following the initial injury she noted pain over her elbow and weakness in her same hand. She complained of numbness and tingling in her ring and little fingers.

90 A 55-year-old man has noticed a burning or stinging sensation antero-lateral aspect of his thigh. This is aggravated by walking or standing; it is relieved by lying down with the hip flexed. He has a full range of movement in the leg although it is painful, he is able to weight bear and walk.

PART II

Answers to Practice Papers

Answers and notes

Multiple choice questions (single best answer)

1 d. An echocardiogram is the most important next step in the management of this gentleman. This will aid in the decision about anticoagulation. If an echocardiogram shows a structurally abnormal heart then the risk of thrombus formation is small and warfarinisation would be unnecessary. Whilst AF can commonly be managed in the community, it is appropriate to refer for ECHO. Rate control is unnecessary in this scenario as its upper limit is 90 beats per minute.

2 d. This gentleman can be safely discharged without follow-up. The troponin results represent a 12-hour test by which time if there was cardiac damage the levels would have peaked. This combined with the fact that there are no ischaemic changes on the ECG make the risk of a cardiac event minimal. Having ruled out a cardiac cause for his chest pain a gastrointestinal cause is most likely given the associated nausea. There is no indication to start this gentleman on aspirin.

3 e. Measuring digoxin levels in this lady will detect any potential toxicity which would account for her symptoms. This case actually showed digoxin toxicity and a binding agent was administered. There is no indication to insert a pacing wire in this lady as her heart rate is being maintained at 40 beats per minute although there is complete heart block. Having stopped this lady's digoxin, her heart rate increased to approximately 120 beats per minute and ultimately she had a permanent pacemaker inserted. Amiodarone is indicated in refractory tachycardias.

4 a. Ventricular septal rupture is a rare but serious complication of myocardial infarction. The event occurs 2–8 days after an infarction and often precipitates cardiogenic shock. Dressler's syndrome is a pericarditis that develops between 2 and 10 weeks post myocardial infarction or cardiac surgery. One theory is that it is an inflammatory response secondary to an autoimmune reaction to myocardial neoantigens.

5 a. This lady had no history of alcoholism and no signs of outflow tract obstruction. The most likely cause of her dilated cardiomyopathy is viral. The commonest viruses implicated in this condition are coxsackie A and B, influenza A and B adenovirus and echovirus among others.

6 d. Whilst measuring the blood pressure in all limbs raises the suspicion of aortic dissection, the most diagnostic investigation is a CT chest. Other diagnostic investigations include MRI and a trans-oesophageal echocardiogram. There are no diagnostic ECG changes associated with dissecting aortic aneurysms and liver function tests are of no use in confirming the diagnosis.

7 c. This clinical picture is typical of diabetic ketoacidosis (DKA) occurring secondarily to a preceding infection. In times of stress, such as post-operatively, in the case of infection or inflammation or after an event such as a myocardial infarction, blood glucose levels may rise due to an increase in the stress response and release of gluconeogenic hormones. Insulin requirements may increase remarkably during these periods and close blood glucose control is important to establish. Education of patients with type I diabetes mellitus is key to preventing DKA and these patients should be taught to increase the frequency of their blood glucose monitoring and increase insulin appropriately in line with any increase in blood glucose. Failure to do this will result in glucose levels rising but the lack of insulin leads to increased production of glucagon, resulting in increased amounts of gluconeogenesis, glycogenolysis and lipolysis. A combination of the osmotic diuresis leading to dehydration and tissue hypoxia (leading to lactic acid production through anaerobic metabolism) and lipolysis leading to increased production of ketone bodies (which are inherently acidic) results in a florid metabolic acidosis, which may be severe enough to be life-threatening. Treatment involves replacing any fluid losses with 0.9% normal saline (up to 6 L may be required in a 24-hour period) and commencement on a constant infusion of insulin at, for example, 6 units/hour in order to suppress ongoing ketogenesis (which will occur for some hours after blood glucose has been controlled). Monitoring of the blood glucose and urinalysis for ketones is imperative to guide management and when the blood glucose drops to below 15 mmol/L then the infusion can be halved to 3 units/hour and 5% dextrose solution written up instead of saline as fluid replacement. Once the blood glucose is under adequate control, the urine is free from ketones and the patient is eating and drinking normally then consideration of normal insulin regimen is appropriate. If the patient is not yet fully established on eating and drinking then conversion to an insulin sliding scale (similar to but NOT the same as the insulin infusion as infusion rates are allowed to vary between 0.5 and 6 units) may be a step-down until oral intake is established. Potassium replacement should also be considered as although levels may appear normal acutely, when insulin infusion is started and resolution of acid–base deficits occur then potassium levels will inevitably fall and must be replaced accordingly.

8 a. Hypothyroidism may manifest with a plethora of features including constipation, bradycardia, hypothermia and confusion among other physical signs of thyroid dysfunction. Thyroid function tests should always be taken whilst investigating the cause of confusion in an elderly patient not otherwise known to be confused as extremes of both hyper- and hypofunction may lead to confusion. General reduction in mobility may be the root cause of falling in patients with hypothyroidism and should prompt investigation of thyroid dysfunction before more specialised falls investigation is performed. Electrocardiography may well reveal a sinus bradycardia, which along with an element of postural hypotension may well contribute to falling, however, the cause of bradycardia should be investigated. Echocardiography may be useful in detecting any clinically significant valvular disease, of which the most relevant to falls is aortic stenosis. The triad of symptoms typically associated with aortic stenosis (syncope, angina and dyspnoea) are often subtle in the elderly and often the only sign of severity is a fall leading to admission. CT scan of the head is part of the screen for confusion and reversible causes of dementia but may also reveal a subdural haematoma that may be contributing to or resulting from head injury sustained during a fall. In the presence of such florid clinical indices of thyroid dysfunction this should be considered only after blood tests have returned normal and the cause of confusion is still undiagnosed. Addison's disease (primary adrenocortical failure) may present in many different ways, however, the classical presentation is of hypotension, hyperkalaemia, hyponatraemia with nausea and vomiting. The short synacthen test is a specific test for Addison's disease and measurement of the cortisol level at baseline before and 30 minutes after injection of **syn**thetic **ACTH** (hence the name!). A rise of greater than 500 nmol/L at 30 minutes post-injection excludes Addison's disease. Treatment is of the underlying cause and replacement of steroids with prednisolone or hydrocortisone if oral intake is compromised.

9 e. Acute glaucoma, one of the most important ophthalmological emergencies, presents with a fixed dilated and often oval-shaped pupil.

Features of ophthalmological disease are as follows:

- *Acute glaucoma*: Entire eye is red, both conjunctival and ciliary vessels are injected. Pupil is fixed, dilated and oval in shape, the intraocular pressure is high.
- *Iritis*: Redness is most marked around the cornea and does not blanch on pressure. The pupil is small and fixed.
- *Conjunctivitis*: Conjunctival vessels injected, blanch on pressure. Pupil is normal and reactive.
- *Subconjunctival haemorrhage*: Bright red sclera with rim around limbus, pupil is normal.

10 b. Hypertension is a common cause of retinopathy and the history alone may aid in making a diagnosis that is further confirmed on fundoscopy. Classification schemes for hypertensive retinopathy wax and wane in popularity and may exist in the normal population as well as overlap with other syndromes such as diabetic retinopathy. The Scheie classification provides a simplified format from which to work from:

- *Grade 0*: Hypertensive but no visible retinal abnormalities
- *Grade I*: Arteriolar narrowing
- *Grade II*: Arteriolar narrowing with focal constriction
- *Grade III*: Diffuse narrowing with retinal haemorrhage
- *Grade IV*: Papilloedema and hard exudates

The changes seen in diabetic retinopathy (DR) are often classified by the degree of retinopathy seen. However, this system is more useful clinically as local treatment, e.g. laser photocoagulation may be influenced by the degree of retinopathy. The following classification represents a simplified format as schemes are in constant flux:

- *Background DR*: Microaneurysms (dot) and microhaemorrhages (blot) and hard exudates.
- *Pre-proliferative DR*: Cotton-wool spots and extensive blot haemorrhages.
- *Proliferative DR*: Neovascularisation.
- *Macular disease:* Hard exudates encroaching on fovea or macular oedema.

Age-related macular degeneration (ARMD) can occur as 'dry' or 'wet' degeneration with the defining feature being the presence of choroidal neovascularisation (leading to 'wet' ARMD). Although dry ARMD is by far the more commonly encountered type, wet ARMD is the more rapidly progressive and requires attention due to the accompanying visual deterioration that is seen. CMV retinitis usually occurs in the immunosuppressed and is sometimes seen in AIDS patients. It manifests as cotton-wool spots with flame haemorrhages often given the name 'pizza–pie' fundus because of its appearance. Ankylosing spondylitis usually presents with uveitis (inflammation of the components of the uveal tract; namely the iris, ciliary body and choroids) and is thought to occur in autoimmune disorders due to immune complex deposition in the uveal tract.

11 a. Approximately 45% of breast cancers occur in the upper outer quadrant of the breast. A quarter of cancers occur in the retro-areolar region with the lower inner quadrant being the least common site of tumours.

12 e. The majority of breast cancers are hormone sensitive. They are classified as oestrogen receptor positive or ER+. For cancers that are hormone sensitive treatment may be commenced with medications such as tamoxifen, which is an oestrogen receptor antagonist. With this in mind, risk factors for breast cancer can be thought of as those that increase the duration for which the body is producing hormones, e.g. those with an early menarche and late menopause. There is some controversy surrounding dairy produce in diet and whether there is any association with the development of breast cancer. There is at present no firm evidence to suggest that there is an association. Other risk factors for breast cancer include past history, use of oral contraceptives, never having breastfed and a family history.

13 b. Although all the investigations should be considered depending upon the chronicity of the swelling, the most important is to perform a joint aspiration. It is indefensible to miss a septic arthritis by not performing a diagnostic and simple tap in light of the above clinical signs. Septic arthritis will completely destroy a joint in a short space of time and the patient will head down the path of total joint replacement and potential litigation. Fluid should be sent for microscopy to look for organisms, cells and crystals (*Note*: gout and pseudogout), culture and sensitivities. Blood cultures are merited preferably prior to antibiotic therapy in light of the features of systemic infection, however, these should not be done in preference to aspiration. Imaging of the knee joint is useful in due course to see the extent of damage if resolution is not achieved with antibiotic therapy.

14 d. Rheumatological disease exhibits a predilection for the female sex. Ankylosing spondylitis is one of the few conditions that goes against this trend being approximately 6 times more common in males than females in early teenage years and twice as common in males by 30 years of age. Typically the patient is a young male presenting with morning stiffness, reduced back movement with backpain and pain over the sacroiliac joints. Rheumatoid arthritis is unlikely for reasons of sex and age. Prolapsed intervertebral discs may present with symptoms of back and hip pain but would be again unlikely (but not infeasible) in a healthy 23-year-old man. Facet joint arthritis presents in middle-to-old age with pain especially on bending backwards as the facets rub against each other.

15 b. Rectal examination is avoided in neutropenic patients as trauma to the ano-rectum is easily manifested and may provide an easy access route to the bloodstream for gastrointestinal flora. Where possible these patients should be nursed in isolation in a side-room with full barrier nursing precautions. These patients should be subjected to the minimal number of examinations and procedures and clinical staff should also be restricted to essential members only.

16 d. There is no association between iron deficiency anaemia and peripheral neuropathy. This finding is associated with a vitamin B12 deficiency. There are approximately 500 million cases of iron deficiency anaemia worldwide – it most commonly affects pre-menopausal women. The small bowel is responsible for absorption of iron, which is stored in the body in the form of ferritin. Signs of iron deficiency include koilonychias (spoon-shaped nails – both fingers and toes), angular stomatitis and glossitis. Other signs are associated with anaemias in general including fatigue and pallor.

17 d. Sickle cell disease is most commonly seen in patients of African, Arabian or Southern European descent. Carriers have one normal and one sickle gene and usually remain asymptomatic. Those individuals homozygous for the sickle chain suffer with sickle cell disease. The red blood cells are of abnormal, sickle shape and therefore 'clog' smaller blood vessels resulting in ischaemia of distal tissues and associated pain. Clinical features include pallor as a result of the anaemia. Splenomegaly is seen in early disease but, as it progresses the spleen shrinks as due to the lack of blood supply. Bone crises are often predisposed by infection, cold or hypoxia, therefore the initial management of a sickle crisis is to apply oxygen and provide some symptomatic relief. Pigment gallstones are seen in the condition due to the haemolysis of the red blood cells. Leg ulcers are not a feature of this condition.

18 a. Endogenous depression, i.e. depression that occurs without an easily identifiable precipitant, was classically thought to be more resistant to treatment than exogenous (reactive) depression. This artificial classification, however, has lost favour among psychiatrists as the aetiology of depression becomes more multifactorial. Depression can be sub-classified according to severity and the components required to fulfil the diagnostic criteria for a major depressive episode are described below:

At least five of the following, during the same 2-week period, representing a change from previous functioning; these must include either (1) or (2):

1. Depressed mood.
2. Diminished interest or pleasure (anhedonia).
3. Significant change in weight.
4. Insomnia or excessive sleepiness.
5. Psychomotor agitation or retardation.
6. Suicidal ideation or planned suicide.
7. Fatigue or loss of energy.
8. Feelings of worthlessness.
9. Reduced ability to concentrate.

The above symptoms must also not be associated with signs of mania or excessive elevation of mood (leading more towards a diagnosis of bipolar affective disorder), they must cause clinically significant distress of impairment of functioning and organic causes for symptomatology must be ruled out. Symptoms must also not be associated with a grief response or bereavement. Females have been shown to be more prone to medication overdose and deliberate self-harm behaviour with males favouring more violent modes of suicide.

A lack of a confiding relationship has previously been described as a vulnerability factor for depression along with early maternal loss, greater than three children under 14 years at home and unemployment. These features are part of the Brown and Harris model of depression and have been postulated to be associated strongly with the development of depression.

Organic causes of depression or any change in mood or mental status must be ruled out prior to a diagnosis of psychiatric disease. This may include CT scan of the head and should include as routine blood glucose evaluation, thyroid hormones, vitamin B12 and folate levels, infection screen (including

167

syphilis and, if indicated, HIV) and electrolyte and full blood count. Thyroid disease is the second most common endocrine disorder (after diabetes) and can present insidiously in the elderly population with features of depression or mood alteration.

19 **c.** Section 5(2) refers to a provision by the Mental Health Act for detention of an individual in the hospital against their own wishes for assessment of a mental health condition and is valid for 72 hours. It requires only one responsible medical officer and should only be used as a temporising measure until formal psychiatric evaluation can be carried out.

It would not be an appropriate course of action to allow this man to be discharged, either against medical advice (option D) or with follow-up with a community psychiatrist (option E), as he is likely to be a danger to himself or others and has already exhibited behaviour that would merit at least a brief period of assessment if not psychiatric treatment as an inpatient.

A Section 3 order refers to a detention order for a period of up to 6 months per Section 3 (i.e. it can be renewed) for treatment of a psychiatric condition. It is typically seen converted from a Section 2 where the assessment has been made and the decision to start treatment deemed appropriate. It requires two medical recommendations to be held valid.

Cuff and restraint under common law is not an appropriate modality to use in this case where a psychiatric diagnosis is suspected and would have to be justified on a case-by-case basis under the direct decision by a consultant physician.

20 **c.** In older males, a dilated abdominal aorta is relatively common finding. Other risk factors include with a family history of the complaint. In approximately 10% of cases an associated popliteal artery aneurysm will be found. Smaller aneurysms (below 4 cm) are considered to be benign and grow at a rate of 1–2 mm per year. The most feared complication of AAA's is rupture. Approximately 5% of aneurysms over 6 cm rupture spontaneously. Resection is usually advised in those aneurysms 5–6 cm in diameter. Complications of this surgery include renal failure since the renal artery ostia is often compressed during the procedure when the aorta is cross-clamped. Other complications include MI as coronary artery disease is usually present in those people with aortic compromise. As a result of cross clamping of the aorta the back pressure on the heart increases, which increases the workload of the heart. This, coupled with the metabolic stress that occurs when the legs are reperfused, may precipitate an MI.

21 d. Polycythaemia is commonly found in COPD patients and other respiratory diseases where gas transfer is reduced. Chronic hypoxia stimulates the production of erythropoietin from the kidneys, which acts on the bone marrow to augment the oxygen carrying capacity of the blood. Usually this is the most important derangement that is found in the full blood count in the absence of an exacerbation.

22 a. This gentleman has a ventricular septar defect. This is an unusual but serious complication of MI, confirmed by echocardiography, and requires surgery to close the defect. On auscultation a pansystolic murmur is heard, which should raise suspicion, and the shortness of breath without radiological changes is caused by increased release of atrio-natriuretic peptide caused by increased pressure in the right atrium. Aortic regurgitation would give a diastolic murmur and heart failure would produce characteristic changes on the chest X-ray. Dressler's syndrome is a late complication, occurring weeks to months after the initial insult and presents with recurrent pericarditis and pleural effusions associated with fever which doesn't fit this clinical presentation.

23 b. This boy has a classical history of a testicular torsion. This is usually torsion of the spermatic cord in a structurally abnormal testis. It is possible for it to occur in a structurally normal testis although, it is less common. This constitutes a surgical/ urological emergency. Often there is a history of mild trauma or previous attacks of pain due to the torsion and spontaneous untwisting. The supply of the testis is from T10 sympathetic pathway which is why abdominal pain occurs. These patients require emergency surgery to correct and stabilise the torsion. On occasions when the torsion has compromised the testicular blood supply for a long duration of time ischaemia may result which then requires an orchidectomy and treatment.

24 c. Testicular tumours are commonly found incidentally after minor trauma to the scrotum, the mass often mistakenly attributed to the trauma itself. Torsion of the testicular apparatus such as the hydatid of Morgagni is often heralded by pain and more rarely a blue spot on examination of the scrotum. In this particular case the diagnosis is made more suspicious by the scar in the groin, possibly attributed to previous surgery for undescended and maldescended testes, which are associated with testicular tumours. As a final point, seminoma is more commonly found in patients over 30 years of age than teratomas.

25 a. Dermatitis (eczema) is a common problem that often affects individuals whose line of work involves immersion in irritant substances such as bleach, shampoo, chemicals, washing up liquids and similar agents. Therefore one can predict with some accuracy a period of resolution from their dermatological problem when they are away from the workplace and hence irritant, such as during holiday periods. This type of dermatitis is sometimes referred to as extrinsic eczema to differentiate from intrinsic or atopic eczema. Lichen planus is typically associated with characteristic fine white lines that lie over the papules (Wickham's striae) and may affect the wrist. A chemical burn is a possibility, however, this does not usually present with an itchy rash. Porphyria cutanea tarda is a rare form of porphyria manifest as cutaneous photosensitivity. Psoriasis typically favours the extensor surfaces and usually presents as a non-itchy silver scale on an erythematous base.

26 c. Dermatitis herpetiformis forms crops of itchy blisters that are commonly found on elbows, knees and scalp. The itch can drive people to suicide and can be usually very effectively and with much gratitude relieved by oral dapsone. Dermatitis herpetiformis is associated with coeliac disease and as the risk of lymphoma is greatly increased by having both conditions, regular surveillance is recommended. Psoriasis does commonly affect the elbows but usually does not present with itch and eczema may present in such sites and with pruritus but is not strongly associated with coeliac disease. Scabies should always be kept in mind when considering itch, usually in children in the web spaces of the hands and feet. Track marks from the burrowing *Sarcoptes scabiei* mite can often be seen and harvested for microscopic diagnosis.

27 d. This girl is a legal minor in the eyes of the law and under common law is in the responsibility of her parents. However, a landmark legal case in 1985 (Gillick v West Norfolk and Wisbech Area Health Authority) brought to court by the parents of a teenage girl who was prescribed contraception without the know-ledge of her parents clarified the legal standpoint on medical treatment for those under the age of 16 years. This standpoint is often referred to as Gillick competence (or the Fraser guidelines after the representative of the House of Lords who conceived the guidelines) in reference to this test case and reasons that young people in England and Wales (and Northern Island) under the age of 16 can consent to medical treatment if they have sufficient maturity and judgement to enable them fully to understand what is proposed. A similar law called the The Age of Legal Capacity (Scotland) Act 1991 exists in Scotland.

The Fraser guidelines are, however, open to interpretation by the agent assessing whether a minor is Gillick competent. Thus it is the duty of the doctor or health care provider responsible for m172edical care and treatment of that minor to assess whether the ability to understand, retain and act upon information in an informed manner is present in those under the age of 16 years. If deemed the case then the minor assumes the same rights as any competent adult seeking medical treatment.

In this case referral to a family planning clinic is appropriate as it is both the girl's wish and will serve to provide support, education and contraceptive advice if sexual activity continues. Counselling about sexual intercourse and contraceptive options is of vital importance in increasing the awareness of the merits and disadvantages of teenage pregnancy and the risk of sexually transmitted infection and blood-borne virus exposure.

Offering a sexually transmitted infection screen should occur in conjunction with counselling as she has been engaging in unprotected intercourse and most importantly she should also be encouraged to discuss the pregnancy and her feelings regarding sex with her parents. However, it must be stressed that any information shared with a health care professional can only be passed on to her parents with her express consent (if deemed Gillick competent).

28 **a.** In a young fit person the two most sensible treatment options include a surgical repair or a below knee cast with the foot in equinus position. After surgery, the re-rupture rate is 2–5% whilst it is 8–10% for those treated conservatively. The commonest site for rupture is 4–8 cm above the point of insertion. Characteristic signs of tendo Achilles rupture include difficulty in walking and standing on tip toes. There may also be a visible gap in the tendon and a positive Simmons test (no plantar flexion on squeezing the affected calf). If there is any doubt clinically, an ultrasound scan may be used to confirm the diagnosis. Conservative treatment is most appropriate for elderly people whilst younger and more active patients are usually managed with surgical repair. Infection is the biggest surgical complication involved with this procedure and since the Achilles tendon is quite superficial any wound infection may result in disrupting the integrity of the tendon repair.

29 **a.** The common peroneal nerve consists of branches of L4–S1. Its motor supply is to the anterior compartment of the calf

including tibialis anterior and extensor hallucis longus. The sensory component supplies the 1st web space and the dorsum of the foot and front side of the leg. This nerve winds around the head of the tibia and in certain tibial plateau fractures its integrity may become compromised.

30 a. Sensitivity is defined as the number of disease and test positive (true positive) divided by the number of all the people with the disease. Represented as a formula this can be expressed as **a/(a + c)**. The table below can be used as reference for the following answers:

Test	Disease	
	Positive	Negative
Positive	a	b
Negative	c	d

A test that has a high sensitivity is one that is appropriate to use as a screening test for a population as it will pull up few false negatives (high se**N**sitivity = few false **N**egatives) as most of the people who are disease positive will be 'caught' by the test as positive.

A test that has a high specificity, by comparison, should be used once enough individuals have been screened and will 'catch' those individuals who are disease and test negative (i.e. true negatives). This is good for weeding those people out who tested falsely positive in the screening test but are reassured to find out they are truly negative. It can be expressed as **d/(b + d)**.

Positive predictive value refers to the number of true positives who tested positive for the disease and can be expressed as **a/(a + b)**. As the accuracy of any test will increase with population size it follows that the positive predictive value of a test will increase the higher the prevalence of disease.

Negative predictive value refers to the number of true negatives who tested negative for the disease and can be expressed as **d/(c + d)**.

There were actually 140 false negatives in this case (box **c**) as these are defined as the number of people who are disease positive who test negative.

Finally this test should not be used as a screening test as the sensitivity is only 80.1% (**a/(a + c)**) which is not high enough to justify use as you would 'miss' approximately 20% of those with the disease as the test would not pick these people up.

31 b. The condition placenta praevia occurs when the placenta abnormally implants in the lower segment of the uterus. Bleeding is usually painless unlike the other common cause of antepartum haemorrhage, abruptio placentae (placental abruption). Physical signs are usually few. Breech or oblique presentation is occasionally seen due to the mechanical obstruction to birth canal outflow. Routine ultrasound scans may over-estimate the prevalence of this condition as the lower segment grows cephalically late in the last trimester and it is estimated that up to 10% of placentae are low-lying before 37 weeks. Cervical cancer would otherwise be a diagnosis not to be dismissed, however, as cervical smears are usually recommended as part of antenatal care, this makes this option unlikely. Placenta accreta is usually encountered at Caesarean section, often with catastrophic effect, and does not usually present with antepartum haemorrhage.

32 c. This lady has suffered a deep vein thrombosis. Risk factors for deep vein thrombosis include:
- Past history
- Pregnancy
- Malignancy
- Antiphospholipid syndrome
- Oral contraceptive pill use
- Nephrotic syndrome
- Recent surgery
- Pelvic mass
- Recent childbirth
- Obesity

Whilst she has no past history she is pregnant and therefore has a pelvic mass! In pregnancy, patients may be reluctant to take anticoagulants. The diagnosis should be confirmed as soon as possible and if for any reason there is a delay, treatment dose of a low molecular weight heparin should be administered.

33 c. Cystic fibrosis is characterised by a defect in a chloride channel transporter and is usually due to single amino acid substitution at position 508. Children usually suffer from multiple recurrent chest infections (usually due to *Pseudomonas*) failure to thrive and malabsorption. Cystic fibrosis should be at the forefront of a differential diagnosis of any chest problems and failure to thrive in any infant. PAS positive macrophages refers to a finding in Whipple's disease caused by the Gram positive rod *Tropheryma whippelii*. Whipple's disease usually causes malabsorption in men over 50 years old. Cobblestone appearance is a typical finding on barium enema in Crohn's disease – a disease affecting any part of the gastrointestinal system, unlike ulcerative colitis. A double bubble on abdominal X-ray is occasionally seen associated with Down's syndrome due to duodenal atresia. Abnormal bone marrow cytology refers to the possibility of a haematological malignancy such as acute myelogenous leukaemia and unlikely to present in this manner.

34 b. The growth of male breast tissue, known as gynaecomastia, is a normal finding in the neonate due to maternal oestrogens and in the pubertal boy and elderly male due to the changing ratio of testosterone to oestrogens in these age groups. This is not a typical finding that would be consistent with non-accidental injury and therefore a referral to social services would be inappropriate. Referral to a breast surgeon and needle aspiration are also unjustified in this case and may even be deleterious to growing breast tissue. Short course prednisolone is also unwarranted and is not indicated in cases of gynaecomastia.

35 d. The transverse colon is spared many of the complications that are commonly seen in the sigmoid colon; the site of most pathology in the gastrointestinal tract. A host of conditions including diverticulitis, volvulus, colorectal carcinoma and angiodysplasia to mention but a few afflict this area. Ruptured aortic aneurysms are most often seen in older men, however, the clinical picture of upper abdominal pain, raised inflammatory markers and a high amylase in a clinically unstable patient should prompt investigation to rule out this fatal condition. Pancreatitis is one of the most likely causes of the above clinical picture and an amylase less than the often quoted limit of 4 times normal (360 IU/L) does not exclude this common condition.

36 c. Rigler's sign is a radiographic finding of bowel perforation. It manifests as a dual-enhanced image of the bowel due to the presence of air in the peritoneum and in the lumen of the bowel. Murphy's sign is positive when pain is elicited over the right upper quadrant when two fingers are placed here and the patient asked to breathe in. An inflamed gallbladder will cause the patient to catch his or her breath. Rovsing's sign relates to pain felt in the right iliac fossa when pressure is applied to the left iliac fossa and is associated with appendicitis. Kerr's sign is pain felt in the shoulder tips associated most classically with ruptured ectopic pregnancy. This pain is referred pain from blood irritating the diaphragm and emphasises the common embryological relationship between the motor innervation of the diaphragm (C3, C4 and C5) and the sensory dermatome supplying the shoulder tips (C4). Trousseau's sign in the context of abdominal disease relates to crops of tender nodules affecting blood vessels (*thrombophlebitis migrans*) often associated with pancreatic malignancy.

37 d. Bile leak is a recognised complication of hepatobiliary surgery and presents within days post-operatively. Bile is a potent irritant to the peritoneum causing a chemical biliary peritonitis associated with rising biliary enzymes and bilirubin. Conservative management will often suffice for minor leaks, however, surgical intervention is the definitive treatment in severe cases. Accidental ligation of the common bile duct is a rare but catastrophic complication of cholecystectomy, however, this is not routinely seen in cyst fenestration. Cholecystitis presents with a similar clinical picture but does not usually present with such marked derangement of liver enzymes without the co-existent bile duct involvement seen in biliary colic. Propofol is commonly used as an anaesthetic induction agent and although associated with hepatotoxicity in large doses would not normally cause significant hepatic injury. Biliary sepsis is always a high risk with hepatobiliary surgery but presents characteristically with relatively normal liver enzymes and signs of clinical sepsis.

38 a. Pulmonary embolus is an often overlooked risk of laparoscopic procedures. During surgery the peritoneum is insufflated with carbon dioxide to a pressure of around 15 mmHg. Occlusion of the venous system draining through the abdomen including the great vessels has been reported to increase the incidence of post-operative venous thromboembolism. Thromboembolic deterrent stockings (TEDS) are recommended for 4 weeks with daily injection of subcutaneous low-molecular weight heparin for any patient who has recently undergone laparoscopic procedures. Pulmonary embolus is associated with pleuritic chest pain, tachycardia, the often quoted, rarely seen deep S wave in lead I, deep Q wave in lead III and inverted T wave in lead III (S1,Q3,T3), with haemoptysis or silently. Beware the elderly on beta-blocking medication who do not mount a tachycardia; a useful warning sign of pulmonary embolus!

39 b. Fibrin degradation products (D-dimer) is a test useful only in the process of ruling out a pulmonary embolus. A negative result predicts a high likelihood of absence of pulmonary embolus; a positive result is almost meaningless diagnostically. D-dimers are expected to rise post-operatively and thus should not form the first line of investigation for a suspected pulmonary embolus. Arterial blood gases and electrocardiography are invaluable for the investigation of dyspnoea for both quantifying the respiratory compromise and in stratifying the differential to either cardiac or respiratory causes. Chest radiographs may demonstrate pneumonic processes or pneumothoraces and form part of the standard investigation of breathlessness. CT-PA forms the most definitive imaging in cases of suspected pulmonary embolus but may return equivocal results in the presence of pre-existing lung pathology.

40 c. Inguinal hernias present the greatest diagnostic challenge when defining the subtype of hernia; indirect hernias were often said to be controlled by pressure over the internal (deep) inguinal ring at a point 1–2 cm above the femoral pulse once reduced. However, this clinical distinction is frequently inaccurate in even the most experienced hands. A more useful definition is that direct hernias pass medially to the inferior epigastric artery with indirect hernias passing laterally. This can be neatly summed up as 'MDs don't Lie' (**M**edial **D**irect, **L**ateral **I**ndirect). Confusion between inguinal and femoral hernias can be avoided by remembering that inguinal hernias present above and medial to the pubic tubercle with femoral hernias presenting below and lateral. Spighelian hernias are located at the lateral border of the posterior rectus sheath, passing through the arcuate line to present as a mass in the lower abdominal wall. Ventral hernias are often seen in the elderly and are associated with a widening of the recti muscles (divarication of the recti).

41 b. Acute exacerbations of asthma can be defined as severe or life-threatening. Criteria for diagnosis are as follows:
Severe attack
- unable to complete sentences
- respiratory rate of greater than 25/minute
- heart rate greater than 110 beats per minute
- PEFR of less than 50% of predicted
Life-threatening
- cyanosis, very poor respiratory effort
- silent chest
- bradycardia and hypotension
- PEFR <33% predicted

Arterial blood sampling will show normal or high PCO_2 and PO_2 less than 8 kPa.

In any case of asthma exacerbation a chest X-ray should be ordered to exclude a pneumothorax and to look for a concurrent pneumonia. The principles for management of exacerbations can be remembered by the mnemonic 'O SHIT';

O: Oxygen

S: Salbutamol

H: Hydrocortisone (or prednisolone)

I: Inhaled steroids

T: Theophylline (be aware of risks of toxicity – if not already on regular theophyllines will need a loading dose)

Magnesium is now used in acute asthma and the use of theophyllines is reducing. Check with your trust about local policy.

42 **e.** Whilst this lady has a strong history of asthma it is important to exclude other causes of shortness of breath. Anaphylaxis refers to a severe allergic reaction including both dermal and systemic signs and symptoms. The full-blown syndrome includes urticaria with occasional angioedema with hypotension and bronchospasm. Anaphylaxis is mediated by IgE and symptoms and signs are caused by rapid onset of increased secretion from mucous membranes, increased bronchial smooth muscle tone, reduced vascular smooth muscle tone and increased capillary permeability occur after exposure to an offending substance. Pneumothorax is a collection of gas in the pleural space resulting in collapse of the lung on the affected side. A tension pneumothorax can be a life-threatening condition caused by air within the pleural space that is under pressure. This causes displacement of mediastinal structures which in turn compromises cardiopulmonary function.

Tracheal obstruction or a massive pulmonary embolus will understandably cause acute onset shortness of breath. Stridor may be a clue in airway obstruction and a history of risk factors should be sought in a suspected pulmonary embolus. An upper respiratory tract infection should not present acutely.

43 **e.** Pulmonary embolus and deep vein thrombosis risk should be assessed in all patients who present with pleuritic pain and shortness of breath. Patients post-surgery, especially hip surgery, obese patients, malignant disease, immobility and the oral contraceptive pill all increase the likelihood of a venous thromboembolism. Carotid massage would be completely contraindicated in this woman as she is hypotensive. It is useful as a first-line manoeuvre in cases of supraventricular tachycardia

once the absence of a carotid bruit has been established. Frusemide is useful in cases of heart failure in the presence of relatively normal renal function. CT with pulmonary angiography is the gold standard for diagnosing but not treating pulmonary embolus but is not even an option in this case due to this woman's unstable condition.

44 **b.** Intramuscular adrenaline injection of 1 mL of 1:1000 adrenaline is the recommended treatment for suspected anaphylaxis. Note that this dose differs from the 1:10000 intravenous (i.v.) injection dose of adrenaline used in cardiac arrest. The clues to a severe allergic reaction are manifold from the history; severe shortness of breath occurs secondary to oedema of the upper airway and larynx and his medications reveal an atopic predisposition. Laryngeal mask airway and endotracheal intubation would be possibilities if adrenaline did not work as a first line or if airway control was an issue. Nebulised salbutamol and i.v. hydrocortisone would provide some relief for airway oedema but are not as effective as adrenaline in the acute management of anaphylaxis.

45 **b.** This question is slightly controversial as there are two possible answers that might be considered depending on the clinical situation. This patient has two main problems; as he is drowsy he is not likely to protect his airway and thus is at risk of aspiration, and on clinical examination he has evidence of a right-sided tension pneumothorax. Most clinicians would consider attempting a procedure such as needle thoracocentesis to drain a tension pneumothorax before securing an airway. A nasopharyngeal airway is contraindicated due to the complex facial fractures as the risk of basal skull fracture is high. An emergency tracheostomy is a last resort attempt to secure an airway and can be avoided by early intubation if airway management is likely to become difficult. Chest drain insertion is not the recommended procedure for releasing a tension pneumothorax.

46 **b.** Advanced Parkinson's disease can result in many features including a mask-like facial appearance and a difficulty in swallowing. This patient suffered an aspiration pneumonia. The commonest site for an aspiration pneumonia, or indeed inhalation of a foreign body, is the right lower lobe of the lung. This is due to the anatomy of the right main bronchus being more vertical than the left due to the positioning of the heart. Parkinson's disease is not known to be closely associated with heart failure.

Atypical pneumonias are usually widespread and provide more generalised signs than those described above.

47 c. INR (International Normalised Ratio) is derived from the prothrombin time, which is then normalised against a laboratory standard to give values that are interpretable and standardised wherever the tests are taken. The INR is a very specific and sensitive indicator of liver damage and is the investigation of choice when assessing liver function (although many laboratories persist with using the incorrect liver function test terminology when assaying levels of liver transaminases). Albumin is also a product of liver synthesis and can be expected to fall with chronic liver diseases. Glycaemic control is also regulated in a large part by the liver and hypoglycaemia due to impaired gluconeogenesis and glycogen storage is often a complication of patients with advanced liver impairment. AST and ALT are useful markers of acute liver insult such as hepatitis, however, they are not well correlated with the degree of liver failure. Alkaline phosphatase and bilirubin are often associated with obstruction of the biliary system and will often rise in obstructive jaundice preferentially to the transaminases. Fibrinogen is a useful indicator of consumption and turnover of clotting products and can be low in disseminated intravascular coagulation (DIC) and venous thromboembolism (VTE).

48 b. This woman has developed *Clostridium difficile* diarrhoea, which is associated with pseudomembranous colitis. It is particularly a complication of clindamycin use but few antibiotics are completely free of this side-effect. Treatment is with either metronidazole or vancomycin for more seriously ill patients. Her blood results can be explained by dehydration due to fluid and electrolyte loss from the gastrointestinal tract. Intravenous potassium replacement is rarely indicated in patients with hypokalaemia and in fact in inexperienced hands may be extremely dangerous due to cardiac arrhythmias. Diuresis is not indicated as this woman is in negative fluid balance and the addition of amoxicillin is unlikely to be effective at treating *C. difficile* diarrhoea. Blood is not needed in this case for fluid replacement; 0.9% normal saline is adequate.

49 d. Autoimmune hepatitis (AIH) tends to affect young- to middle-aged women and may present acutely with features of hepatitis or more insidiously with features of chronic liver disease. Extra-hepatic involvement is common with rash, arthralgia and arthritis accompanying more constitutional features of hepatitis such as nausea, malaise, vomiting and loss of appetite as well as weight loss. An interesting finding is that many women experience amenorrhoea and the clinical picture of a young woman of childbearing age with vomiting, loss of appetite and some abdominal pain can easily lead to misdiagnosis if an accurate history is not taken. Antibody screens are useful in making the diagnosis and a dichotomy is classically described between those individuals with Type I and Type II AIH:

- *Type I*: Involvement of antinuclear antibodies (ANA) with or without antismooth muscle antibodies (SMA).
- *Type II*: Mainly children involved and with liver/kidney microsomal Type I antibodies (LKM1).

Budd–Chiari syndrome presents with acute epigastric pain and shock and is due to occlusion of the hepatic vein. It presents rapidly and would not fit the clinical picture in this case. Viral hepatitis is an option to be considered in any young person with a tender right upper quadrant especially in the face of mild jaundice and hepatomegaly and risk assessment should be carried out for blood-borne viruses and possibly hepatitis serology. McArdle's syndrome is a glycogen storage disease (Type V) and presents with muscular pain after exercise due to deficiency in myophosphorylase. A muscle biopsy is diagnostic. A useful mnemonic for remembering the rare disorders of glycogen storage is 'Very Poor Carbohydrate Metabolism' standing for Von Gierke's disease, Pompé's disease, Cori's disease and McArdle's disease.

50 **a.** Pharyngeal pouches occur more commonly in men than women and in the elderly. The features described above are classically associated with the presence of a pharyngeal pouch. There have been instances of rupture of the pouch, most usually at oesophogastroduodenoscopy (OGD) if there has not been a significant suspicion of pouch disease, however, most cases are diagnosed early and surgically amenable to excision and repair. The pouch forms at an anatomical weakness between the inferior pharyngeal muscle complex posteriorly, known as Killian's dehiscence. Diagnostically is it best seen on contrast swallow where the pouch is clearly delineated. Plummer–Vinson syndrome describes iron-deficiency anaemia and dysphagia caused by the formation of a keratinised web. Features associated with iron deficiency such as koilonychia (spoon-shaped nails) and atrophic glossitis may be rarely seen. The post-cricoid web is a direct but very rare consequence of severe iron-deficiency anaemia. Chagas' disease was described by a Brazilian physician who described the characteristic symptoms of achalsia (failure of the oesophageal cardia to relax)

in the South American population with *Trypanosoma cruzi* infection. Contrast swallow shows the level of obstruction often with hugely dilated and poorly functioning proximal oesophagus. A failure of neuromuscular co-ordination is thought to be the pathogenesis behind the disease. Mallory–Weiss tear often follows a large meal and binge-drinking leading to a small linear tear in the oesophageal mucosa. Oesophageal carcinoma presents with progressive dysphagia for solids then liquids often with florid constitutional signs of cancer.

51 b. ERCP would be the next most appropriate investigation as this man has the symptoms and blood test picture most likely to be primary sclerosing cholangitis (PSC). The association between ulcerative colitis and PSC is well recognised and up to 75% of patients with PSC may have inflammatory bowel disease. Liver biopsy is a useful investigation to confirm the diagnosis in cases with equivocal or borderline investigative results and shows a characteristic 'onion-skin' appearance to the intrahepatic biliary system. ERCP in most cases will make the diagnosis with a 'beaded' appearance due to alternating section of dilatation and stricture of the bile ducts. CT scan may detect areas of liver damage due to chronic backpressure from strictured bile ducts but is far less superior at imaging the biliary tree than magnetic resonance cholangiopancreatography (MRCP). Colonoscopy is useful for detecting inflammatory bowel conditions in patients who present with abdominal pain and change of bowel habit but may have additional benefit in screening for colorectal cancer, which is increased in risk by PSC. Plain abdominal radiography is only of benefit in the diagnosis of complications of inflammatory bowel conditions such as bile duct fistula (aerobilia) and bowel obstruction due to stricture as the most important.

52 c. The clinical picture is one of carcinoid syndrome secondary to a carcinoid tumour. The syndrome of facial flushing, watery diarrhoea, abdominal pain and cardiac abnormalities imply hepatic metastases of a carcinoid tumour. Common sites in the bowel are terminal ileum, rectum and appendix (25% of all tumours), however, involvement of other organs such as ovaries or testes have been reported. Diagnosis is elegantly made from the clinical picture and 24-hour collection of urine for levels of 5-HIAA, a metabolite of 5-HT (serotonin) that is postulated to be responsible for the cardiac manifestations of the disease and profuse watery diarrhoea. 24-hour urine collection for protein is useful in cases

181

of renal disease where the amount of proteinuria can be quantified. Urine and plasma osmolalities are usually taken together in the diagnosis of disorders of free water clearance such as the syndrome of inappropriate ADH (SIADH). A low plasma sodium is seen in the face of inappropriately high urine osmolality indicating free water retention. Fluid restriction may be used to bring the level of sodium up slowly. Too rapid correction of plasma sodium is associated with the development of central pontine myelinolysis – a catastrophic shrinking in the size of brain cells due to rapid osmolarity shifts, which may be fatal. 24-hour urine collection for the presence of VMA (metabolites of catecholamines) may be helpful in making the diagnosis of phaeochromocytoma, a rare catecholamine-producing tumour. 90% of tumours are in the adrenal medulla, 90% benign and 90% of these unilateral.

53 b. This gentleman provides a good history that raises suspicion of subarachnoid haemorrhage (SAH). He requires an urgent CT scan of his brain to rule this out and to assess for raised intracranial pressure. This is usually indicated in order to proceed with a lumbar puncture to assess for xanthochromia as up to 10% of SAH can be missed on CT scan alone. An MRI scan of this gentleman's brain would provide a detailed view of his cerebral parenchyma, although this is not the first-line investigation in this case. The history given includes no mention of fever, therefore looking for a systemic infective cause with blood cultures is unnecessary. Neurological observations and regular analgesia, although important, are unlikely to aid with the diagnosis and therefore are not first-line considerations.

54 c. Lesions of the cerebellum provide characteristic signs that can be remembered by the mnemonic 'DANISH P':
D: dysdiadochokinesis
A: ataxia
N: nystagmus
I: intention tremor
S: slurred speech
H: hypotonia
P: past pointing
This lady's lesion is in the cerebellar vermis as she has bilateral signs of cerebellar disease. Lesions of the bilateral basal ganglia would be incredibly unusual and provide Parkinson's-like features including a rest tremor. A lesion of the left temporo-parietal lobe would provide a dysphasia (assuming this is her dominant hemisphere) and some visual field defects in addition

to hemisensory neglect. Lesions of the frontal lobe would result in personality changes and dysphasia – not in keeping with the clinical details in this case.

55 **c.** Of the listed investigations, CT scan is the most important to obtain. This lady is displaying signs of a vascular event; distinguishing between an infarct or haemorrhage is vital and this can be done by CT scan. Although an INR level will give us vital information about her anticoagulation state, in the short term this is not imperative. A carotid duplex scan could be a helpful adjunct to a cardiovascular examination in identifying a cause of an ischaemic episode if that transpires to be the case. Electrocardiogram and echocardiogram would again identify a cardiac cause of any emboli if the CT scan showed an infarct, however, these are not first-line investigations.

56 **b.** This patient has Wilson's disease. It is an autosomal recessive disorder affecting the lenticular nuclei (globus pallidus and putamen) and the liver, hence the description of hepatolenticular degeneration. Copper deposits can also be seen in the cornea–scleral junction. Copper and caeruloplasmin screening should reveal the diagnosis which can be confirmed with the positive family history. Wilson's disease should be considered in patients with acute mental state changes or impaired mental development for their age. Porphyria is most likely to present with colicky abdominal pain, vomiting and fever. It is a low penetrant autosomal dominant condition. Glycogen storage disorders e.g. Hunter's syndrome, usually present as gargoylism in children. Presentation of Parkinsonism at this age, unless drug-related, is rare and the symptoms and signs are not identified in this case.

57 **a.** Superficial temporal arteritis is 'never' seen in patients this age. It is a disease of the over 55s and is more prevalent in women than men. There is a 25% association with polymyalgia rheumatica and symptoms of scalp and temporal artery tenderness, e.g. on brushing hair, pain whilst eating and most drastically sudden blindness in one eye. Thus any suspicion of superficial temporal arteritis should prompt immediate twice daily 40–60mg prednisolone until the diagnosis has been disproven. All the other causes of headache are commonly experienced in the general practice setting and could reliably be attributable for the pattern of symptoms exhibited by this patient.

58 **d.** Papilloedema is congestion of the optic disc invariably associated with raised intracranial pressure. It is most often bilateral.

General features reflect the underlying disease process but a choked disc is characteristic, though differentiation from papillitis may be difficult.

In the acute setting vision is rarely affected but peripheral vision may be lost in chronic cases where it is frequently accompanied by transient visual obscurations. Papilloedema results from raised intracranial pressure in which the subarachnoid space surrounding the optic nerve is patent e.g. papilloedema is not necessarily a consequence of raised intracranial pressure.

Causes include:

- Intracranial space-occupying lesions – tumours, especially of the posterior fossa due to restricted space; cerebral abscesses; subdural haematoma.
- Any condition that results in hydrocephalus in an adult, e.g. subarachnoid haemorrhage, meningitis, head injury.
- Venous sinus thrombosis due to congestion.
- Benign intracranial hypertension – most likely in patients with visual complaints but otherwise normal.
- Malignant hypertension – bilateral with other signs of hypertensive neuropathy.
- Central retinal venous occlusion, ischaemic optic neuropathy, optic neuritis – unilateral with sudden loss of vision.
- Chronic carbon dioxide retention.
  Other rare causes include:
- Metabolic:
  - Hypoparathyroidism
  - Diabetic ketoacidosis
  - Chronic carbon dioxide retention
  - Obesity.
- Haematological – anaemia, leukaemia.
- Toxic – tetracycline, lead, oral progestational agents, corticosteroid withdrawal.
- Spinal cord tumours.

59 e. The condition described is typical of retroperitoneal fibrosis (peri-aortitis). It is an autoimmune condition where there is progressive fibrosis surrounding the aorta, into which the ureters become embedded causing renal obstruction, failure and retention. Methysergide has a particular association and may still be seen in use for resistant migraine. Paracetamol can lead to acute tubular necrosis as an adverse side effect and acyclovir may cause crystal deposition in cases of dehydration. Gold injections should also be monitored regularly for renal side-effects by follow-up urinalysis for proteinuria. Rosiglitazone must be used with caution in patients with pre-existing renal impairment but itself has few renal side-effects in normal kidneys.

60 **d.** Tuberculosis should always be in the forefront of the differential diagnosis of a patient who has recently come from a developing country, who exhibits weight loss and fever. This presentation is not classic for tuberculosis, however, the presence of a constitutional upset with a sterile pyuria is good enough cause to investigate for the disease. Treating for a urinary tract infection with antibiotics or antifungals is not correct without first excluding growth of alcohol and acid fast bacilli (AAFB) in culture specimens. An intravenous urogram may be necessary down the line to investigate any specific blockage to the urinary tract but a chest X-ray is mandatory for any suspicion of tuberculosis so prompt treatment and barrier nursing precautions can take place if necessary. Cystoscopy is unlikely to be helpful as there has been no mention of any haematuria and may be considered at a later stage if indirect imaging is inconclusive.

Extended matching questions

61 **b.** This lady is suffering from a pneumonia; this can be associated with chest pain. Risk factors for her developing chest infections include the fact that she has a history of lung disease and that she resides in a nursing home. Sedentary lifestyles are more often associated with acquiring infections particularly in institutionalised patients.

62 **e.** Bornholm's disease is a post viral illness that is associated with costochondritis. Patients describe a chest pain that can be recreated by sternal pressure, similar to Tietze's syndrome or idiopathic costochondritis, but on further questioning its incidence closely follows a viral illness.

63 **g.** The clue in this scenario is the recent addition of diclofenac into his medication list. The history obtained from this gentleman suggests a diagnosis of GORD or gastro-oesophageal reflux disease. Exacerbation of his symptoms on lying flat suggest a gastric association and deficiency in the distal oesophageal sphincter. The nausea associated with this pain could be associated with cardiac pain but in the context of this history we can be reassured that the likely cause of this gentleman's pain is GI in origin.

64 **h.** Acute onset chest pain which is described as radiating to the back is characteristic of aortic dissection. Aortic dissection

is defined as separation of the layers within the aortic wall. Tears in the intimal layer result in the propagation of dissection (proximally or distally) secondary to blood entering the intima-media space. Aortic dissection is more common in males than in females, with a male-to-female ratio of 2:1. The condition commonly occurs in persons in the sixth and seventh decades of life. Patients with Marfan's syndrome present earlier, usually in the third and fourth decades of life.

DeBakey classified aortic dissection into three types, as follows:
- *Type I*: The intimal tear occurs in the ascending aorta, but the descending aorta is also involved.
- *Type II*: Only the ascending aorta is involved.
- *Type III*: Only the descending aorta is involved:
  - Type IIIA involves the descending aorta that originates distal to the left subclavian artery and extends as far as the diaphragm.
  - Type IIIB involves the descending aorta below the diaphragm.

The pain of aortic dissection may be distinguished from the pain of acute myocardial infarction by its abrupt onset, although the presentations of the two conditions overlap to some degree. Aortic dissection should be strongly considered in patients with symptoms and signs suggestive of myocardial infarction but without classic ECG findings.

65 c. Risk factors for pulmonary embolus include immobility, malignancy, post-operative period for abdominal or pelvic surgery, lower limb fractures, previous thrombo-embolic disease, pregnancy and hip or knee replacements. In addition to these there are further minor risk factors including long distance travel, use of combined oral contraceptive pill or hormone replacement therapy. In the case in question, this lady is 1 week in the post-operative period for having a knee replacement. The mention in the case of right calf swelling, progressing to chest pain exacerbated by inspiration is a classical description of a pulmonary embolus.

A ventilation/perfusion scan or a CT pulmonary angiogram should be organised to confirm the diagnosis and treatment dose anticoagulation should be commenced as soon as the diagnosis is suspected and if confirmed this should be replaced with warfarin.

66 a. Cushing's syndrome manifests clinically with a plethora of clinical signs due to excess amounts of corticosteroid. The typical clinical picture is of an obese patient who exhibits a moon-face appearance, abnormal fatty pads over the neck and upper back leading to the classical buffalo hump with easily bruised and paper thin skin. Hypertension and diabetes mellitus are commonly found due to both the mineralocorticoid and gluco-corticoid effects of excess corticosteroid and a picture of hyper-natraemia and hypokalaemia provides a clue to the pathology in the face of a strong clinical suspicion. Cushing's syndrome can be as a result of Cushing's disease, which describes the above clinical findings as a consequence of a primary pituitary neoplasm (usually adenoma). Other ACTH-dependent causes may be due to an ectopic focus of ACTH secretion such as a small-cell car-cinoma of the lung. ACTH-independent causes include a primary adrenocortical tumour such as an adenoma or commonly exogen-ous steroid use such as that seen often in those requiring steroid immunosuppression for transplants or autoimmune disease.

67 **g.** Hypothyroidism may present in the elderly with very non-specific signs and should be considered in the differential of any-one presenting with confusion (so-called part of the 'dementia' screen) and general deterioration with no readily identifiable cause. One of the most common endocrine disturbances along-side diabetes mellitus, it should not be missed as a cause of a range of symptoms from neurological signs, typically bradyki-nesia, reduced deep tendon reflexes and parasthesias from nerve entrapment (especially carpal tunnel syndrome) to abdominal pain from chronic constipation to mental disturbance manifest as confusion and apparent memory impairment. Other subtle signs of hypothyroidism include loss of the outer one-third of the eyebrows with male-pattern frontal balding, hypothermia (leading to the aptly named 'granny's tartan' – erythema *ab igne* from sitting close to or being in close contact with a source of heat such as a fire, electric heater or hot-water bottle), brady-cardia and dry, coarse skin. Thyroid function tests are usually diagnostic and demonstrate a low free T4 with a compensatory high TSH in primary hypothyroidism. Very occasionally a low TSH and a low free T4 may be seen in the context of panhypopi-tuitarism and assay of levels of sex hormones, ACTH and other pituitary hormones will confirm the diagnosis.

68 **c.** Diabetes mellitus can often present in a similar fashion to other endocrine diseases and thus it is important that inves-tigations be interpreted in the correct fashion. Loss of weight, fatigue, polydipsia and polyuria are features of not only dia-betes mellitus but also diabetes insipidus (DI) (resulting from to loss of free water due to an inability to secrete or respond to vasopressin and thus be able to concentrate urine). Occasionally

hysterical polydipsia manifests with the above clinical features and can be difficult to clinically distinguish from DI. In this case performing urine electrolyte and osmolality studies can differentiate between these two very different conditions; in DI there is secretion of free water and thus urine osmolality is very low, however, in hysterical polydipsia urine osmolality is normal as intake is matched by output keeping an overall isotonic balance to osmolality. Clues in the scenario suggesting a diagnosis of diabetes mellitus are the concurrent infection (that raises stress hormone levels e.g. cortisol causing an increase in blood glucose levels), the high urine osmolality (due to high glucose load as the renal tubular threshold for glucose absorption has been exceeded) and the very high plasma osmolality. This can be approximated thus:

$$P_{osm} \sim 2(Na^+) + K^+ + urea + glucose \quad \rightarrow \quad units = mOsm/L$$

Plugging in the values for sodium, potassium and urea leaves the remaining component (glucose) at 20.1. This high glucose in the absence of any previous history of diabetes mellitus suggests a type II manifestation of high blood sugar; hyperosmolar hyperglycaemic state (previously hyperosmolar non-ketotic coma, HONK). Urine dipstick will confirm the presence of heavy ketonuria (suggestive of diabetic ketoacidosis (DKA) or an element of HONK/DKA overlap) and an arterial blood gas would demonstrate the pH. As a general rule, any event such as surgery, illness or even myocardial infarction can manifest clinically in addition to the primary event with features of high blood glucose control, which may then progress to hyperosmolar hyperglycaemic state or DKA.

69 **b.** The diagnosis of acromegaly can often be very subtle with those closest to the patient often bringing the changes to attention. It is often helpful to look at old photographs if there is a suspicion of acromegaly as coarsening of features, protrusion of the jaw (prognathism) and change in clothing or shoe size may all point to a retrospective diagnosis. Most often due to a pituitary adenoma (80% macroadenoma, 20% microadenoma) visual symptoms may be a complaint alongside headache and even bedside visual field testing may reveal a defect, commonly a bitemporal hemianopia (tunnel vision). Sausage fingers (leading to an inability to wear rings), greasy coarse skin and a thickening of the forehead are all signs of growth-hormone excess that characterises acromegaly. Trans-sphenoidal hypophysectomy is usually employed as a treatment modality, sometimes in conjunction with medical therapy to reduce the

size of a very large macroadenoma or surgically incompletely resected tumour.

70 e. Phaeochromocytoma is a rare tumour of the sympathetic nervous system notable for the production of catecholamines. Tumours may be adrenal or extra-adrenal and occur in both children and adults. The 'Rule of 10' mnemonic is a helpful way of remembering that phaeochromocytomas are **10%** ectopic, **10%** malignant and **10%** multiple. Symptoms may often be mistaken for anxiety attacks or cardiac in origin as palpitations, tremors, severe anxiety with no basis and chest pain may all be manifestations of the tumour. Severe hypertension is commonly associated and this may prompt more serious investigation of otherwise subtle symptomatology. Plasma metanephrines (metabolic products of catecholamine pathways) is the most sensitive investigation but a useful screening tool is the 24-hour urine collection for metanephrines and catecholamines. Imaging modalities should be used only on the basis of a strong clinical suspicion and/or biochemical evidence of a catecholamine disturbance as the incidence of adrenal mass (so-called incidentaloma) found on imaging has been estimated to be around the order of 7% in the elderly population. MRI scanning of the abdomen is the preferred and most sensitive and specific modality and thus should be employed after positive biochemical tests have been confirmed.

71 b. Rheumatoid arthritis affects females 3 times more commonly than males. Its peak age of onset is between the ages of 30 and 50 years old. It can be described as a symmetrical polyarthropathy affecting both small and large joints. Common symptoms are swollen, painful, stiff hands and feet, worse in the mornings. Patients may also describe a recent history of constitutional symptoms and fatigue. Patients with suspected rheumatoid arthritis should always be referred to a rheumatologist for commencement of disease modifying drugs as soon as the diagnosis is confirmed in order to reduce the amount of joint damage sustained.

72 a. In acute gout there is often severe pain, redness and swelling in the affected joint. The metatarsophalangeal joint of the big toe is most commonly affected. Deposition of sodium monourate crystals in the joint space are responsible for the symptoms and attacks may be precipitated by trauma, surgery, starvation or commencement of diuretics. Risk factors include a high protein diet, alcohol and obesity. Aspirin is known to increase serum urate. Allopurinol can be used to reduce the level of urate in the circulation but it must not be commenced within 3 weeks of an acute attack as it can precipitate another incident.

73 h. This patient is suffering from arthritis mutilans – telescoping of the joints in her ring finger on her right hand. This arthritis is a form of psoriatic arthropathy, associated with the skin condition psoriasis. There are several similarities in this skin condition to rheumatoid arthritis. It is, therefore, important to consider psoriasis in any new patient presenting with rheumatoid features as the joint conditions may present before the skin lesions.

74 f. At the age of 16 years ankylosing spondylitis is 6 times more common in males than females. By the age of 30 it is twice as common in males. Typical presenting symptoms are morning back stiffness and progressive loss of spinal movement. Other features include hip and knee involvement and plantar fasciitis, as eluded to in this case study. Diagnosis is clinical but strongly supported by radiology, e.g. squaring of the vertebrae, formation of a 'bamboo spine' and obliteration of the sacroiliac joints. This is a rare example of a rheumatological condition being more common in males than females.

75 c. Osteoarthritis is the commonest joint condition; it is usually primary but may be secondary to any joint disease or joint injury. Its mean age of onset is 50–60 years old. Pain is defined as being worse after periods of activity and towards the end of the day, with some eventual joint deformity and reduction of movements. Radiologically there are four main features; loss of joint space, subchondral sclerosis, cyst formation and marginal osteophytes. Treatment is mainly NSAIDs for pain relief and reduction of risk factors and exacerbating factors.

76 d. *Cryptosporidum parvum* is a protozoal infection that can cause a severe diarrhoea in immunocompromised individuals. Protozoal cysts adhere to the gut wall and cause a florid secretory diarrhoea that requires large volume fluid resuscitation. The organism can be found in cattle and can cause a self-limiting diarrhoea in immunocompetent individuals. Treatment is mainly supportive as antibiotic therapy has not been proven to be effective.

77 e. *Cryptococcus neoformas* is a fungal infection usually associated with meningitis in HIV. The clinical signs may be masked by the damped immune response seen in immunocompromised individuals and thus the fever, neck stiffness and photophobia associated with inflammation of the meninges may be impaired or even lacking. *Cryptococcus* may be diagnosed by India Ink staining of a sample of CSF at lumbar puncture and carries a 20% mortality even with treatment.

78 b. Candidiasis is often seen in diabetics, those on immunosuppressive therapy and those with immunodeficiency. The most common manifestation is oral candidiasis with white plaques in the mouth and oropharynx. Oesophageal candidiasis presents with odynophagia (pain on swallowing – usually retrosternal) and dysphagia due to the pain. Treatment is usually with fluconazole or another associated 'azole' by mouth for a couple of weeks. Severe cases may merit using amphotericin with caution ('amphoterrible' – coined because of severe nephrotoxic side-effects).

79 c. Infection with the protozoan *Toxoplasma gondii* can cause encephalitis and cerebral abscesses of which the latter may catastrophically be misdiagnosed as primary cerebral tumour or stroke. The symptoms are those of a space-occupying lesion, may cause fitting, focal neurological deficit, confusion and personality change, and may be difficult to distinguish from a cerebrovascular event. MRI is the investigation of choice in imaging suspected toxoplasma infection and can prove to be spectacularly superior to CT scanning in defining numbers and character of lesions. Treatment with pyrimethamine in combination with sulfadiazine and folinic acid for at least 6 weeks can produce remarkable reversal of the clinical state.

80 a. Pneumocystis Jerovici pneumonia (formally called *Pneumocystis Carinii* Pneumonia (PCP)) is one of the most common life-threatening infections in HIV/AIDS. It can act as a benchmark for the severity of immunosuppression as it is rarely seen with CD4 counts higher than $200/mm^3$. Prophylaxis when CD4 counts drop below $200/mm^3$ is given and co-trimoxazole (Trimethoprim and Sulfamethoxazole) is the agent of choice. Chest signs may be clinically absent but the usual scenario is an HIV positive individual who is in frank respiratory compromise with hypoxia, tachypnoea, tachycardia with fine crepitations throughout the chest. Treatment is with high-dose co-trimoxazole for up to 3 weeks with systemic corticosteroids for severe disease (defined as a P_aO_2 of less than 9.5 kPa).

81 h. Lithium carbonate is a frequently used drug for both prophylaxis and treatment of mood disorders and has been termed a 'mood-stabiliser'. Classically used as a first-line agent in the long-term treatment of bipolar disorder (manic-depression) it helps maintain euthymia and reduces up- and downswings of mood. Side-effects of lithium can be severe and drug monitoring must be undertaken on a regular basis. Lithium toxicity can be precipitated by electrolyte derangements, most notably hyponatraemia, and may lead to nephrogenic diabetes insipidus characterised by an inability to concentrate water in the kidney and leading to dehydration and polydipsia that is resistant to desmopressin.

82 e. Eye movement desensitisation and reprocessing (EMDR) has been used with some success in those suffering from post-traumatic stress disorder (PTSD) following violent acts especially sexual abuse and trauma from combat. EMDR usually takes place over multiple sessions and involves the assessment of a patient for EMDR therapy including whether they are emotionally stable enough to start the process of therapy. Subsequent therapy sessions involve identifying a negative thought or image relating to the trauma and a positive thought or belief. The remainder of the therapy involves uncoupling the negative thought process by typically following the therapists fingers across the visual field multiple times and to express the thought processes experienced at the time. Other modalities such as music or other tactile stimuli can be employed instead of eye movements. The aim of the process is to slowly replace the negative emotion experienced during sessions with the positive belief identified at the beginning of therapy. Closure of sessions involves written reflection of events between sessions and evaluation of the effectiveness of the self-calming measures.

Other modalities used in the treatment of PTSD involve the use of selective-serotonin reuptake inhibitors (SSRIs) and beta-blocking medication to reduce the symptoms of hyperarousal.

83 a. Schneider's first rank symptoms describe the spectrum of symptoms experienced by those with schizophrenia and are as follows:
1. Auditory hallucinations
2. Thought insertion
3. Thought withdrawal
4. Thought block
5. Thought broadcast
6. Somatic hallucinations
7. Lack of control over bodily function e.g. controlled by external forces
8. Delusions (fixed unshakeable beliefs)

Treatment involves the use of neuroleptics, either the older classes such as haloperidol or risperidone (with their risk of extra-pyramidal side-effects, e.g. parkinsonism and sedation profile) or the newer classes of neuroleptics such as olanzipine, clozapine and quetiapine. Haloperidol and risperidone are commonly used in the acute management of psychosis with the newer agents more useful for longer-term management. Clozapine must be monitored frequently for the serious side-effect of agranulocytosis; defined as a white blood cell count less than 500/mm^3.

84 g. Anxiety attacks are often associated with situations such as speaking in public or being in a public place and share similar characteristics to the specific phobias. Agoraphobia (the fear of being in a public place) is one of the most commonly associated phobias with anxiety. Generalised anxiety disorders have no readily identifiable precipitant and anxiety attacks can occur daily over long periods of time. In this case the woman is exhibiting a panic disorder, manifest as anxiety when performing in public. There are many modalities used to counteract anxiety such as selective serotonin reuptake inhibitors, other classes of antidepressants and benzodiazepines (which should only be used as a last resort in intractable anxiety due to the dependence forming effects of benzodiazepines). Simple measures, however, are often overlooked and these include breathing exercises, dietary modifications including avoiding all caffeine-containing products and relaxation techniques. These should be at least considered as a first line before instituting medication, which may eventually become a long-term and unnecessary crutch.

85 d. Electroconvulsive therapy (ECT) is a highly effective form of treatment for severe depression that is refractive to medical therapy and especially useful in the treatment of depression associated with delusional symptoms. The process involves undergoing a short course of general anaesthesia with a muscle relaxant (to prevent muscle damage and rhabdomyolysis associated with rapid muscular contraction during the procedure) then passing of current via two electrodes across the brain. The effect is similar to a tonic–clonic seizure in both electrical brain activity and clinical effect with post-ictal amnesia and confusion being infrequent non-anaesthetic related side-effects. The reversal of mood is extremely rapid with the use of ECT and can produce profound effects in a short space of time making it an effective therapy for those at severe risk of self-harm or suicide in which antidepressant medication may take too long to have effect.

86 c. Gardeners expose themselves to many organisms if durable gloves are not worn and infections of the nailbed and surrounding area are common. These conditions are occasionally confused with fungal infections of the nailbed and scrapings for mycology can be taken if there is any doubt. Another common infection spread characteristically following rose-thorn pricks is with *Sporothrix* spp. This usually presents with characteristic tracks that spread distal to proximal.

87 b. Glomus tumour typically presents as a mass under the nail with severe pain as the most common feature. The bluish hue is another feature of this rare tumour that can resemble a subungval melanoma. Looking for other signs of melanoma can often be useful in differentiating between these two conditions.

88 e. Self-harm injuries commonly occur on the forearms and are more common in the female population. Injury to the radial and median nerves is most common in injuries to the wrist, the median nerve being especially vulnerable to slash injuries due to its relatively superficial course at the carpal tunnel. Radial nerve injury typically presents with an inability to extend the hand leading to wrist drop. The aide memoire 'BEST' (**b**rachioradialis, **e**xtensors of the forearm, **s**upinator and **t**riceps) describes the muscle of the forearm supplied by this nerve.

89 h. This injury is one of the most commonly injured bones of the carpal row, thought to be due to the higher stresses imposed on the scaphoid due to its unique position spanning both proximal and distal rows of the carpal bones. Falling on an outstretched hand is the mechanism of injury usually encountered in this type of injury, occasionally complicated by neurovascular compromise as with any fracture. Tenderness in the anatomical snuffbox forms a useful clinical reckoner if scaphoid fracture is suspected.

90 g. Associated with a diverse variety of conditions such as diabetes mellitus, acromegaly, rheumatoid arthritis and pregnancy, carpal tunnel syndrome (CTS) manifests with tingling and numbness that patients often describe as being relieved by shaking out their hands. Pain is typically complained of at night, and can be exacerbated by tapping over the carpal tunnel with the wrist extended (Tinel's test) or by stressing both wrists together into forced flexion (Phalen's test) and form a useful clinical screen for CTS. It is thought to be due to fluid retention in the case of pregnancy, diabetes and acromegaly although the exact mechanism is not known.

Answers and notes

Multiple choice questions (single best answer)

1 c. This patient needs to be admitted for an open reduction and internal fixation of the fracture. The key feature in this history is the rotation of the fragment. If the fracture was undisplaced and not rotated this could be managed in a backslab and followed up in fracture clinic however, since there is associated rotation the patient requires surgical management to achieve a successful outcome. On examination of this gentleman's hand it was noted that he was unable to form a fist due to swelling and pain (not uncommon with unrotated fractures either) but there was obvious rotation of his affected little finger.

2 c. The investigation most likely to be diagnostic is the MRI of the spine. Whilst the bone scan will be useful if the MRI scan does show metastases (which, in this case it did) alone it will not be diagnostic. Whilst it is important to exclude sinister causes of this gentleman's pain it is also important to exclude common causes of low back pain including discitis and disc prolapse, all of which may be identified on MRI or CT scan. This gentleman was found to have metastases in his spine and returned to a tertiary centre to have both chemotherapy and radiotherapy.

3 c. This case presents a difficult ethical dilemma that is not infrequently encountered and can require extremely sensitive handling of the situation. An adult that is unconscious or otherwise incompetent to make a decision with respect to understanding, weighing up the options and retaining information in order to make an informed decision about their medical care presents difficultly in deciding what is in the patient's best interest. A discussion with family members may sometimes help inform the decision; however, there is no legal requirement (for an otherwise competent adult) for assent from the family or close relatives before making decisions about medical care in situations where that adult cannot consent to treatment.

Refusing to perform surgery without blood is indeed a surgeon's prerogative as a splenectomy following trauma may be dangerous without the back-up of blood products and may ultimately cause more harm than good. However, this is not the right course of action as without surgery the prognosis is poor. Using crystalloid replacement is similarly not correct for the reasons above.

The brief clinical indicators point to a ruptured spleen in a hypotensive road traffic accident victim in whom delaying surgery any longer than is necessary would be seriously detrimental to the prognosis and would be labelled as medically unsafe.

Awaiting a court order in an emergency situation would take too long and would not allow the appropriate timely intervention (emergency surgery) to occur thus this should not be considered.

As the child is 14 years of age and a legal minor the parents have a legal right to dictate what medical treatment is appropriate for their child. However, in the case of emergency or life-threatening situations this may be overcome by the need to do what is in the patient's best interest. The four pillars of ethics are beneficence, non-maleficence, autonomy and justice, and should always be borne in mind when addressing ethical situations. Applied to this case the surgeon would be covered from a legal and ethical standpoint to act in the patient's best interest and take the child to surgery, even if this is against the religious view of the parents. Further justification is that religious values of parents are not intrinsically inherent to children and should not be assumed to represent the true wishes of the child in a situation such as this. A sensible strategy would be to take the onus from the parents by stating that clinical need dictates this course of action and if there was any other way to proceed without transfusion it would have been explored. Often this abdicates the feeling of blame and responsibility that comes with making an active decision by taking the decision out of their hands.

4 **c.** Molluscum contagiosum is caused by a poxvirus and is most commonly seen in children. Lesions are typical in appearance and present as discrete papules sometimes with a surrounding area of mild erythema due to an eczematous process. A distinctive feature of molluscum contagiosum is the presence of a central core of keratin, which can be expressed from the lesions. They are treated conservatively and will resolve on their own or can be squeezed between two fingernails to express the central keratin plug. Varicella zoster does give a similar picture; however, the absence of significant itch, blistering vesicles

and distribution in a particular dermatome makes the diagnosis unlikely. Herpes simplex is found in two subtypes: HSV 1 affecting the oral and buccal mucosa causing 'cold sores' and HSV 2 affecting primarily the genital tract (although both types can be found almost anywhere in the body). The lesions are transmissible through direct contact, e.g. kissing, and may be painful and ulcerated with small eruptive vesicles. The lesions will settle spontaneously although in the immunocompromised or elderly a prolonged course may occur. Eczema presents as an itchy rash with typical erythema and excoriation of the skin from scratching. Lesions are neither papular nor discrete entities and characteristically affect flexor surfaces. Pityriasis versicolor is a skin condition affecting primarily young adults and is due to *Malassezia* yeasts, a normal skin commensal. Areas of macular hypopigmentation are seen in persons of dark skin colour with a faint brownish colour in those persons of light skin colour. Microscopic examination of skin scrapings reveals the yeasts clumped in short balls and longer hyphae.

5 d. Arthropathy is a condition that is usually associated with psoriasis and may in fact sometimes be the first presentation of psoriasis in a patient with no obvious skin lesions. The arthropathy can mimic many other rheumatological conditions including rheumatoid arthritis and osteoarthritis, however, usually presents in one of four patterns:
1. Distal interphalangeal joint involvement.
2. Rheumatoid-like joint changes.
3. Large joint involvement.
4. Seronegative-type joint changes.

Up to 10% of psoriatics will suffer with some kind of joint change associated with skin disease. Eczema can be broadly classified into exogenous, i.e. usually due to an allergic or irritant stimulus, and endogenous, i.e. no identifiable precipitant. The latter classification further subdivides into atopic eczema, eczema associated with venous insufficiency, eczema affecting the sebaceous glands, discoid eczema and asteatotic eczema, which tends to affect the elderly (especially those who are subject to hospital and nursing home washing and bathing). Eczema responds to emollients to keep the skin from drying and atopic eczema usually benefits from topical steroid cream. Secondary bacterial infection can manifest in broken eczematous skin and a topical steroid and antibacterial combination therapy or even systemic antibiotics may be employed to both eradicate the infection and return the skin to a more balanced level of hydration.

6 d. This investigation is useful in the screening for two common urological conditions: prostate cancer and benign prostatic hyperplasia (BPH). Epidemiological evidence suggests BPH is more common in the Afro-Caribbean population and may be linked to higher testosterone levels. Suprapubic catheterisation is a useful therapeutic and diagnostic procedure for those whose urethral catheterisation is contraindicated, such as urethral stricture or pelvic trauma where there is a risk of urethral rupture. In an elderly gentleman presenting with such symptoms, it is usually advisable to perform a digital rectal examination, prostate-specific antigen, renal function and urinalysis as part of routine management.

7 e. The condition described is typical of retroperitoneal fibrosis (peri-aortitis). It is an autoimmune condition where there is progressive fibrosis surrounding the aorta, into which the ureters become embedded causing renal obstruction, failure and retention. Methysergide has a particular association and may still be seen in use for resistant migraine. Paracetamol can lead to acute tubular necrosis as an adverse side-effect and acyclovir may cause crystal deposition in cases of dehydration. Gold injections should also be monitored regularly for renal side-effects by follow-up urinalysis for proteinuria. Rosiglitazone must be used with caution in patients with pre-existing renal impairment but itself has few renal side-effects in normal kidneys.

8 d. This lady is suffering an allergic reaction to the antibiotics. Despite having had five previous doses and no known drug allergies these symptoms of facial flushing and tingling in her hands are characteristic of an allergic reaction. More severe cases of allergy/anaphylaxis may result in shortness of breath and chest pain. Although this was not the case here, these should always be noted as important negatives in the patients notes. It is important to stop all antibiotics in this case to assess the response to steroids and antihistamines as there may be another underlying cause for these symptoms and failure to identify this could lead to malpractice cases.

9 a. This lady needs to continue rehabilitation before being discharged home. Being a recurrent attender should pose the question of whether there is an underlying social issue. This lady, although medically fit, would not benefit from being immediately discharged under GP care as this option has been available to her but she has repeatedly chosen to call an ambulance. Remaining in hospital until she feels ready to leave would lead to a number of problems both financially and physically in terms of acquiring hospital infections and taking up an acute bed. Being assessed by social services is a realistic option, although in reality this takes time and means an extended stay in hospital whilst the process is completed. Placement in a local cottage hospital is a good compromise; it allows continued rehabilitation with physiotherapists whilst being less at risk of developing further infections.

10 **b.** Signs of an ischaemic limb include the **6 P's**:
- **P**allor
- **P**ulseless
- **P**araesthesiae
- **P**ainful
- **P**aralysis
- **P**erishingly cold

From the history we know that this lady is suffering from the pallor and pulselessness described above. She has a present femoral pulse but not below that level which suggests an embolus at the mid-femoral level. The symptoms are not indicative of arterial insufficiency and there has been no mention of an abdominal mass to suggest an abdominal arterial aneurysm. In cases of venous ulceration you would expect to see changes in the skin, including breakdown of the epidermal level which is not described here.

Potential sources of emboli in this case include the left atrium, heart valves and from the aorta among others.

This lady went on to have an embolectomy and post-operative management with unfractionated heparin. Unfortunately due to her age and her concomitant chest problems her outcome was not as good as desired and she died 36 hours post-operatively.

11 **e.** Panic disorders are seen 2 to 3 times more commonly in females than males and are diagnosed according to strict criteria involving sensations of choking, tingling or numbness, chest tightness and shortness of breath, fear of losing control and a variety of other perceived symptoms. In addition to the presence of these symptoms a diagnosis of panic disorder is only valid if there is an additional persistent worry for a period greater than 1 month about recurrence of attacks, the consequences of having another attack and a significant behavioural modification as a result of a panic attack, e.g. avoiding public places. Panic disorders exhibit a bimodal distribution in prevalence with peaks seen in late adolescence and then again in the mid-30s.

There have been a wide variety of medical co-morbidities associated with panic disorders: irritable bowel syndrome, COPD, cardiomyopathy, hypertension, migraine headache, mitral valve prolapse to name a few of the more studied examples. Agoraphobia is often seen with panic disorder and is estimated to be present in between 30% and 50% of cases of diagnosed panic disorder.

Treatment modalities used for panic disorder include cognitive behavioural therapy involving exposure and subsequent desensitisation to panic-inducing stimuli, respiratory training to help break the cycle of reinforcement of panic-induced hyperventilation and medical therapy usually in the form of antidepressant medication with selective serotonin reuptake inhibitors as first-line followed by tricyclic antidepressants as a second-line modality.

12 c. PTSD is defined as a pathological anxiety reaction that develops following an extreme traumatic stressor (often an act of physical violence) witnessed or experienced by an individual. Features manifest as mood disturbance, a re-experiencing of the event, hypervigilance (exaggerated startle reaction) and avoidance of stimuli (e.g. location) associated with the event. It is differentiated from the very similar condition of acute stress disorder by the duration of symptoms. PTSD symptoms usually occur a few months from the sentinel event and can last for anywhere between less than 3 months to greater than 6 months. Acute stress disorders typically occur within 1 month of a traumatic event and last for less than 1 month from onset.

Depressive symptoms make a diagnosis of depression a differential to consider; however, there are only a few of the symptoms of a depressive episode listed in the clinical vignette and the addition of nightmares associated with a history of a traumatic event alongside the features of a pathologically heightened sense of awareness (hypervigilance and exaggerated startle response) make this diagnosis unlikely.

Schizoid personality disorders present with behavioural manifestations that are typically detached from close relationships, aloof and exhibiting signs of anhedonia (inability to enjoy oneself). Rarely seen in the clinical setting this diagnosis forms part of the Cluster A (odd, eccentric) classification of personality disorders along with schizotypal and paranoid personality disorders.

GAD describes a chronic anxiety state characterised by disproportional worry about a wide range of life events that cause impairment to normal social functioning. The pertinent features associated with GAD are of anxiety that occurs for most days for greater than 6 months and manifest with greater than three somatic symptoms such as sleep disturbance, poor concentration and mood disturbance.

13 b. This clinical picture represents acute lymphocytic leukaemia. The child is in the right age category, approximately 4–8 years of age. Symptoms of this condition may be split into bone marrow failure, systemic symptoms and local symptoms. Systemic symptoms include malaise and weight loss with sweats or anorexia being the most common. Acute myeloid leukaemia commonly presents in the elderly approximately aged 70 years old. A chest X-ray may be helpful in the diagnosis, a mediastinal mass is occasionally seen. For confirmation of the diagnosis a trephine bone marrow biopsy is required.

14 c. It is chronic myeloid leukaemia that involves the translocation of the so-called Philadelphia chromosome.

15 a. Hodgkin's lymphoma typically presents with a picture of painless localised lymphadenopathy with systemic features associated with malignancy of weight loss, fevers, night sweats and lethargy. Often seen in young men around the age of 20 years there is a second peak in middle age. Almost pathognomonic of Hodgkin's lymphoma is the interesting association of pain upon drinking alcohol and this sometimes may be the primary complaint of those presenting with the disease. The pathological hallmark of Hodgkin's lymphoma is the Reed–Sternberg cell, sometimes referred to as owl's eyes.

Infectious mononucleosis is caused by the Epstein–Barr virus and commonly presents insidiously with fatigue and malaise with a sore throat being the second most common symptom. Penicillin derivatives such as amoxicillin should be avoided in the treatment of infectious mononucleosis as they may cause a maculopapular rash.

Non-Hodgkin's lymphoma is typically classified into low-grade, intermediate-grade and high-grade depending on the clinical behaviour of the tumour. Presenting most often with peripheral lymphadenopathy there may be involvement of bone marrow causing abnormal blood counts and constitutional features of cancer are common reported symptoms.

Polycythaemia rubra vera is a disorder affecting the totipotent haematopoeitic stem cells and causes a varying degree of overproduction of erythrocytes, leucocytes and platelets. Often causing vascular thromboses patients may present with stroke, myocardial infarction, deep vein thromboses or pulmonary emboli. Arterial thromboses are, interestingly, seen 3 times more commonly than venous thromboses.

MDS actually describes a group of haematopoeitic disorders that many authors group as a form of pre-malignancy.

Characterised by either a hypercellular or hypocellular bone marrow with abnormal forms seen on peripheral blood smear this disorder is likely underestimated in the population over 70 and may be increasing in incidence due to the relative increase in blood tests taken on arrival to hospital as compared to years ago. Clinically the symptoms of anaemia or thrombocytopaenia may be the only clues to an abnormal marrow and is often the mode of diagnosis in the majority of elderly patients presenting to hospital with nebulous constitutional upset.

16 **b.** The symptoms and biochemical markers of renal failure and lung involvement, i.e. haemoptysis should raise the concern of hepatopulmonary diseases such as Goodpasture's syndrome. A proliferative glomerulonephritis associated with pulmonary infiltrates causing haemoptysis (sometimes massive in nature) are the pathological hallmarks of this aggressive disease. Antibodies to basement membranes affecting both glomeruli and alveoli are the typical antibodies exhibited by patients with Goodpasture's syndrome. Anti-neutrophil cytoplasmic antibodies (ANCA) are more strongly associated with systemic vasculitides such as Wegener's granulomatosis (PR3-ANCA), microscopic polyangiitis and Churg–Strauss disease (MPO-ANCA). Anti-SCL 70 is classically associated with systemic sclerosis, anti-mitochondrial antibodies often seen in cirrhosis of liver and biliary tree and rheumatoid factor associated with rheumatoid disease and associated syndromes, e.g. Felty's syndrome. It is worth noting, however, that no antibody is entirely specific or sensitive to a particular disease and there are many patients without any disease who will exhibit positive antibody titres.

17 **e.** Carpal tunnel syndrome (CTS) is commonly associated with rheumatoid arthritis but lesser known but important other associations include dialysis, pregnancy, diabetes mellitus and hypothyroidism. Symptoms are always in the distribution of the median nerve and are characteristically described by patients to affect them at night, relieved by shaking the hands out and the symptoms of which can be often brought on in clinic by Tinel's test (tapping over the extended wrist) and less reliably by Phalen's test (forced flexion at the wrist). Treatment options in chronological order of trial should include wrist splinting, local steroid injection (symptomatic relief only) then consideration of surgical decompression of the carpal tunnel indicated in cases of (a) prolonged symptoms and (b) neurological symptoms, e.g. thenar eminence wasting. Plain radiographs of the wrist and hand are unlikely to be of any use in the management of CTS,

however, may provide useful baseline views for assessing radiographic progression of rheumatoid disease.

18 **d.** Investigation of breast lumps involves triple assessment. The gold standard for this varies in accordance with the age of the patients.

All patients require:

- Clinical assessment.
- Imaging (either mammogram or ultrasound).
- Cytology/histology.

The imaging is dependent on the patient's age. For patients under the age of 35 years old an ultrasound is the most appropriate form of imaging due to the ductal and dense nature of the breast tissue. After the age of 35 years, breast tissue becomes increasingly fatty which is better imaged with mammography. In patients with breast implants it may be necessary to consider CT scanning.

19 **c.** There is radiological evidence of an abscess which will require drainage. In the first instance a needle aspiration under local anaesthetic is the most appropriate treatment. In the event that this is unsuccessful due to the pus being too thick or not achieving symptomatic relief an incision and drainage should be considered. This treatment should always be followed up with a course of antibiotics, usually flucloxacillin or erythromycin if penicillin allergic. Patients should be advised to continue to breastfeed. Although this may provide discomfort it will aid the healing process and in addition it is safe to do so whilst being on antibiotics. In all cases pus should be sent off to exclude an inflammatory carcinoma.

20 **c.** Marfan's syndrome is an inherited connective tissue disorder that affects the expression of the fibrillin gene leading to defects in the connective tissue of the ocular, skeletal and cardiovascular system. Mitral valve prolapse, tall, spindly stature, ectopia lentis (lens dislocation) as well as aortic involvement such as aortic-root dilatation, aortic regurgitation and aortic dissection are associated with the syndrome. William's syndrome is a neurodevelopmental disorder with cardiovascular abnormalities and typical facial appearances. Hypercalcaemia is also commonly seen. Most importantly in this syndrome is the association of supravalvular aortic outflow obstruction, which may be severe enough to cause sudden death. Down's syndrome is a disorder of mental development, behaviour and associated with characteristic features including a single palmar crease, upslanting palpebral fissure and a flat nasal bridge. Ocular involvement

is legion ranging from refractive errors as the most common to congenital cataracts. Lens dislocation, however, is a relatively rare event. Turner's syndrome is a disease affecting females and presents with short stature and signs of ovarian dysfunction. Widely spaced nipples and a webbed neck are often quoted features of this disease and genetic analysis reveals a 45 X0 karyotype. Reiter's syndrome is a rheumatological manifestation of the triad of conjunctivitis, urethritis and arthritis, and classically occurs following a sexually-transmitted infection although this can be seen after a bout of infectious diarrhoea. It is a seronegative arthropathy, so-called because rheumatoid factor is negative in these patients and is grouped with reactive arthropathy, enteropathy-associated arthropathy and ankylosing spondylitis.

21 **d.** Sjögren's syndrome (keratoconjunctivitis sicca) manifests as dryness of the mucous membranes leading to dry eyes, dry mouth (xerostomia) and occasionally dryness of the tracheobronchial tree. Investigations include the Schirmer test, which assesses the amount of tear production from the eye with a reduction to less than 5 mm of tearing after 5 minutes on a strip of filter paper suggestive of the condition. Erythrocyte sedimentation rate and autoantibodies, especially anti-Ro and anti-La (SS-A and SS-B) are frequently raised in Sjögren's syndrome. Anterior uveitis is associated with the seronegative arthropathies, a group of arthritic conditions so-called because they do not exhibit a positive rheumatoid factor. Classified into enteropathy-associated arthritis, reactive arthritis (including Reiter's syndrome), psoriatic arthritis and ankylosing spondylitis are commonly associated with extra-articular features such as inflammation of the (anterior) uveal tract comprising iris, ciliary body and choroid. Symptoms of anterior uveitis include pain in the affected eye, tear production, blurred vision and occasionally photophobia. Acute glaucoma can present in a similar fashion to anterior uveitis and must be differentiated if appropriate treatment can be instituted. One of the true ocular emergencies it presents with an acutely painful, red eye with both conjunctival and ciliary vessel injection. The pupil is fixed, dilated and oval in shape and the intraocular pressure is high. Beta-blockade, acetazolamide and topical steroids form the mainstay of treatment. Subconjunctival haemorrhage presents with an acute red eye consisting of bright red sclera with a rim around the limbus. The pupil is normal, which allows differentiation from the other causes of red eye. Retinal vein occlusion commonly occurs in elderly hypertensive patients and presents with an acute deterioration in visual acuity. It can be detected on fundoscopy as

either a wedge deficit on the retina (due to a branch retinal vein occlusion) or when central presents with dot and blot haemorrhages or florid retinal haemorrhages leading to the description of the appearance as a 'stormy sunset'. Photocoagulation is the treatment of choice in preventing the neovascular complications of retinal vein occlusion; however, no medical therapy has been demonstrated to be curative once the event has occurred.

22 e. Cushing's disease is associated with hyperglycaemia due to the glucocorticoid effect of cortisol and associated steroids. Cushing's disease describes a specific disease of hypercortisolaemia due to excess ACTH from a pituitary tumour. It is a subdivision of Cushing's syndrome, which describes glucocorticoid excess usually due to excess ACTH (90%) of which the majority (90%) are due to ACTH-producing pituitary tumours. Other causes of excess ACTH leading to Cushing's syndrome include ectopic production from certain lung and carcinoid tumours and rarely over-administration of ACTH. Primary causes of Cushing's syndrome include steroid use, adrenal tumours and alcohol abuse. Addison's disease can be thought simplistically as the opposite of Cushing's syndrome as primary adrenal failure leads to low levels of circulating corticosteroids. Thus hypoglycaemia, hypotension and hyperkalaemia and hyponatraemia occur. Liver failure tends to present with hypoglycaemia due to impaired liver function leading to poor glycogen production (resulting in low 'glucose' stores during periods of fasting) and impaired fatty acid metabolism. Insulinomas are classically associated with severe hypoglycaemia due to excess production of insulin and may be biochemically tested for by assay of c-peptide levels (which are cleaved from insulin precursors to release physiologically active insulin). In cases where exogenous insulin may be abused thus mimicking the effects of insulinoma, c-peptide levels can be taken; they will be high in insulinoma and within normal limits or low in exogenous insulin administration (as c-peptide is not present in synthetic insulin). Gliclazide is a sulphonylurea that is similar in structure to sulpha antibiotics. The mechanism of action as a hypoglycaemic agent was discovered when malnourished and starved patients were given sulpha antibiotics leading to hypoglycaemic attacks and acts by increasing endogenous insulin production (sulphonylureas squeeze the pancreas!). Sulphonylureas should be used with caution in the elderly because of the decreased awareness for hypoglycaemic attacks and thus inability to counteract the effects (e.g. by taking sweet foods/drinks). The duration of action of the sulphonylureas is long and therefore any diabetic presenting to hospital with hypoglycaemia on sulphonylurea tablets must be either admitted for blood glucose observation for a 24-hour period until the effect has worn off or in exceptional circumstances where they themselves or those around them are able to measure the blood glucose and know how to counteract any hypoglycaemia, may be allowed to return home but with a low threshold to return to hospital if there is any doubt about the effectiveness of treatment.

23 **c.** Clues from the vignette include the fact that the patient is asking for other therapeutic options other than tablets and the fact that the T4 level is elevated in the face of a high thyroid-stimulating hormone (TSH), which in the absence of a secondary cause for hyperthyroidism (e.g. hypothalamic or pituitary disease producing high TSH) is discordant with the clinical state. The most likely explanation is chronic undertreatment of hypothyroidism leading to a raised TSH as the pituitary tries to compensate for low levels of T4 followed by over-replacement prior to the clinic appointment in order to try to give the biochemical appearance of compliance. Subclinical hypothyroidism presents with a T4 that is in the normal range but at the low end of the spectrum with a raised TSH. Treatment of subclinical hypothyroidism depends on the clinical state and often these patients are followed up with regular interval blood tests to assess the need for thyroxine replacement. Sick euthyroid syndrome is often seen biochemically as a low TSH and low T4 (and T3) and occurs in the absence of any pre-existing thyroid or hypothalamo-pituitary disease. It can occur for a number of reasons including gastrointestinal and cardiovascular disease and is defined from intrinsic thyroid dysfunction by the resolution of abnormal thyroid tests with resolution of the underlying non-thyroid illness. Inadequate replacement with thyroxine would lead to a low T4 and a high TSH (simply slightly 'milder' biochemical indices of hypothyroidism than frank untreated hypothyroidism) and the opposite would lead to high T4 associated with a depressed TSH (by the negative feedback mechanism).

24 **e.** Whilst all of the options are correct, the most important is to complete a primary survey. Once this has been done the full extent of the situation will become clear and it will then be more appropriate to ask for help and order further investigations.

25 **e.** Erythema nodosum has no association with infective endocarditis. Retinal haemorrhages are seen in the form of Roth

spots. Vasculitis accounts for Osler's nodes, splinter haemorrhages, Roth spots and Janeway lesions.

26 **b.** Furosemide is a loop diuretic. When given i.v. furosemide can reduce arteriolar vasodilatation which is a beneficial action independent to their diuretic effect. ACE inhibitors have an adjunct affect when used in combination with diuretics but in this situation optimisation of the diuretic therapy is the first step in management of this patient. Whilst bumetanide is a useful drug it is a loop diuretic and there is limited benefit of adding this into his treatment regime. Metolazone is a thiazide diuretic and is known to cause a profound diuresis. It has a role in severe hear failure resistant to large doses of loop diuretics.

27 **b.** Cocaine is known to cause spasm of coronary arteries and its abuse should always be suspected in cardiac sounding chest pain in a young person. Amphetamines are also known to cause cardiac arrhythmias.

28 **d.** This case is describing Marfan's syndrome. It is associated with mitral valve prolapse and a dilated aortic root. The prolapse gives a mid-systolic click followed by a systolic murmur heard at the apex. Associations of Marfan's syndrome also include lens detachment and a marfarnoid habitus where arm span is characteristically longer than height.

29 **b.** Serum potassium is important to monitor in patients on digoxin as hypokalaemia can potentiate the effects of digoxin leading to toxicity.

30 **c.** Ibuprofen and other non-steroidal anti-inflammatory drugs (NSAIDs) should be avoided if possible in anything other than mild renal failure (arbitrarily defined as a glomerular filtration rate of between 20 and 50 mL/minute). The mechanism of action of the NSAIDS is to inhibit cyclo-oxygenase enzymes thus decreasing the amount of prostaglandin production (PGE_2 and PGI_2 especially). Prostaglandins are involved in the inflammatory cascade but additionally have effect on the maintenance of renal blood flow, especially at the site of the glomerular afferent arterioles. Thus the decrease in production of prostaglandins in patients who are susceptible to changes in renal homeostasis (such as those with renal impairment) can cause decompensation of function. Alternative analgesic modalities should be sought that can safely be used in patients with suboptimal renal function.

31 **b.** Post-streptococcal glomerulonephritis is associated with streptococcal upper respiratory tract infections and usually

presents anywhere between a week and 3 weeks post-infection. Haematuria, often described as dark or smoky rather than frank blood, is frequently encountered. Oedema, especially of the periorbital region, is a common presentation in children with post-streptococcal glomerulonephritis and accompanies proteinuria, hypertension and oliguria. Treatment is usually supportive with spontaneous resolution being the rule. Minimal change glomerulonephritis is the most common cause of the nephritic syndrome in children. Symptoms are similar with oedema, hypertension and association with upper respiratory tract infection; however, thromboembolic events due to loss of anti-clotting products in the urine make the diagnosis more likely. Corticosteroids form the mainstay of treatment. Henoch–Schönlein purpura is a vasculitis of small vessels that affects young males twice as frequently as females and manifests as punctate bleeding points associated with abdominal pain and gastrointestinal bleeding. Characteristic 'bruising' occurs over the buttocks and lower limbs and may sometimes be mistaken for non-accidental injury in a child. Berger's disease is the commonest primary glomerulonephritis worldwide. Immune complex deposition is thought to be part of the pathophysiology of Berger's disease with ensuing glomerular damage and renal failure. Treatment may be supportive only if the degree of renal failure is mild. Rapidly progressive glomerulonephritis describes a pathological reduction in glomerular filtration rate over a short space of time and may be associated with anti-glomerular basement membrane antibodies, immune complex deposition or vasculitis-associated disease. Immunosuppression is the treatment modality of choice.

32 **d.** Hyperkalaemia is associated with CRF and is most important in the setting of acute on when levels can be rapidly elevated due to a sharp fall in glomerular filtration rate CRF. Treatment of acute severe hyperkalaemia (potassium level above 6.5 mmol/L or electrocardiogram changes) is managed firstly by intravenous injection of 10 mL of 10% calcium gluconate as cardioprotection. Secondly infusion of e.g. 10 units of short-acting insulin with 50 mL of 50% dextrose over 30 minutes will shift potassium intracellularly. Correcting the underlying cause, e.g. hypovolaemia may stabilise the potassium level, however, depletion of total body stores of potassium may be indicated and can be achieved by using calcium resonium. Other electrolyte abnormalities may be a dilutional hyponatraemia secondary to fluid retention, hyperphosphataemia and associated hypocalcaemia due to reduced renal hydroxylation of vitamin D with uraemia and metabolic acidosis due to impaired hydrogen ion excretion.

Neurological manifestations of CRF include restless legs syndrome, peripheral neuropathy and non-specific signs such as dizziness and headache associated with dialysis.

33 c. Frusemide is an example of a loop diuretic and has action at the loop of Henlé. Other loop diuretics include ethacrynic acid and bumetanide. The mechanism of action is one of inhibition of the sodium/potassium/chloride co-transporter in the thick ascending limb of the loop of Henlé and inhibits reabsorption of the above electrolytes at this site. Renal losses of sodium of up to 15–20% are seen causing a loss of concentrating power at the loop and thus loss of free water. Acetazolamide is a carbonic-anhydrase inhibitor acting at the proximal convoluted tubule causing increased excretion of sodium bicarbonate with resultant loss of sodium, potassium and free water. The effect is self-limiting as levels of bicarbonate fall thus producing a temporary diuresis. Osmotic agents are not commonly used in the treatment of fluid overload and are more useful in the management of raised intracranial pressure; however, mannitol is an example of an osmotic agent that acts on the parts of the nephron freely permeable to water (proximal convoluted tubule, descending limb of the loop and collecting tubule). Water is drawn into the tubular lumen by osmosis with relatively marginal effect on sodium loss from the kidney. Thiazide drugs such as bendrofluazide and the newer agent indapamide act at the distal convoluted tubule to reduce sodium and chloride reabsorption. Potassium loss is significant with the thiazide diuretics and is due to a relative increase in the electrolyte gradient in the collecting duct essentially flushing away potassium. Spironolactone, amiloride and triamterene are examples of potassium-sparing diuretics with spirono-lactone being especially useful in conditions of hyperaldo-steronism such as Conn's disease (primary aldosteronism) and hepatic cirrhosis.

34 b. Oliguria is not an indication for dialysis itself and the cause should be investigated and treated, e.g. hypovolaemia. Manifestations of oliguria such as fluid overload refractory to treatment or build-up of toxins such as urea and nitrogenous compounds may, however, influence the decision to dialyse. A useful mnemonic for remembering the indications for dialysis is 'AEIOU' standing for **A**cidosis, **E**lectrolyte abnormalities, **I**ngestions, **O**verload and **U**raemic symptoms. Severe or worsening metabolic acidosis with a pH < 7.2 and persistent hyperkalaemia >7 mmol/L are good markers of the need for dialysis. Fluid overload, e.g. pulmonary oedema, that is likely to cause respiratory embarrassment and/or cardiovascular instability may be adequately managed with dialysis when medical therapy has failed. In the setting of acute overdose, especially with metabolic derangement as may be seen with aspirin overdose, dialysis can be a useful means of stabilising a patient until adequate acid–base homeostasis is achieved.

35 **c.** In early disease there are no clinical findings. With disease progression myoclonus and gait disorder may be seen but very unlikely to be present at the onset of the condition. A CT scan of the brain may show diffuse cortical atrophy in late disease but again in early disease there are often no radiological signs. Two of the commonest features to develop are memory impairment and language dysfunction, and dominant inheritance is seen in some families with an approximate age of onset of 50–60 years. Whilst insight remains depression is a common feature. As the disease progresses and insight is lost depression understandably becomes a less common feature.

36 **c.** In a case such as this one a diagnosis of a subarachnoid haemorrhage needs to be excluded. From the history it sounds as though the patient is quite well but she is describing the characteristic history of the worst pain ever experienced with no exacerbating or relieving factors. Subarachnoid haemorrhage can be fatal if it is not diagnosed and discussed with the neurosurgical team promptly. In many cases it can lead to fluctuations in the Glasgow Coma Scale requiring intensive monitoring and nursing. Whilst meningitis is important to rule out, the history is not classical for this. Subdural haemorrhages are most commonly seen in the elderly or in those patients who abuse alcohol. Benign intracranial pressure is most commonly seen in younger patients (20–40 years), usually females, particularly those with a raised body mass index.

37 **d.** *Bacillus cereus* is often associated with refried rice and is the culprit behind diarrhoea and vomiting that occurs soon after ingestion of food colonised by the bacterium. A mnemonic to help remember the association between *B. cereus* and rice is 'Eat refried rice? Be serious!' The onset of symptoms can be very rapid, anywhere between 1 and 5 hours from ingestion. *Clostridium botulinum* can be found in many processed foods and has been associated with 'floppy baby syndrome'. This is due to the release of botulinum toxin usually associated with babies who have been fed honey and subsequently suffer vomiting and even paralysis. Rotavirus is another important cause of diarrhoea in children and is often responsible for outbreaks of

playground diarrhoea. It is self-limiting and will resolve with adequate fluid rehydration and rest. *Cryptosporidium parvum* is a fungal infection commonly associated with HIV infection and usually resolves unless the patient is severely immunocompromised, i.e. CD4 count < 200. Treatment is supportive as there are no effective antimicrobial agents of proven value. *Escherichia coli* is possibly one of the more notorious causes of infective diarrhoea and has many subtypes. Enterotoxic *E. coli* is frequently associated with travel to different climates and cultures and has been aptly named 'traveller's diarrhoea'. As with almost all the types of diarrhoea the treatment is fluid rehydration. Antibiotics are not used unless there are signs of systemic compromise.

38 e. Budd–Chiari syndrome is due to obstruction of the hepatic vein causing back-pressure and eventual damage to the liver. Approximately one-third of cases have no identifiable cause; however, associations between hypercoagulable states have been well described in the literature. Oral contraceptive pill, polycythaemia rubra vera as well as haematological and intra-abdominal malignancy may all predispose to this catastrophic syndrome. Diagnosis is usually by venous phase CT scan, which delineates the filling defect in the hepatic vein and even inferior vena cava. Ultrasound of the liver may be a useful non-invasive bedside investigation to demonstrate retrograde flow in the portal system due to outflow obstruction and hence strengthen the diagnosis. Viral hepatitis may present similarly but usually with jaundice and right upper quadrant pain with or without a palpable liver. Gross ascites and signs of portal hypertension are not usually manifest without chronic liver disease and this goes against an acute infectious cause. Epstein–Barr virus infection can cause hepatomegaly and may occur post infectious mononucleosis but similarly to viral hepatitis does not usually cause a picture of chronic liver disease. Wilson's disease is a rare inherited disorder of copper metabolism causing hepatolenticular degeneration and deposition of copper in liver and basal ganglia. It causes both movement disorders and liver failure in those not identified and treated early. Deposition of copper in Descemet's membrane in the eye causing Kayser–Fleischer rings is pathognomonic of this disease. $\alpha 1$-antitrypsin deficiency affects both lungs and liver causing emphysema and chronic liver disease. $\alpha 1$-antitrypsin is a protease involved in damping down inflammatory cascades and plays an especially important role in the protection of alveoli from protease damage in the lungs. It is associated with chronic liver disease and hepatocellular carcinoma in adults in approximately one-fourth of all $\alpha 1$-antitrypsin deficient patients. **211**

39 c. This man is suffering from Crohn's disease (CD). The combination of clinical pattern and colonscopic appearance makes the diagnosis unlikely to be ulcerative or other types of colitis. Aphthous ulceration is often one of the earliest signs on colonscopy and occur anywhere from mouth to anus thus differentiating CD from ulcerative colitis (UC), which occurs proximally from the rectum occasionally involving the terminal ileum (backwash ileitis). CD can be thought of as a transmural inflammatory process with multiple skip lesions associated with a cobblestone pattern. The mnemonic, 'a thick old Crone skipping down a cobblestone pavement', sums up the histological and colonscopic appearance of CD neatly. Anal and perianal diseases are also a hallmark of CD very rarely seen in UC; this man is likely complaining of an anal fissure causing severe pain on passing stool and thus strengthens the diagnosis. Barium follow-through is an extremely useful investigation in eliciting small bowel involvement of disease and the pathological hallmark of small bowel CD of rose-thorn-type ulceration may be seen.

40 b. A typical regimen for the management of diabetic ketoacidosis (DKA) is outlined below:
1. Start an infusion of 50 units of short-acting insulin in 50 mL of 0.9% sodium chloride at a high rate (e.g. 6 units/hour) with 5 L fluid replacement with 0.9% sodium chloride.
2. Once blood glucose levels are below 15 mmol/L convert to 5% dextrose fluid replacement and halve infusion rate (e.g. 3 units/hour).
3. Monitor urine for ketones and once ketones are negative or very low and the patient is eating and drinking normally stop the insulin infusion.
4. If the patient is not eating normally convert insulin infusion to sliding scale with hourly blood glucose measurement.
5. Potassium is driven into cells by insulin and will thus appear initially high due to lack of insulin but will rapidly drop with sliding scale. Titrate up to 40 mmol/hour against the serum potassium.

The rationale for large volume fluid rehydration is that high levels of blood glucose cause a massive osmotic diuresis and may be associated with vomiting. Fluid losses through the kidneys and gastrointestinal tract lead to serious dehydration. High levels of insulin infusion are used to suppress ongoing ketogenesis, which will happen hours after the blood glucose levels have been brought down and thus urinary monitoring of ketones is vital to guide requirements to sliding scale. Metabolic acidosis will respond to fluid rehydration and will correct with the breakdown of ketone bodies, a byproduct of free fatty acid metabolism. Type I diabetics eating and drinking normally should be given subcutaneous insulin 30 minutes pre-prandially with insulin infusion stopped 1 hour after the meal to ensure adequate insulin cover during the transition. Basal bolus insulin or intermediate-acting insulin will not be adequate to suppress ketogenesis, which is key in correcting the metabolic acidosis and thus should not be used in the acute management of DKA.

41 d. This woman is exhibiting the symptoms and signs of diverticulitis. Left iliac fossa pain associated with a high white cell count, raised inflammatory markers and constitutional upset makes the diagnosis likely. A tender palpable mass in the abdomen is occasionally found on clinical examination but is not an indication for surgery as many can be managed conservatively with antibiotics such as cefuroxime and metronidazole. If an abscess is suspected that is resilient to medical therapy, CT-guided percutaneous drainage is a relatively safe and feasible option. CT scanning of the abdomen is a very useful imaging modality that carries none of the complications, e.g. perforation that direct visualisation of the bowel does. Recent trials of risk factors for diverticular perforation have identified a possible role for opioid and non-steroidal anti-inflammatory drug (NSAID) analgesia in the development of such complications. Long-term use of opioid analgesia has been shown to increase intracolonic pressure and hence possibly increase the risk of mechanical perforation of diverticulae. NSAIDs have been linked to an alteration in mucosal blood flow via prostaglandin inhibition leading to a consistently identified risk of perforation in up to 20% of diverticular complications. This should, however, not preclude the use of NSAIDs but guide sensible prescribing of this often feared analgesic agent.

42 d. Normal portal venous pressure is between 8 and $15\,cmH_2O$. Portal hypertension occurs when there is outflow obstruction to the portal system and can be evidenced by clinical manifestations and ultrasonographically, with reversal of flow along the portal vein. Obstruction can be classified as pre-hepatic, (e.g. portal vein thrombosis secondary to neonatal umbilical infection), hepatic (e.g. cirrhosis) or post-hepatic (e.g. tumour compression). As there is a rich collateral supply to the abdominal viscera, a substantial rise in portal pressure will cause the formation of porto-systemic anastomoses. The most clinically significant of these are oesophageal varices, which can present with life-threatening gastrointestinal bleeding. Splenomegaly can occur secondary to backpressure through the splenic vein and may cause leukopaenia, thrombocytopaenia and anaemia.   **213**

Diaphragmatic varices can complicate surgery at the time of liver transplantation and may cause subphrenic haematomas that may become secondarily infected and form abscesses.

43 a. The arterial blood gas (ABG) results provided in this question are all within the normal range. The patient has an adequate PO_2 without retaining carbon dioxide. These results suggest that 35% of oxygen is adequate for this patient; lower levels may not provide adequate oxygenation and higher levels may lead to CO_2 retention. A baseline ABG will have already been performed on air and therefore this is not necessary to repeat. It is important to repeat a blood gas sample on 28% oxygen as this may also provide suitable results. Having established the most appropriate oxygen concentrations it is sometimes useful to measure saturations after exercise to ensure that no drop is seen in the level of oxygenation. This patient went on to have lung function tests, which in addition to a $PaO_2 < 7.3\,kPa$ on air meant that he satisfied the criteria for long-term oxygen therapy.

44 e. Examination skills can be learned by rote to a large extent although an experienced candidate will be slick in their approach. Interpretation of clinical findings proves to be more of a challenge for students. In this case we are provided with three pieces of clinical information:
↓ chest expansion unilaterally.
↓ breath sounds on the affected side.
↓ percussion note on the affected side.

These features are all leaning towards a diagnosis of an extensive collapse or pneumonectomy. A lobectomy would be unlikely to provide such dramatic signs as the remainder of the lung normally expands to fill the void left by removal of a single lobe. Characteristic findings of a pleural effusion would be ↓ chest expansion on the affected side, stony dullness to percussion with bronchial breathing above the effusion. Other scenarios are widely available in clinical textbooks although there is no substitute for clinical practice for compounding your knowledge!

45 a. Flow volume loops can be difficult to interpret for the inexperienced student. The x-axis represents time, whilst the y-axis is a measure of both inspiratory and expiratory flow (the negative deflection is the inspiratory component whilst the positive is expiratory measured in litres per second.). Flow volume loop **a** shows a typical loop of a person that does not suffer with respiratory disease. The expiratory curve shows maximal peak expiratory flow and the straight line joining up to the inspiratory curve suggests a non-collapsible airway. Curve **b** represents a patient suffering with emphysema. The expiratory curve shows early airway collapse, the inspiratory phase is reduced in volume compared with our normal patient. Curve **c** represents fixed upper airways obstruction whilst **d** represents variable upper airways obstruction and curve **e** shows a restrictive pattern.

46 d. *Streptococcus pneumoniae* is the commonest cause of community-acquired pneumonia. Students are often under the misconception that the organism most likely to be responsible for community-acquired pneumonia is *Staphylococcus aureus*. This is responsible for most hospital-acquired pneumonias. *Haemophilus influenzae* is the second most common organism responsible for community-acquired pneumonia. Patients suffering from chronic obstructive pulmonary disease are most likely to get chest infections caused by Moraxella catarallis due to their underlying lung condition.

47 c. Antibiotic use in community-acquired pneumonia varies with GP preference. The recommended antibiotic for a simple case is amoxicillin (provided that the patient is not allergic to penicillins). Amoxicillin is derived from ampicillin which is better absorbed, producing higher plasma and tissue concentrations, and whose absorption is not affected by the presence of food in the gut. Augmentin is a compound preparation of amoxicillin and the beta-lactamase inhibitor clavulanic acid. The clavulanic acid protects the amoxicillin from the penicillinases produced by virtually all staphylococci and therefore this should not be given as first-line therapy since *Staphylococcus* is not one of the most common infective organisms. Metronidazole provides cover for anaerobes and works by breaking DNA strands. Erythromycin may be used in patients with allergies to penicillins.

48 a. While several other species of genus *Legionella* have been identified, *L. pneumophila* is the most frequent cause of human legionellosis and a relatively common cause of community-acquired and nosocomial pneumonia in adults. The organism can be found in natural aquatic habitats (freshwater streams and lakes, etc.) and artificial sources (cooling towers, potable water distribution systems). *Legionella* organisms are cleared from the upper respiratory tract by mucociliary action. Any process that compromises mucociliary clearance (e.g. smoking) increases risk of infection. *Legionella* organisms may infect other parts of the body including the lymph nodes, brain, kidney, liver, spleen, bone marrow and myocardium.

Staphylococcus aureus is usually a hospital-acquired pneumonia and pneumococcal pneumonia will usually present as a lobar infiltration.

49 b. There are two significant congenital diaphragmatic abnormalities that usually require intervention: (1) large central tendon defects and (2) herniation through the foramen of Bochdalek. Congenital herniation of abdominal contents through the foramen of Morgagni are usually small and insignificant and usually require no further treatment. Trauma to the diaphragm can occur with both blunt or penetrating injury to the abdomen and usually affect the relatively unprotected left hemidiaphragm. The liver usually takes the brunt of right-sided injury resulting in relative right hemidiaphragm sparing. These usually require urgent surgical intervention as fulminant respiratory distress is likely to occur. Embryologically the diaphragm is made up of the **s**eptum transversum, **p**leuroperitoneal membrane, **m**esentery of the dorsal oesophagus and the **d**orsal body wall, neatly summed up by the mnemonic 'Several Parts Make Diaphragm'.

50 a. Being of female sex affords a certain amount of resistance to the development of duodenal ulceration and this is markedly seen during pregnancy. Steroid use has been shown to predispose to the formation of ulcers by mechanisms that involve both a disturbance in acid regulation and secretion and interference with the normal protective mucosal layer of the stomach. Cushing's ulcer is the eponymous name given to the development of acute peptic ulceration secondary to head injury, major surgery or acutely stressful conditions, and a strong association between ulcer formation and severe burns has also been described (Curling's ulcer). These findings form the basis for the routine use of proton pump inhibitors such as omeprazole as part of the gastrointestinal prophylaxis of the critical care bundle in situations of acute stress.

51 e. Post-operative ileus is a common recognised sequel of abdominal surgery where handling of the bowel leads to a period of inactivity. It is commonly seen in open as opposed to laparoscopic procedures due to the greater manipulation of the bowel required in this type of approach. The initiation of oral intake is often subjective and will depend on factors such as the length of operation, the difficulty of the procedure, i.e. a case of ruptured appendix will normally accompany a greater period of bowel inactivity than an intact but inflamed appendix. Anastomotic leak is a serious complication more often seen during large bowel procedures due to the relatively poor blood supply to this part of the gastrointestinal tract. It is usually heralded by a tense, rigid abdomen, absence of bowel sounds and a patient who is unwell. Adverse reactions to anaesthetic agents are relatively common, however, usually present soon post-operatively or soon after induction of anaesthesia. Small bowel obstruction can be a long-term complication of any abdominal surgery, however, is almost never the cause of such a clinical picture so soon after appendicectomy.

52 d. The prescription of anti-emetic medication should always be with caution; the cause for vomiting should be assessed and a diagnosis made before starting anti-emetics. Serious causes for vomiting, e.g. gastrointestinal obstruction, must be excluded. Erect chest radiographs are useful if perforation is suspected; however, in this case the clinical index of suspicion is low and would not be a useful investigation. Abdominal radiographs are useful only in cases of suspected gastrointestinal obstruction, as a crude assessment of renal tract stones (a KUB – kidneys, ureter, bladder radiograph is far superior) and often as a useful method of confirming constipation in elderly patients who complain of abdominal pain and difficulty in passing stool! Nasogastric tube passage would be an option if vomiting were severe or unlikely to settle with anti-emetics. However, it would not be necessary to feed a patient like this via nasogastric tube in the short term and thus would be an unnecessary hindrance to recovery of normal oral intake. Proton pump inhibitors such as omeprazole are not required in a young patient without documented peptic ulcer disease and in this example would not afford any significant benefit in the immediate management of vomiting caused by post-operative ileus.

53 a. The diagnosis is strongly suggested by two salient features in the history: the presence of high blood glucose in an elderly man with no previous history of diabetes mellitus and jaundice. Compression of the distal end of the common bile duct by the head of the pancreas causes backpressure leading to jaundice. The presence of new-onset diabetes mellitus in the elderly should always be treated with suspicion and a diagnosis of diabetes mellitus should never be made until an attempt to rule out malignancy has been undertaken. Cholangiocarcinoma does present with weight loss, jaundice and deranged liver enzymes; however, the presence of raised blood glucose with a painless hepatomegaly is more suggestive of head of pancreas cancer. Choledocholithiasis (literally stone in biliary tree) can cause an intermittent jaundice and right upper quadrant pain, however weight loss and hepatomegaly suggest a more sinister cause. Hepatitis is usually associated with tender hepatomegaly and does not usually accompany raised blood glucose.

54 b. Chest radiography is the investigation most likely to aid with diagnosis of the cause of breathlessness. The history is consistent with an element of heart failure with peripheral as well as pulmonary oedema; however, a large unilateral pleural effusion should raise suspicion of a localised respiratory lesion, e.g. infection or malignancy. An echocardiogram will not be useful diagnostically as the clinical signs point to a degree of heart failure and an electrocardiogram, although a useful screening tool for suspected pulmonary embolus and signs of cardiac disease, can be performed later once localised disease has been ruled out. Pleural tap and drainage are the most useful diagnostically and therapeutically, however, in the non-acute situation radiographic confirmation of the diagnosis and extent of pleural effusion is useful. Finally, there is a tendency to start antibiotics empirically in elderly patients without accurate history of diagnosis. The minimal history and examination are not strongly suggestive of pneumonia and it is sensible to await chest imaging before considering antibiotics.

55 e. Scaphoid fracture. This injury is one of the most commonly injured bones of the carpal row, thought to be due to the higher stresses imposed on the scaphoid due to its unique position spanning both proximal and distal rows of the carpal bones. Falling on an outstretched hand is the mechanism of injury usually encountered in this type of injury, occasionally complicated by neurovascular compromise as with any fracture. Tenderness in the anatomical snuffbox forms a useful clinical reckoner if scaphoid fracture is suspected.

56 a. This history is representative of Crohn's disease. It is a chronic inflammatory condition of the GI tract, it is characterised by transmural granulomatous inflammation. Crohn's disease may affect any part of the gut from the mouth to the anus, but favours the terminal ileum and proximal colon. Unlike ulcerative colitis there are parts of the bowel that are unaffected in between lesions. Ulcerative colitis does not have skip lesions; 15% of patients have a positive family history and there is an increased risk in smokers of 3–4 times. Extra-intestinal signs include erythema nodosum, clubbing, conjunctivitis, episcleritis and arthritis among others. Investigations include blood tests, sigmoidoscopy and biopsies and small bowel enema. Exacerbations are managed with intravenous steroids and rehydration with topical treatment if necessary.

57 e. This lady is suffering with toxic shock syndrome. It was first described in 1978 and is caused by the exotoxin *Staphylococcus aureus*. In extreme cases the condition may progress onto *Streptococcus* multi-organ failure. Other clinical symptoms include a fluctuation in the level of consciousness and a widespread erythematous macular rash. The biggest clue to the diagnosis comes from the history of recent menstruation and useful investigations include vaginal examination, blood tests for U&Es, LFTs, clotting screen, FBC and arterial blood gas. Other useful tests include an ECG and a chest X-ray to exclude other causes of these symptoms.

58 d. *Gardnerella vaginalis* produces an offensive brown discharge, it causes an inflammation of the vagina in women or the glans penis in men. It often results in dysuria. Both chlamydia and gonorrhoea result in urethritis. Whilst most infections can be distinguished by colour or quality of discharge the most reliable method is by taking appropriate swabs.

59 d. The prevalence of disease is defined as the number of active cases in a defined time divided by the total population surveyed. The number of people with the disease is 20,000 people in that year with the total population in the same period being 140,000. Incidence is defined as the number of new cases diagnosed in given time period divided by the total population in that time period. Thus option **b** (500/140,000) describes the incidence of the disease.

Option **e** (250/140,000) describes the mortality rate specific to that disease. A similarly calculated figure is the absolute mortality rate (sometimes referred to as the death rate), which describes the total number of deaths per population.

60 e. An upper motor neurone paralysis is usually seen as a result of a stroke. It results in weakness of the facial muscles but spares the muscles of the forehead due to their dual innervation. The facial nerve arises from its origin in the pons and travels past the cerebello-pontine angle through the petrous part of the temporal bone to emerge via the stylomastoid foramen into the parotid gland where it divides into branches. Along its course it traverses with the chorda tympani and the nerve to stapedius, therefore if there is a lesion in the petrous temporal bone the facial weakness is accompanied by hyperacusis and loss of taste on the affected side.

Bell's Palsy is by far the commonest cause of a lower motor neurone lesion and is a diagnosis of exclusion. It is believed to result from a viral infection and results in swelling of the nerve in the petrous temporal bone. The absence of symptoms in any of the other cranial nerves helps to secure the diagnosis. Management involves time and most patients make a full and spontaneous recover over a period of months.

Extended matching questions

61 d. This scenario is describing a dislocation of the hip. This is commonly caused by trauma to the leg including a dashboard injury during a road traffic accident or injury involving a motorbike. From the examination the important features to remember are the positioning of the leg, although shortening is seen in both fractures and dislocations, internal rotation is characteristic of posterior dislocations of the hip. In cases of fractures or dislocations patients may well experience difficulty in weight bearing after the injury and therefore this does not distinguish one from the other. The other possible diagnosis in this case is a peri-prosthetic fracture, this will usually be clearly visible on X-ray if it is present.

62 a. This child is suffering with an irritable hip. Many hip conditions in children have similar presentation during their early stages and thus are difficult to distinguish. The commonest cause responsible for this condition is a transient synovitis which usually resolves within a couple of weeks. In a child of this age it is important to consider other paediatric conditions including Perthes' disease and slipped upper femoral epiphyses although both of these would have some positive findings on X-ray. Although his hip joint does not feel hot nor does it look erythematous the possibility of a septic arthritis needs to be investigated. This is done by a battery of blood tests including inflammatory markers and aspiration of the joint. In children, and particularly in the case of a hip joint this aspiration is best done under general anaesthetic in the operating theatre. The fluid obtained should be urgently sent to microbiology for microscopy, Gram staining and culture.

63 b. This patient has suffered a fractured neck of femur. This diagnosis should always be considered in elderly patients with a history of falls, particularly in those patients who are unable to weight bear due to pain. There are different types of neck of femur fractures and their management varies in accordance with the type of fracture sustained.

Fractures may be either intracapsular or extracapsular.

Intracapsular fractures

These are is divided by the level of the fracture line in the neck:

- Subcapital
- Transcervical
- Basal

In this group, the proximal fragment often loses part of its blood supply and hence the union of this fracture is difficult. This is a serious injury in the elderly patient. In the very old and debilitated person, it can precipitate a crisis in the precarious metabolic balance. It can become a terminal illness due to uraemia, pneumonia, bed sores, etc., and be fatal.

Extracapsular fractures

These are all grouped as trochanteric fractures of various types.

Patients with intracapsular fractures are managed by hemiarthroplasty whilst extracapsular fractures are managed with a dynamic hip screw.

64 e. This lady has suffered a peri-prosthetic fracture. In patients undergoing any kind of procedure involving insertion of prostheses this is a potential risk. It is believed that some of these fractures are caused at the time of insertion although, they are too small to be picked up at the time, it is only when they become symptomatic they are discovered. It is a particular complication with the resurfacing prosthesis – should this happen the management involves removing the prosthesis and inserting a more traditional hip replacement. For patients complaining of such symptoms so soon after surgery peri-prosthetic fractures should be considered as a potential differential diagnosis.

65 h. In this scenario the diagnosis is of a septic arthritis until proven otherwise. He has a fever and severely limited range of movement in the affected joint which are characteristic findings of a septic joint. It is normally said that the joint should be hot and swollen though in the case of the hip it is not possible to assess these findings due to the depth of the joint itself. The raised white cell count and inflammatory markers confirm the diagnosis and the ultimate way to do this is by aspirating a sample from the joint. In the case of the hip this is often done under general anaesthesia. In this particular case, if the metalwork has become infected it is more than likely that it will need to be removed and occasionally replaced.

66 a. Cocaine is a pre-synaptic reuptake inhibitor effectively increasing the synaptic concentrations of dopamine, noradrenaline and serotonin at higher doses. Dopamine is involved in the so-called 'reward' pathways of the brain and hence higher levels lead to the feeling of euphoria and 'high' that is produced by cocaine use. Cocaine is also a vasoconstricting drug and this action can be seen with disastrous effect in those individuals who swallow packets of cocaine with subsequent eruption of the packets in the gastrointestinal tract. Massive local vaso-constriction can occur leading to ischaemic segments of bowel as well as systemic absorption leading to tachycardia (due to increased sympathetic drive), myocardial ischaemia due to vasoconstriction and tachycardia (termed rate-related ischae-mia) that may manifest as angina and increased risk of stroke due to hypertension and localised ischaemia due to vasocon-striction followed by reperfusion injury.

The local anaesthetic effect of cocaine (it was for many years used as a topical anaesthetic agent) when applied systemically can cause conduction defects in the myocardium and arrhyth-mias and these must be borne in mind when treating patients with suspected cocaine overdose. Aspirin must not be used in the acute management of angina-like pain as the risk of cerebral haemorrhage post-vasoconstriction is high and bleed-ing can be catastrophic.

67 i. Marijuana (*Cannabis*) is the most commonly abused illicit substance in the United States. It has a variety of actions that vary from euphoria, an altered perception of space and time, hallucinations, anxiety and paranoia to drowsiness and with chronic use the development of an 'amotivational syndrome' characterised by a lack of interest in social and occupational life and a lack of energy. The mechanism of effect of marijuana is still largely unknown although the putative active agent is delta-L-tetrahydrocannabinol (THC), correlating to large num-bers of diverse THC receptors found scattered throughout the brain. Long-term effects include orthostatic hypotension and tachycardia and smoking marijuana has been linked with the development of a lung disease similar to chronic obstructive pulmonary disease. Effects on the central nervous system are controversial but appear to include a type of atrophy that may be related to long-term use. Frequently seen are the injected conjunctiva of marijuana use.

68 g. Chronic alcohol use has been linked to various vitamin and essential mineral deficiencies due to both a lack of dietary intake and secondary to vomiting. Most notable are the effects of a lack of thiamine and vitamin B12, which are involved in the development of Wernicke's encephalopathy and Korsakoff's psychosis and when chronic can lead to subacute degeneration of the spinal cord (vitamin B12). This lady is exhibiting signs and symptoms of Wernicke's encephalopathy – a triad of ataxia, ophthalmoplegia and confusion, and may progress to the irreversible Korsakoff's psychosis manifests as confabulation and memory deficits. The ECG changes are most likely due to hypomagnesaemia, occasionally seen in alcoholics, those with malabsorption syndromes and diabetics. The widened QT interval has been linked to a risk of developing torsade de pointes and correction of the electrolyte deficit should be part of the standard of care for the acute management of complications of chronic alcohol abuse.

69 **f.** Opioids are responsible for a plethora of adverse effects if abused the most serious of which is respiratory depression. This can often be so severe as to cause a life-threatening depression that may occur whilst the patient retains a level of consciousness. Miosis, nausea, vomiting, constipation, itch and hypotension are some of the other effects that are suggestive of opioid overdose. Florid respiratory depression may manifest clinically as a very low respiratory rate causing a drop in pH as CO_2 is not cleared and a loss of consciousness (hence the high CO_2 and low pH suggesting a respiratory acidosis in this scenario). Easily reversed by opioid antagonists such as naloxone and naltrexone the clinician must not be lulled into a false sense of security by the apparent improvement in the patient's clinical state as the effects of some of the longer-lasting opioids (such as methadone) and large doses can quickly overcome the effects of such antagonists.

70 **d.** PCP is a powerful dissociative hallucinogen originally used as an anaesthetic agent until the post-anaesthesia side-effects associated with the drug precluded its use. When abused it has been associated with psychosis, violence and agitation, tachycardia and high temperature and anxiety. Neurological signs such as vertical or horizontal nystagmus are common as is hypertension. Tachypnoea and irregular breathing patterns have been described in PCP users and rarely muscular rigidity syndromes and dystonias are seen. Treatment modalities aim to reduce absorption via the gastrointestinal tract when ingested and to reduce the agitating effects of the drug. Benzodiazepines are a safe antidote to control the behavioural symptoms associated with use and are preferable to antipsychotic agents, which carry the risk of causing neuroleptic malignant syndrome,

seizures and malignant hyperthermia. Rhabdomyolysis is a side-effect of muscular rigidity syndromes and merits testing of creatinine kinase levels and careful monitoring of renal function with aggressive fluid therapy if suspected.

71 **f.** Bacterial vaginosis, although a cause of vaginal discharge, is not usually classified as a sexually transmitted infection as it can present unrelated to sexual intercourse. The terminology vaginosis is used as there is usually no inflammation of the vagina, separating this condition from diseases causing vaginitis. A change in the normal pH of the vagina is thought to play a role in the alteration of the normal flora and encourages overgrowth of bacteria such as *Gardnerella vaginalis*, *Mycoplasma hominis*, *Mobiluncus* spp. and anaerobes such as *Bacteroides*. Microscopy of vaginal epithelial cells reveals the presence of 'clue cells', which are squamous vaginal cells on which the causative bacteria are attached.

72 **g.** Gonorrhoea typically presents in men with a yellow purulent discharge from the urethra with associated dysuria and irritation. However, *Neisseria gonorrhoea* has a predilection for epithelium of the cervix, rectum, conjunctiva and pharynx depending upon exposure to such sites. In women the presentation is much more subtle and insidious. Up to 50% of women may be asymptomatic with gonorrhoea and may eventually present with altered vaginal discharge, dysuria and intermenstrual bleeding with fertility problems as a long-term consequence of severe untreated infection. *Neisseria gonorrhoea* exists as Gram-negative intracellular diplococci and are easily recognisable on microscopy. Treatment involves using fluoroquinolones such as ciprofloxacin or ofloxacin for uncomplicated disease, amoxicillin (sometimes with probenecid) in penicillin-sensitive areas or ceftriaxone in areas of high penicillin resistance.

73 **a.** *Candida albicans* is an extremely common non-sexually transmitted infection of females and males. In females it can cause a very itchy vulvovaginal rash (pruritus vulvae) with a creamy white curd-like discharge from the vagina. In men infection with *Candida albicans* may occasionally arise due to cross-infection from a partner but more usually is the manifestation of an underlying disorder such as immunosuppression, diabetes or overuse of broad-spectrum antibiotics. In this case the patient was a known diabetic and some would argue that the routine workup of male patients presenting with balanitis (infection of the head of the penis) should include investigation of undiagnosed

diabetes. Treatment can be obtained over the counter as either a topical antifungal pessary or cream or as an oral tablet.

74 c. *Chlamydia trachomatis* is a common sexually transmitted infection with up to 5% of the UK population of sexually active women infected. It is often clinically silent until the long-term consequences are discovered and a retrospective diagnosis is offered. Some authorities report figures as high as 80% for asymptomatic infection in women with approximately half of all infected males demonstrating no clinical symptoms. Well-recognised sequelae of infection with *Chlamydia trachomatis* are infertility (due to salpingitis and pelvic inflammatory disease) and Reiter's syndrome – a triad of conjunctivitis, arthritis and urethritis. Diagnosis of *Chlamydia trachomatis* is complicated by the fact that it is an obligate intracellular bacterium and thus complex cell culture, direct fluorescent antibody and DNA testing form the mainstay of diagnostic techniques.

75 b. TV is a sexually transmitted infection that causes inflammation of the vagina (vaginitis) and can often be confused with bacterial vaginosis (BV) a non-sexually transmitted infection that does not affect the vagina itself. The discharge is classically described as a 'champagne discharge' as it is green-yellow and frothy and may accompany a 'strawberry cervix' – so-called as the cervix is often dotted with small haemorrhagic areas. Diagnosis is with dark-ground microscopy on a wet prepar-ation and treatment involves metronidazole 400 mg twice daily for a week.

76 a. Reiter's syndrome presents classically with a triad of urethritis, conjunctivitis and arthritis. It is sometimes sub-classified as part of reactive arthritis, which presents similarly after a gastrointest-inal infection. Reiter's syndrome typically affects young males with a sexually transmitted infection such as non-specific urethritis. Joint involvement is limited usually to a few large joints.

77 g. Psoriatic arthropathy may present with a range of arthritis patterns, the most common of which is arthritis affecting the distal interphalangeal joints. Evidence of nail changes is very strongly suggestive and manifest as nail pitting, nail dystrophy and onycholysis (lifting of the nail from the nail bed). For reasons still not entirely clear, between 5% and 8% of individuals with psoriasis develop a seronegative arthritis. Radiologically, the erosions of psoriatic arthropathy are central in the joint and present with thinning of the distal end of a phalanx (pencil) in a relatively spared proximal end of the adjacent phalanx (cup) giving a pencil-in-cup appearance.

78 h. Enthesopathy is an inflammation at the junction of ligament or tendon and bone and it occurs more frequently with seronegative arthritides than other arthritides, e.g. rheumatoid arthritis. Typically presenting as plantar fasciitis or Achilles tendonitis patients usually complain of pain and stiffness at the affected site. The pathogenetic basis of enthesopathy is still not known; however, molecular mimicry and cross-reaction between infective organisms and joint components are thought to play a role.

79 d. Ankylosing Spondylitis (AS) is more common in males than females and presents with back pain, morning stiffness, decreased thoracic excursion, chest pain as well as extra-articular features such as uveitis, enthesopathy and rarely aortitis. A reduction in back flexion to less than 5 cm as assessed by Schoeber's test in a young male with sacroiliac pain is almost diagnostic of ankylosing spondylitis. Radiological changes are marked with local erosion of bone at the junction of spinal ligament and bone with bone healing at these sights (syndesmophyte formation) causing ankylosis (fusion) of the vertebrae. AS and other spondyloarthritides are all associated with the HLA-B27 subtype.

80 b. Enteropathic arthropathy can be seen in between 10% and 15% of sufferers of ulcerative colitis and Crohn's disease. As with many of the seronegative arthritides the joints are affected in an asymmetrical pattern with the large lower limb joints preferentially affected. Interestingly the arthritis symptoms may occur some time before the gastrointestinal disturbance. Gastrointestinal bypass surgery has also been linked to the development of an arthritis picture similar to that associated with inflammatory bowel disease and is thought to be due to the introduction of antigens normally protected from the immune system by changes in the normal mucosal uptake of the gastrointestinal tract as a consequence of surgery.

81 f. Although there are several conditions that could mimic this history the most serious is a Wilm's tumour. They arise from the kidneys and may present with haematuria. Due to the nature of their presentation, these tumours can often become large before producing any symptoms or signs. Any patient with a suspected malignancy or suggestion of a mass should be sent for appropriate imaging, either CT scanning or ultrasound with an appropriate surgical referral made in anticipation of the result.

82 a. This vignette is describing a case of intussusception. It affects children between the ages of 6 months and 4 years old and results in abdominal pain. Since the affected children are young they often appear to be unwell, occasionally vomit and characteristically pass red currant jelly-like stool. Other clinical features include a fever and a palpable abdominal mass. Abdominal X-rays may appear to be entirely normal or may show an absent caecal shadow. Diagnosis may be confirmed or indeed managed by air or barium enema, it characteristically reveals a coiled spring or sudden termination of barium. These patients should be urgently referred to the surgical team.

83 **d.** The case in question is describing volvulus. This occurs when a segment of bowel rotates on its mesentery resulting in obstruction and abdominal distension with associated pain. There is an association with congenital malrotations but it can occur in other scenarios including adhesions from previous surgery or Meckel's diverticulum. The best management involves a high index of suspicion with rapid abdominal X-ray and surgical referral in order to preserve viable bowel.

84 **b.** This is a case of pyloric stenosis. It is most common in first born males and most frequently occurs between the ages of 2 and 10 weeks. Vomiting is characteristically projectile in nature with progressive dehydration and constipation. The vomiting is unaltered food and in severe cases a hypochloraemic acidosis may be seen. On examination a palpable mass in the epigastrium may represent the thickening of the pylorus – it is most easily felt during a feed. The diagnosis can be confirmed on ultrasound scan and surgical management is necessary to relieve the obstruction.

85 **e.** Acute appendicitis should always be considered in a child presenting with acute abdominal pain with fever. Although in this case it is important to be cautious that her symptoms do not relate to her reproductive tract. Further probing in the history revealed commencement of the pain in the centre of the abdomen some 24 hours earlier with radiation of the pain down to the right iliac fossa. Gynaecological causes of pain tend to originate in the appropriate iliac fossa. To confirm the diagnosis an ultrasound scan should be obtained as this can be useful in excluding diagnoses such as ovarian cysts in addition to confirming appendicitis.

86 **a.** The mechanism of action of atropine is via blockage of the vagus nerve and subsequently enhances sinus node automaticity and atrioventricular conduction:
- Atropine causes blockade of parasympathetic activity at both the sinoatrial (SA) node and the atrioventricular (AV) node

it may increase sinus automaticity and facilitate AV node conduction.
- Dosages of atropine for adults in asystole, or pulseless electrical activity with a rate less than 60 beats per minute, is 3 mg i.v..

Atropine may increase myocardial oxygen demand and unmask sympathetic overactivity.

87 e. The dose of magnesium sulphate is 8 mmol (4 mL of a 50% solution) for refractory ventricular fibrillation if there is any suspicion of hypomagnesaemia, especially if the patient is on potassium-losing diuretics.

Other indications are for the use of magnesium are:
- Ventricular tachyarrhythmias in the presence of possible hypomagnesaemia.
- Torsade de pointes.
  Digoxin toxicity.

88 c. The use of amiodarone in shock-refractory VF is believed to improve survival. Experts believe that in VF or pulseless VT resistant to three shocks there is a role for amiodarone. Initially 300 mg intravenously should be given before continuing with shocks. The UK Resuscitation Council suggests that a further dose of 150 mg may be given for recurrent or refractory VF/VT followed by an infusion of 900 mg over the next 24 hours.

89 f. Adenosine slows conduction across the atrioventricular (AV) node but has limited effect on myocardial cells, this makes it very effective for terminating paroxysmal supraventricular tachycardias associated with re-entrant circuits. Adenosine has a short duration of action and therefore the affect of the drug may be short-lived. Induction of AV nodal block can reveal underlying atrial rhythms in those patients presenting with narrow complex tachycardias, it slows down the ventricular response. Side-effects of administration of adenosine include episodes of severe bradycardia.

90 h. Flecainide is a potent blocker of sodium channels and therefore slows conduction. The effect of flecainide can be seen on the ECG as lengthening of the PR interval and widening of the QRS complex.

Flecainide is known to be negatively inotropic and may result in bradycardia and hypotension. Other side-effects documented include blurring of vision and oral paraesthesiae.

PAPER 3

Answers and notes

Multiple choice questions (single best answer)

1 a. Alport's syndrome is an inherited disease of the kidney affecting young boys between 5 and 20 years of age. Inheritance is in three forms: X-linked dominant, autosomal dominant or autosomal recessive. The clinical presentation is one of asymptomatic haematuria with progressive sensorineural deafness and eye disorders (lenticonus). Treatment is to support the progressive renal failure. Renal transplantation may be considered, however, there is a risk of anti-glomerular basement membrane nephritis even after transplantation. Anderson–Fabry disease is an X-linked-recessive disorder of trihexoside deposition. Clinical features include a burning sensation in distal limbs associated with a characteristic blue hued rash (angiokeratoma corporis diffusum). Goodpasture's syndrome is a pulmonary–renal syndrome manifest as pulmonary haemorrhage and massive haemoptysis associated with proliferative glomerulonephritis. Linear anti-glomerular basement membrane deposits are seen on immunofluorescent staining of biopsy specimens. Treatment involves aggressive immunosuppression with or without plasmapheresis. Wegener's granulomatosis is a necrotising granulomatous vasculitis affecting the respiratory tract and kidney. Typically sinusitis with epistaxis, haemoptysis and renal failure all co-exist. Autoantibody assay returns a positive anti-neutrophil cytoplasmic antibody (c-ANCA), which responds to corticosteroid and cyclosphosphamide. Von Hippel–Lindau syndrome is an oncologic vascular disorder manifest in many different organs with renal cysts and tumours, phaeochromocytoma, retinal angiomas and haemangioblastomas of brain and spinal cord being most frequently seen. Clinical clues to the diagnosis are often posterior fossa symptoms of dizziness, ataxia and headache in young adults often with retinal detachment detectable on fundoscopy.

2 d. Myeloma should always be kept in mind when considering the differential diagnosis of an elderly patient with back pain and renal failure. The simple and non-invasive urine test for Bence–Jones protein, the light-chain fragment of the B-cells overexpressed in myeloma, makes this investigation one that should not be overlooked in the diagnostic work-up of patients with renal failure. The mechanism of renal failure in myeloma is thought to be a directly toxic effect of light chains on the nephrons and leads to the characteristic 'flea-bitten' appearance of myeloma kidney. Paget's disease is a disorder primarily of bone remodelling leading to alternating osteoclastic bone resorption followed by abnormal osteoblastic woven bone formation. Symptoms usually include bone pain, excessive warmth over the affected bony sites due to hypervascularity, bony deformity and neuropathy due to nerve compression (especially the vestibulocochlear nerve). Sarcoidosis is characterised by the presence of non-caseating granulomata and is most classically a disease of the respiratory system, however, renal involvement is seen in rare cases. Hyperparathyroidism can lead to a raised calcium and is usually seen as the byproduct of failing kidneys. However, chronic hyperparathyroidism itself may manifest as renal stones, uraemia and eventual renal failure. Bony involvement is common and may be seen as an erosive arthropathy, subperiosteal bone resorption at the phalangeal tufts or a 'rickets-type' picture. Osteosarcoma presents typically with pain and soft tissue swelling and classically Codman's triangle is seen on radiographs, indicative of periosteal tenting from underlying bone. Radiographic appearances are usually a mixed lytic/sclerotic picture but purely lytic or sclerotic lesions can be seen.

3 c. Caeruloplasmin and serum copper are useful tests in the investigation of liver disease of unknown aetiology and are sensitive indicators of the presence of Wilson's disease (hepatolenticular degeneration). A renal ultrasound scan is useful to identify any obstruction, scarring from previous infection or altered renal size indicative of long-term renal damage or chronically reduced renal blood flow. Safe and non-invasive to perform this should always be considered in the investigation of renal disease. Complement levels (C3 and C4) as well as double-stranded DNA (dsDNA) and erythrocyte sedimentation rate (ESR) should be used as a screen for systemic lupus erythematosus (SLE, lupus) nephritis. Generally, an elevated ESR and anti-dsDNA and low C3 and C4 levels are associated with active nephritis. Anti-neutrophil cytoplasmic antibodies (ANCA) are useful in the detection of vasculitic diseases affecting the kidney such as Wegener's granulomatosis and Churg–Strauss disease among many. Bence–Jones protein (light-chain fragment) is a simple and effective screening tool for suspected myeloma with associated light-chain nephropathy and should never be omitted from the diagnostic work-up of renal failure.

4 a. Renal ultrasonography should be the first-line investigation of those listed. Other useful investigations to be considered initially should be a urine dipstick, urine pregnancy test and a bedside blood glucose level. Blood pressure is markedly elevated in this otherwise well middle-aged woman and the deterioration in renal function is significant. The additional clue from the history that two relatives suffered strokes at a 'young age' should prompt strong consideration of a diagnosis of autosomal-dominant polycystic kidney disease (ADPKD). ADPKD is associated with cerebral (berry) aneurysms, cysts in other organs such as liver, pancreas and spleen and cardiac valvular defects. Renal failure is progressive and may lead to end-stage renal disease (ESRD). Renal ultrasound scan is a very sensitive and specific tool in detecting cystic abnormalities of the kidneys and may well confirm the suspected diagnosis. CT scan of the head should not be rushed into on the basis of a lack of neurological signs until other simple investigations have been performed and would only be indicated if blood pressure control did not ameliorate symptoms. Renal biopsy is not without serious risks and should never be undertaken unless knowing histology will influence management; 24-hour urine collection for metanephrines is indicated in cases of suspected phaeochromocytoma and along with adrenal CT scanning aids diagnosis of this rare cause of hypertensive crisis. Carotid and vertebral Dopplers are sometimes indicated in cases of stroke secondary to suspected arterial stenosis such as atherosclerotic disease. A history of multiple transient ischaemic attacks (TIA) or strokes in the absence of a good cause such as atrial fibrillation may prompt examination of carotid arterial flow waveform. A similar process may occur in the vertebrobasilar system (so-called posterior circulation stroke) and manifests as symptoms of dizziness, vertigo, nausea and lower cranial nerve abnormalities.

5 c. This question has slightly different answers depending on practice in North America or other parts of the world, however, the main message is the same. Surgical exploration of both kidneys with histopathological diagnosis is the gold standard for focussing future treatment. In Europe imaging modalities may suffice for a firm diagnosis of unilateral versus bilateral disease to be made with an operative approach favoured in borderline cases. In North America there is a trend towards early operative diagnosis with exploration of both kidneys. CT scanning of the abdomen has a role in the diagnosis of a suspected Wilm's tumour, however, staging CT of the chest, abdomen and pelvis must be performed to assess for metastatic spread of tumour. Renal ultrasonography may initially be used to assess for tumour involvement, however, it does not carry the sensitivity nor specificity of CT or MR imaging. Chest radiography is a useful baseline investigation to assess for pulmonary metastases but again if Wilm's tumour is identified then staging CT is performed. Albumin/creatinine ratio is a very useful investigation in the work-up of renal disease of various origins and can detect microalbuminuria (defined as the presence of albumin in the urine of 30–300 mg/day) – one of the pathological hallmarks of early renal disease. Especially useful in the investigation of patients with diabetes and cardiovascular disease it should be performed on a regular basis to guide secondary prevention strategies, e.g. tight blood pressure or glucose control and as a prognostic indicator of the level of renal deterioration.

6 **c.** Drug-induced interstitial nephritis presents acutely typically following commencement of penicillins although it has been described in association with diuretics such as frusemide, non-steroidal anti-inflammatory drugs (NSAIDS) and sometimes with infections. Acute renal failure associated with fever, arthralgia, rash and eosinophils in both blood and urine help to make the diagnosis. Haemolytic uraemic syndrome (HUS) is a vascular disorder with the formation of platelet aggregates. A triad of symptoms are usually seen (i) microangiopathic haemolytic anaemia (ii) thrombocytopaenia and (iii) acute renal failure. It is the commonest cause of acute renal failure in children and usually occurs following a diarrhoeal disorder although many infections may cause HUS. Cholesterol embolus is rarely seen but can be catastrophic when occurring. Clinically manifest with disturbance of renal biochemistry associated with eosinophilia and purpura of limbs usually in those with arterial disease. A net-like rash (livedo reticularis) is sometimes described similar to that seen in systemic lupus erythematosus (SLE) and may aid diagnosis. Acute tubular necrosis is a common and spontaneously resolving cause of acute renal failure and is associated with hypovolaemia, drugs that are nephrotoxic and rhabdomyolysis by a direct insult to the renal tubules from excess myoglobin in the glomerular filtrate. The typical clinical picture is of acute renal failure refractory to rehydration that eventually responds within days to weeks. Treatment is to ensure adequate hydration until tubule function is restored.

7 **e.** Head injuries may result in basal fractures to the petrous temporal bone which can result in damage to the seventh cranial nerve. Although uncommon cranial sarcoid may be bilateral and can affect cranial nerves III, V, VI and VII. Lyme disease is caused

by infection via tics and the infective organism is Borrelia Bergdorfori. The commonest neuropathy associated with this condition is of the facial nerve and can once again be bilateral. Gullain–Barre syndrome is usually symmetrical and ascending in its presentation. In severe cases cranial nerves may be involved although in less severe cases its pathology remains in the limbs and trunk. Medullary infarction results in damage to the nucleus of cranial nerve VII which provides upper motor neurone signs.

8 d. Holmes–Adie pupil is usually large but can be small after pro-longed light exposure. In acute retrobulbar neuritis pupils are of normal size, often an afferent defect may be seen on the affected eye. Amitriptyline overdose gives large pupils due to the anti-cholinergic effect. Unequal pupils or anisocoria is seen in syphi-lis. Pontine haemorrhage gives a bilateral sympathetic lesion probably associated with parasympathetic overactivity resulting in constricted pupils.

9 b. A spastic paraparesis is usually seen in upper motor neur-one lesions. It is a fairly common feature of multiple sclerosis often due to plaques affecting the cervical and thoracic cord. In the case of syringomyelia, the syrinx acts as a mass effect often affecting the cervical cord resulting in upper motor neurone signs most commonly in the legs with a wasting and weakness affecting the trunk and arms in a cape-like distribution. In the case of a meningioma the symptoms are caused by a mass effect. Since the spinal cord terminates at the level of L1-2 any pathology affecting the lumbosacral spine will result in lower motor neurone signs and therefore weakness would be seen most commonly.

10 e. Hypercalcaemia may result in vague limb pains but not muscle cramps. A low calcium may account for twitching or tetany as will hyponatraemia or hypokalaemia. Cramps have been reported in cases of hyponatraemia. Central pontine mye-linolysis usually results from a rapid correction of hyponatrae-mia, the neurological symptoms that develop are believed to be secondary to oedema of the cells in the pons. Hyperthyroidism is known to result in proximal limb myopathies, tremor, hyper-reflexia and occasionally seizures as can hyponatraemia. A rare complication of hypoglycaemia is hemiparesis. It is occasionally seen in infants and children but is easily treatable with intraven-ous glucose which normally results in a complete recovery.

11 c. The nerve supply to the thenar muscles of the hand is the median nerve whilst, the nerve supply to the intrinsic small muscles of the hand is supplied by the ulnar nerve. A lesion of the ulnar nerve at the elbow would result in damage to the hypothenar and small muscles of the hand but would have no effect on the thenar eminence. Syringomyelia provides weakness and muscle wasting in a cape-like distribution and wasting in the arms is a fairly common peripheral symptom of ALS. Whilst osteoarthritis of the lower cervical and upper thoracic spine is uncommon, it does occur and would result in similar problems to those defined in this case.

12 **a.** Creutzfeld–Jakob disease is caused by a mutation in a naturally occurring in a prion protein. A typical presentation is by a progressive dementia and psychiatric symptoms. The new form of the disease is thought to be much slower in its onset developing over the course of a few years rather than a few months. Although a link to infected meat is a suspected cause this has not been confirmed but there is evidence to suggest that infection may be transmitted by surgical procedures and corneal transplants. Whilst imaging may provide diagnostic information tonsillar biopsy provides a tissue diagnosis.

13 **a.** CEA may be raised in gastrointestinal cancers, especially colorectal carcinoma. As with all tumour markers it can be raised in a variety of cases, notably pancreatitis, cirrhosis and smoking, and must be interpreted within the clinical context. Tumour markers should never be used as a diagnostic tool; the use of markers is to add weight to an already strong clinical index of suspicion and to help guide investigation of possible sites of neoplasm. CA19-9 is also associated with colorectal cancer, however, it may also be raised in pancreatic cancer. AFP is most specific for hepatocellular carcinoma but also may rise in germ cell tumours as well as other liver disorders. NSE is specific for small cell carcinoma of the lung and HCG is raised in pregnancy (depending on your point of view possibly the most benign cause of a distended abdomen) as well as germ cell tumours. CA 153 is raised most commonly in breast disorders including cancer and benign breast disease.

14 **b.** HIDA scan is a nuclear medicine scan involving intravenous injection of a ^{99m}technetium-labelled derivative of iminodiacetic acid. It is an invaluable scan in the investigation of bile duct leakage post-operatively. The radionuclide is excreted by the liver into the biliary system and through into the duodenum. Imaging is taken serially after injection and will define the gallbladder to duodenum in hours. Identification of leaks is evident as nuclear uptake in areas external to the biliary

system. HIDA scan has an additional purpose in the identification of acute cholecystitis and has a sensitivity of around 96% and a specificity of around 94%. The easily performed and non-invasive ultrasound examination of the gallbladder has, however, rendered HIDA obsolete as a first-line investigation for the diagnosis of cholecystitis. Plain abdominal radiograph will not detect a bile leak, however, it may be useful in showing air in the biliary tree as may occur with conditions such as choledochal fistula seen in gallstone ileus and with gas-forming organism infection of the biliary tree. CT scan of the abdomen will detect hepatic abnormalities such as cysts, tumours and collections but is poor at visualising the biliary system and will not demonstrate bile leak. ERCP is both a diagnostic and therapeutic tool for imaging the biliary and pancreatic tree, however, is not as sensitive as HIDA as demonstrating bile leak.

15 d. This clinical picture points towards a lung abscess. Most frequently, the lung abscess arises as a complication of aspiration pneumonia caused by mouth anaerobes. Abscesses can be primary or secondary in origin. A primary abscess is infectious in origin, caused by aspiration or pneumonia in the healthy host whilst a secondary abscess is caused by an underlying condition (e.g. obstruction), spread from an distal site, bronchiectasis and/or an immunocompromised state. It is possible to classify accesses by the infectious organism, e.g. *Staphylococcus* lung abscess and anaerobic or *Aspergillus* lung abscess.

In this clinical scenario the important factors to identify are the swinging fever and the recurrence of cough with foul smelling sputum shortly after a chest infection. These are both factors that should raise suspicion of an abscess. In addition, the X-ray findings of a walled cavity should raise the possibility of the diagnosis. Empyema is different as it is inflammatory fluid and debris within the pleural space. It may result from an untreated pleural space infection which subsequently progresses collection in the pleural space.

16 b. Bronchiectasis is the abnormal and permanent distortion of one or more of the conducting bronchi or airways, most often secondary to an infectious process. It can be catagorized as a chronic obstructive pulmonary lung disease manifested by airways that are inflamed and easily collapsible, which in turn results in air flow obstruction and impaired clearance of secretions. It may be congenital or acquired, although the congenital form is normally diagnosed during childhood. The condition results in destruction of muscular and elastic components of the bronchial walls, which impairs mucociliary clearance and predisposes to recurrent infections.

Impaired clearance of secretions causes colonisation and infection with pathogenic organisms, contributing to the common purulent expectoration noted in patients with bronchiectasis. The result is further bronchial damage and a vicious cycle of bronchial damage, bronchial dilatation, impaired clearance of secretions, recurrent infection and more bronchial damage.

Diagnosis is usually based on a compatible clinical history of chronic respiratory symptoms, such as a daily cough and viscid sputum production, as well as typical findings on CT scan.

17 d. There are many causes of round opacities on chest X-rays. Their location may provide a clue to the likely diagnosis but often it is necessary to revert back to the history and examination for clues. Tuberculosis tends to present in the apices due to the apparent improved oxygenation. Both lung cancer and carcinoid tumour can present anywhere in the lung fields as round lesions.

Sarcoid is a multi-system disorder characterised by non-caseating epithelioid granulomas. Other commonly involved organ systems include the lymph nodes; the skin; the eyes; the liver; the heart; and the nervous, musculoskeletal, renal and endocrine systems. Patients usually complain of non-specific symptoms including weight loss and fatigue. Chest symptoms are fairly common amongst sufferers of the disease.

18 e. Syndrome of inappropriate anti-diuretic hormone secretion is associated with small cell lung cancer. Release of anti-diuretic hormone results in the dilution of the serum, which in turn gives a relative hyponatraemia. Depending on the location of the lung cancer, local spread can include applying pressure onto the superior vena cava resulting in reduced blood return to the heart from the upper half of the body. The superior vena cava is the major drainage vessel for venous blood from the head, neck, upper extremities and upper thorax. It is located in the middle mediastinum and is surrounded by relatively rigid structures such as the sternum, trachea, right bronchus, aorta, pulmonary artery, and the perihilar and paratracheal lymph nodes. It is a thin-walled, low-pressure, vascular structure. This wall is easily compressed as it traverses the right side of the mediastinum.

Clinical features include venous distension of the neck and chest wall, facial oedema, upper extremity oedema, mental changes, lassitude, cyanosis and even coma.

Pressure on the recurrent laryngeal nerve can result in a palsy of the vocal cords and a hoarse voice whilst growth into the sympathetic system can lead to a Horner's syndrome, ptosis, meiosis and anhydrosis on the ipsilateral side.

Pulmonary oedema is not a complication of lung cancer.

19 e. Respiratory failure is a syndrome in which the respiratory system fails in one or both of its gas exchange functions: oxygenation and carbon dioxide elimination. Respiratory failure may be classified as hypoxaemic or hypercapnic and may be either acute or chronic.

Hypoxaemic respiratory failure (type I) is characterised by a low PaO_2 with a normal or low $PaCO_2$. This is the most common form of respiratory failure, and it can be associated with virtually all acute diseases of the lung, which generally involve fluid filling or collapse of alveolar units. Some examples of type I respiratory failure are cardiogenic or non-cardiogenic pulmonary oedema, pneumonia, acute pulmonary embolus and acute exacerbation of asthma.

Hypercapnic respiratory failure (type II) is characterised by a low PaO_2 and a high $PaCO_2$. The pH depends on the level of bicarbonate, which, in turn, is dependent on the duration of hypercapnia. Common causes include drug overdose, neuromuscular disease, chest wall abnormalities and severe airway disorders (e.g. asthma, chronic obstructive pulmonary disease (COPD) and chronic pulmonary emboli).

20 c. Major risk factors for pulmonary emboli include:
- Immobility.
- Abdominal/pelvic surgery.
- Malignancy (abdominal/pelvic/advanced metastatic).
- Lower limb fracture.
- Pregnancy.
- Hip/knee replacement.
- Previous venous thromboembolism.

Minor risk factors include:
- Oral contraceptive pills.
- HRT.
- Long-distance travel.

21 d. Liver failure presents with a plethora of physical signs: jaundice, fluid shift leading to pulmonary oedema and effusion, ascites and peripheral oedema and biochemical derangement of liver function, e.g. increased clotting time, decreased protein/immunoglobulin synthesis, etc. Fluid collections associated with liver failure tend to be transudates rather than exudates (transudates <30g/dL protein; exudates >30g/dL). 'Exudates Exceed 30g/dL protein' is one way of remembering the association. Transudates are mainly associated with *failures*:

1. Heart failure.
2. Liver failure.
3. Kidney failure (nephrotic syndrome).
4. Thyroid failures.

On the contrary, exudates are mainly associated with:

1. *Infection* (e.g. pneumonia, TB).
2. *Inflammation* (e.g. rheumatoid arthritis, SLE).
3. *Malignancy* (e.g. bronchial carcinoma, lymphoma and mesothelioma).

The most likely diagnosis from the pleural tap would be malignancy in this case and must be excluded.

22 **d.** Midline shift is a warning sign of raised intracranial pressure and eventual herniation of brainstem through the foramen magnum. Colloquially known as cerebral compartment syndrome any space-occupying lesion such as tumour, infection, bleeding, etc. may cause a rise in the pressure inside the closed space with catastrophic effect. Modalities used for treating non-surgically amenable causes of raised intracranial pressure include: (1) raising the head of the bed to 30 degrees, (2) osmotic diuresis with mannitol, (3) thiopentone infusion and (4) hyperventilation (rarely performed). Extradural haematoma evacuation is a priority in cases of proven midline shift and/or localising signs (e.g. pupillary inequality). Neuroradiological clipping or coiling of intracerebral aneurysm is not indicated here as the source of bleeding is external to the brain itself.

23 **a.** Respiratory distress is a complication of upper torso burns that must be closely monitored. Surgical escharotomy may be required to release the mechanical restriction to breathing caused by circumferential burns to the chest wall. Infection may result in the intervening period as wound breakdown occurs but does not present such an emergency. Loss of peripheral pulses is again treated with surgical release of constricting tissues most often associated with circumferential burns of the limbs and may influence the decision to transfer an otherwise stable patient to a specialist burns unit rather than at a general treatment centre. Acute stress ulceration (Curling's ulcer) is managed with proton pump inhibition and has been robustly shown

to be effective in treating this complication. Severe dehydration is a close second for the most important complication to be vigilant for in severe burns, however, younger patients can tolerate a larger degree of fluid loss than the elderly. A rough indication to prognosis following burns can be estimated by using the formula below:

patient's age + % burn > 100 = poor chance of survival
e.g. 48-year old + 35% burn = 83
i.e. moderate chance of survival

24 b. The growth of male breast tissue, known as gynaecomastia, is a normal finding in the neonate due to maternal oestrogens, and the pubertal boy and elderly male due to the changing ratio of testosterone to oestrogens in these age groups. This is not a typical finding that would be consistent with non-accidental injury and therefore a referral to social services would be inappropriate. Referral to a breast surgeon and needle aspiration are also unjustified in this case and may even be deleterious to growing breast tissue. Short-course prednisolone is also unwarranted and is not indicated in cases of gynaecomastia.

25 e. Ureteric obstruction is confirmed clinically by an intravenous urogram (IVU). In up to 90% of cases the causative stone can be seen on X-ray of the kidneys, ureter and bladder (KUB) and this is recommended prior to undertaking an IVU as contrast may obliterate from view a small but otherwise radio-opaque stone. Delayed excretion and dilatation of ureter or renal pelvis are useful in making the diagnosis and are frequently seen in this investigation. Reduction in kidney size is not due to obstruction of the outflow tract with the opposite often the case. Perfusion defects can occur in cases of inflow limitation such as renal artery stenosis but will not occur due to outflow obstruction. Bladder residual volumes are rarely seen in cases where a stone has travelled the length of the urinary tract and lodges distal to the neck of the bladder.

26 c. Adhesions post-surgery and strangulated hernias are the most common causes of obstruction of the bowel and therefore are not to be missed when assessing a patient. Classically small-strangulated femoral hernias are missed in obese elderly women. Ulcerative colitis is a disease affecting the colon with the exception of backwash ileitis and would not considered as a cause of small bowel obstruction in this woman. Gastro-colic fistulae can occur in Crohn's disease but more commonly lead to faeculent vomiting than obstruction. Intussusception is a disease affecting typically 5–12-month-old infants. Meckel's diverticulum can lead to small bowel obstruction but this is rare and the most common presentation is one of inflammation.

27 a. He is suffering from rheumatic fever. This infection remains common in the Third World although it is a dreaded complication of a streptococcal sore throat in the West. Diagnosis is made on a group of criteria.

- *Major criteria*:
  - Carditis – tachycardia or new murmurs.
  - Arthritis – usually a migratory arthritis.
  - Subcutaneous nodules.
  - Erythema marginatum – rash with raised red edges and a clear centre.
  - Sydenham's chorea.
- *Minor criteria*:
  - Fever.
  - Raised ESR or CRP.
  - Arthralgia.
  - Prolonged P-R interval.
  - Previous rheumatic fever.

Using the revised Jones' criteria there must be evidence of a recent *Streptococcus* infection and 2 major criteria **or** 1 major and 2 minor criteria.

28 b. This vignette represents a clinical picture of coarctation of the aorta. In this picture there is narrowing of the aortic lumen just distal to the subclavian artery. This results in left ventricular hypertrophy as a result of increased afterload and hypertension secondary to reduced renal perfusion. The reduced blood flow results in the mottled appearances of the lower limbs. Cyanosis does not usually occur in this condition unless the patient is severely anaemic.

29 c. This girl is suffering from pelvic inflammatory disease. This disease ascends from the cervix to the uterus and the fallopian tubes. On examination it is common to find a low-grade pyrexia with lower central abdominal pain. There may be associated nausea and vomiting with tenderness on vaginal examination with cervical excitation commonly exhibited; 90% of there infections are sexually transmitted and the commonest age group to be involved is those between 15 and 20 years of age. The commonest causative organism is *Chlamydia trachomatis* but *Neisseria gonorrhoea* is often implicated. Following pelvic inflammatory disease there is a 5 times increased risk of developing an ectopic pregnancy and infertility.

30 a. 90% of cervical cancers are squamous. Of the remaining 10% the majority are adenocarcinoma. It is a disease that is heavily screened for but symptoms are all too often ignored by those affected. There is a national screening programme in which all women aged 25 years and over (or younger in socially deprived areas) are invited to attend a 3 yearly screening program. There is currently a vaccine under trial for Human Papilloma Virus (HPV) although, it is in the clinical trial stage at present. A common presentation is intermenstrual bleeding or post-coital bleeding which should always prompt an internal examination and speculum. Any patient that has an abnormal looking cervix should be referred to the local gynaecological service for further review and testing.

31 e. The Chi-squared test is most often used in situations where raw data is being examined for effect and is similar to the paired t-test in generating p values, however, the latter is used for comparison of the means of two populations. p value generation describes the number generated by calculation of the squared difference between the observed and expected values as a fraction of the expected values. This value is then converted to a p value relative to the degrees of freedom associated with the number of rows and columns involved.

p values are useful determinates of whether an observation (or set of observations) generated is likely to be due to chance. For example, setting a p value of less than 0.05 is often taken to herald significance (meaning that you are confident that there is only a 5% risk that the data is due to chance events rather than the ordered effect of a true measurable difference). Limits for significance cutoff can be set at higher or lower levels such that in a small population it may only be appropriate to use a cut-off value of less than 0.01, i.e. 1% to attain significance, although this may be in practice difficult to achieve.

Positive predictive values refer to the predictive power of a test and is defined as the number of true positives who tested positive for a disease. It is a useful method of assessing the accuracy of a test and as it is linked to the prevalence of a disease in a population (number of active cases per population per unit time) it will become more reliable with higher prevalences (due to reduction of the statistical error generated by small sample size).

Odds ratio is used to approximate the relative risk of an event occurring and is used most often in examining data from case-control studies.

The Mann–Whitney *U*-test is a non-parametric test that compares two unpaired groups, that is to say that they do not have to follow a normal distribution and the variance within the population from which the data are selected does not have to be equal. The test compares two medians to assess whether the samples are from the same population or not. For simplicities sake it is essentially a non-parametric, i.e. does not have the same constraints on population variance and distribution as the *t*-test but allows a comparison to be made between two data sets.

32 c. Although radiologically the cervical spine X-rays are clear and clinically the patient complains of no tenderness it is important that a CT scan of her neck is organised urgently and her neck is kept immobilised in the meantime. The key feature in this history is the fractured distal radius and iliac wing as well as the history of a fall from a height of approximately 15–20 feet. Having sustained other serious injuries this patient is not in a position to confirm or deny any cervical spine tenderness. In the presence of distracting injuries further imaging should be sought before removal of cervical spine protection. If you ever have any doubts the case should always be discussed with a senior colleague as the consequences of any error is potentially life threatening.

33 d. Loss of pulse is a very late sign of compartment syndrome. If not suspected before this sign is present, the outcome is likely to be poor. Signs of compartment syndrome include:
1. pain in the affected limb disproportionate to the injury,
2. pain on passive movements of the affected limb,
3. pallor,
4. paralysis (often difficult to asses due to presence of cast),
5. paraesthesiae.

If there is any doubt about the integrity of a compartment the intra-compartmental pressure should be measured. As a guide, if it is greater than 40 mmHg urgent treatment, e.g. fasciotomy, should be considered. If you suspect a diagnosis of compartment syndrome senior review should be sought.

34 d. Patients have the right to be fully informed about their diagnosis in order that they may make informed decisions about their medical care. In the case of patients who are assessed to be competent this should always be the principle upon which to act.

In very special situations where the release of a diagnosis is very strongly thought to be seriously detrimental to the health of the patient (and advice from psychiatrists and ethics departments and close communication with the family is strongly advised) then a diagnosis may be withheld from a patient although these cases are few and far between and should only be made by the consultant in charge of that patient's care.

It is required of a doctor who has requested an investigation under implied, verbal or written consent (such as laboratory tests or a chest radiograph, etc.) to disclose the results of that investigation as and when the results become available in a timely manner such that the patient is given adequate time and information to make an informed choice regarding their care. For example, informing a patient that they are to receive a blood transfusion for anaemia on the basis of blood results known the day before surgery 10 minutes from the time of surgery is not appropriate.

Leaving decisions to break bad news to other health care providers who were not responsible for ordering the diagnostic investigation is also not appropriate (e.g. requesting an HIV test on a medical inpatient and asking the GP to break the news of a new diagnosis of HIV).

Additionally, although family members may be involved closely in the care of their relatives with the consent of the patient, it should not be left to the family to disclose results of investigations or aspects of medical care with the patient without a doctor discussing these directly with the patient. The responsibility of a doctor caring for a patient does not extend to the family and the relationship should be confidential and exclusive unless explicitly expressed by the patient themselves. As a useful rule of thumb in the clinical setting, if there is ever any doubt regarding the appropriateness of an interaction then the patient's right to absolute confidentiality to the treating team(s) directly involved in their care must be preserved and consent to extend that confidentiality to include other members must be authorised by the patient themself.

35 **e.** Dapsone is a sulpha-derivative drug that is employed in the effective treatment of dermatitis herpetiformis. Treatment modalities used in the management of psoriasis include agents to keep the skin hydrated such as moisturisers and emollients, cold tar, topical steroids and vitamin D analogues and vitamin A analogues such as tazarotene. Erythrodermic or acute generalised pustular psoriasis is one of the few true dermatological emergencies and should be initially managed with topical treatments and immunosuppressants such as methotrexate and cyclosporin. **243**

Cold tar has anti-inflammatory properties that make this most effective in treating chronic plaque psoriasis, however, patient concordance with treatment is poor. Systemic treatments are also employed to managed chronic stable psoriasis and guttate psoriasis and may consist of ultraviolet light therapy or photo-chemotherapy such as PUVA (**p**soralen plus **u**ltraviolet **A** light), which can be effective in almost all kinds of psoriasis.

36 **a.** The presentation is strongly suspicious for scabies and in this age group should be high on the differential of an itchy rash. Scabies is caused by the *Sarcoptes scabiei* mite, which has a pre-dilection for the epidermis. Typical features of scabies are of an intensely itchy rash, which is caused by a delayed type hyper-sensitivity reaction to the mite itself, with characteristic inflam-matory papules and almost pathognomonic burrows or tracts. Areas commonly affected include the hands and feet with fin-gers, wrists and webspaces, the most often afflicted. Treatment modalities include one or two applications of malathion or per-methrin cream, which are left on the skin for a period of 12 or 24 hours. Aqueous cream is used in the treatment of eczema and whilst it may give some mild symptomatic relief, is not effective in treating scabies. Flucloxacillin 500 mg 3 times daily is usually given in conjunction with another penicillin derivative for cellu-litic infections. If a viral infection was suspected in a young child it may be appropriate to adopt a conservative management pol-icy, however, this will not lead to adequate symptom control and resolution in scabies. Cold tar is a very effective but messy treat-ment option in the management of psoriasis and acts as an anti-inflammatory agent when applied topically to psoriatic areas.

37 **b.** The history above is describing a case of pyelonephritis. The features of the vignette suggesting more than a simple urinary tract infection include the systemic signs of fever, tachypnoea, low saturations and tachycardia. In this case the blood results also showed a raised white cell count with a creatinine of 468 suggesting an acute renal failure secondary to the pyelonephri-tis. This lady made a good recovery with a combination of i.v. fluids and reduced doses of gentamycin and timentin. Since she experiences systemic symptoms oral antibiotics with com-munity follow-up would be an inadequate management plan, although catheterisation and analgesia are important adjuncts to her therapy, alone they are insufficient.

38 **d.** In patients with bowel cancer urinary symptoms are fairly common. The mass effect from the bowel mass exerts pressure

on the urinary system which causes urinary retention. This may subsequently result in a urinary tract infection due to stagnation of urine but the initial symptom is one of difficulty in instigating urination. In those patients undergoing either elective or emergency bowel surgery it is of vital importance that a catheter is inserted to keep the bladder decompressed at all times and to prevent any stagnation in the system. Bowel cancer does not metastasise to the prostate gland and bladder cancer usually results in painless haematuria as a presenting symptom as opposed to dysuria.

39 d. The protein content of the fluid aspirated from the pleural effusion is consistent with a transudate. Causes of transudates can be grouped together as 'failures' e.g. cardiac failure, liver failure (cirrhosis), renal failure (nephrotic syndrome) and thyroid failure (hypothyroidism). Exudates are defined by a protein content greater than 30g/L and caused by infections (e.g. pneumonia), inflammations or malignancies (e.g. bronchial carcinoma).

40 c. Vomiting in meningitis is due to raised intracranial pressure and is central or neurogenic in origin. Patients may offer this clue to the cause of their vomiting by stating that the episode of vomiting came as a surprise to them and was not preceded by a period of nausea. Other causes of neurogenic vomiting are centrally acting drugs and any other cause of raised intracranial pressure such as space-occupying lesion. The other options, whilst feasible, are less likely to be the cause of vomiting in an otherwise healthy young man. NSAID-associated gastritis would be more likely to occur in an elderly patient but more often presents insidiously as an iron-deficient anaemia or occasionally as melaena.

41 d. The case describes a history of a transient ischaemic attack, there is no residual neurological deficit 24 hours after onset of symptoms. Risk factors for TIAs include: male sex, age, smoking, diabetes, hypercholesterolaemia, hypertension and past history of cardiovascular disease. This gentleman had his carotid vessels scanned which showed an 80% stenosis which means that he is at a high risk of developing a further TIA or CVA in the following months. With these findings on carotid scanning the patient should be referred to a vascular surgeon with a view of doing a carotid endarterectomy to reduce the chances of an embolus being dislodged.

42 a. Haloperidol is an extremely useful medication for the acute management of a confused patient with agitation and behavioural symptoms. An alternative agent used to manage behavioural effects of dementia is risperidone, which shares a similar incidence of Parkinsonism side-effects but is more expensive than haloperidol. Given orally, intramuscularly or intravenously these are effective first-line medications for the treatment of acute behavioural crises.

Benzodiazepines should be avoided in demented patients due to the paradoxical exacerbation of behaviour and sedation that occurs. In the acute setting a demented patient should never be assumed to suffer from intrinsic dementia until all organic and reversible causes have been ruled out. A nice mnemonic for tying in the causes of dementia is 'DEMENTIAS' – standing for **D**egenerative diseases (Parkinson's disease, Huntingdon's disease, Alzheimer's disease), **E**ndocrine disorders, **M**etabolic derangement, **E**xogenous factors (heavy metals, drugs, medications), **N**eoplasia, **T**rauma (e.g. subdural haematoma), **I**nfection, **A**ffective disorders (e.g. pseudo-dementia) and va**S**cular (vascular dementia, ischaemic stroke and vasculitis).

Memantine is an NMDA antagonist used in the treatment of cognitive symptoms of Alzheimer's disease. It may be most effective when used in conjunction with cholinesterase inhibitors such as galantamine and rivastigmine. These medications act to increase acetylcholine levels, thought to be the biological correlate responsible for memory and concentration. There is evidence that the cholinesterase inhibitors may ameliorate the so-called secondary (behavioural) component to Alzheimer's disease, however, they are not appropriate for use acutely in the demented patient.

Olanzipine and the other atypical antipsychotic agents are effective agents when used as maintenance of behavioural disturbance, however, are not as predictable in effect when used acutely and thus tend to accede to the 'older' neuroleptic medications such as haloperidol and risperidone.

Sertraline is a selective-serotonin reuptake inhibitor (SSRI) and is a useful adjunct in the treatment of depressive symptoms associated with dementia. It has a good side-effect to treatment profile and may have some benefit for psychotic disturbance as well as mood disturbance.

43 b. The tricyclic antidepressants have a recognisable pattern of toxicity that occurs in overdose, which can be summed up as the 'Tri-C's of toxicity' – **C**onvulsions, **C**oma, **C**ardiac arrhythmias. Patients may present asymptomatically having been found by someone close to the patient or they may sometime self-refer to hospital feeling remorseful of their actions, however, serious side-effects may be delayed for between 2 and 6 hours post-ingestion and careful monitoring should be undertaken of anyone suspected of having an overdose. Cardiac monitoring is essential due to the inhibition of normal cardiac conduction (due to inhibition of the fast sodium channel) leading especially to a prolonged QT interval. Anti-cholinergic effects are also seen commonly with overdose of the tricyclics due to their potent competitive antagonism at central and peripheral muscarinic acetylcholine receptors.

Monoamine oxidase inhibitors (MAOI) such as tranylcypromine when taken in overdose usually manifest with symptoms of catecholamine excess (e.g. sweating, tachycardia, hypertension, tremours and seizures) but arrhythmias are typically uncommon in the setting of pure MAOI ingestion. A well-recognised phenomenon occurring in individuals who are prescribed MAOIs is a hyperadrenergic state resulting from the ingestion of foods containing tyramine such as cheese, red wine and some meats and is due to the build-up of tyramine in the presence of MAOIs (as it is not broken down due to the enzyme inhibition) and acts as a sympathomimetic.

A similar phenomenon known as a serotonin syndrome may occur in individuals co-prescribed MAOIs and selective-serotonin reuptake inhibitors (SSRIs) or even those who overdose with SSRIs (e.g. sertraline) with symptoms of flushing, a change in mental status, sweating and hyperthermia as well as neuromuscular agitation may occur.

Beta-blockade usually causes symptoms of bradycardia and hypotension, which may be life threatening. Other effects less commonly seen are bronchospasm in sensitive individuals and hypoglycaemia in diabetics. The agent of choice to reverse beta-blocker overdose is glucagon, which seems to act independently of the beta receptor to increase heart rate and myocardial contractility.

Digoxin toxicity is manifest by a yellow-green colour disturbance to normal vision, confusion and/or agitation in addition to the distinctive 'reverse tick sign' on electrocardiography. Premature ventricular contractions (PVCs), bigeminy and trigeminy are often encountered signs of digoxin toxicity. Hypokalaemia, hypomagnesaemia and hypernatraemia can all potentiate digoxin toxicity even at normal therapeutic doses and should be considered as a cause of toxicity. Reversal is by use of digibind (a digoxin-binding antibody).

44 a. The diagnosis in this case is of Hodgkin's disease. Approximately 80% of patients with this condition test positive for

Epstein–Barr virus. The condition occurs in young fit people and the elderly. There is an increased risk in those family members of the affected patient. Symptoms are divided into categories A and B where B include constitutional symptoms such as weight loss and night sweats. The diagnosis is confirmed by lymph node biopsy. Treatment depends on the staging and location of the lymphoma.

45 a. The mean age of presentation of myeloma is 65–70 years of age. Myeloma has a clone of cancerous plasma cells which fill the bone marrow and produce a paraprotein M. The production of normal immunoglobulin is suppressed which results in an increased risk of developing infection. Anaemia is a common finding due to chronic disease as is renal failure. Bone marrow normally produces equal amounts of light and heavy chains which make up the immunoglobulin ratio, in myeloma more light chains are produced (Bence–Jones proteins). The median survival is approximately 3 years and disease control is achieved in over half of patients with melphalan. Allogenic bone marrow transplant has been used in small number of young patients with a 25% success rate. Myeloma has a characteristic blood picture including:

↑ **Calcium**
Normal phosphate
Normal alkaline phosphatase

46 b. This question is difficult only because it requires a knowledge of the genetic translocation associated with the more familiar *bcr–abl* fusion gene (Philadelphia chromosome). Genetic translocations are responsible for a large number of genetic predispositions to cancer. Another commonly seen translocation associated with cancer is the t(8;14) *c-myc* activation leading to an increased risk of developing Burkitt's lymphoma. A handy way to remember the chromosomes involved in the Philadelphia chromosome is as follows. Philadel**p**hia chromosome – the 'P' of philadelphia is located at the 9th position and there are 22 letters in the two words put together (hence 9;22). The t(11;22) translocation is commonly associated with a rare bone tumour seen almost exclusively in children and young adults. It is a highly malignant tumour that has a high mortality rate in those who are afflicted.

Robertsonian translocations are a type of genetic transfer of chromosomal material that occurs in association with a number of disorders, most commonly with Down syndrome. Robertsonian translocations can be balanced, in which case there is no loss or addition of chromosomal material and the person carrying that karyotype will be a carrier of Down syndrome and not be afflicted, or unbalanced, resulting in trisomy or monosomy (the latter of which is non-viable). Down syndrome involves trisomy of chromosome 21 and may involve a combination of nearby chromosomes. The translocation t(14;21) is relatively frequently identified as the cause of this disease.

47 c. This question is included to remind the clinician that the management of disease should always remain with the patient as a central focus. The indicators specified may all be associated with disease activity, although the role of early involvement of biological agents is currently being evaluated. Subjectively from a patient's perspective the useful function that is managed comfortably in rheumatoid arthritis is the best indicator of disease activity. Appearances are often deceiving with 'normal' radiographs disguising disabling pain and loss of function whilst long-term deformities of the hands may mask surprising dexterity and adaptation.

48 d. Antiphospholipid syndrome is a spectrum of systemic lupus erythematosus (SLE) often associated with vascular thromboses. The vascular involvement may manifest most strikingly as stroke, myocardial infarction and multi-infarct dementia in a younger population with no obvious identifiable risk factors or more insidiously with migrainous symptoms and recurrent miscarriages. The presence of lupus anticoagulant and anticardiolipin antibodies with the above clinical presentation strongly suggests antiphospholipid syndrome. Reiter's syndrome typically presents with a triad of urethritis, conjunctivitis and arthritis in a young man associated with sexually transmitted or gastrointestinal infections. Systemic sclerosis is a disorder mainly affecting skin, gastrointestinal tract and respiratory system whilst dermatomyositis, as the name suggests, affects skin and muscle mainly. Marfan's syndrome typically affects the aorta and aortic valve, lens of the eye and skeletal system due to mutations in the fibrillin-1 gene.

49 a. The most likely diagnosis in this case is a fibroadenoma of the breast. It is most commonly seen in women age between 15 and 40 years old. Characteristically, fibroadenomas are smooth, firm and well-circumscribed lumps. They may vary in size from 1 to 5 cm and are often very mobile. Along with all other breast lumps these should be investigated using the triple approach and their management, if small, should include reassurance. For larger fibroadenomas management may include excision to restore symmetry to the breasts. Approximately 30% of fibroadenomas shrink and disappear completely. There is no association between fibroadenomas and breast cancer.

50 b. The most likely cause for this gentleman's gynaecomastia is liver failure. The history states that he has suffered with pancreatitis and acute liver failure in the past which suggest that this is likely to be due to hepato-biliary failure. Although it is a physiological change seen in the elderly, this gentleman's condition is most likely to be secondary to further liver problems. There is no evidence that he is suffering with thyroid dysfunction and the history does not state that he is on any medications that are known to cause this condition including digoxin, steroids, methyldopa and anti-androgens.

51 b. Acute glaucoma is a common condition affecting the elderly and one of the few true ocular emergencies that presents acutely. Classified as acute angle-closure and open-angle glaucoma, pain is typically unilateral and may be associated with headache. Blurred vision and visual distortion are symptoms experienced frequently and may be severe enough to reduce acuity to recognition of hand movements only. Dim light,anticholinergic drugs and intrinsic anatomical predisposition such as a shallow anterior chamber all predispose to acute angle-closure glaucoma and may be relieved by drugs reducing aqueous humour production such as beta-blockers and acetazolamide. A few doses of a topical steroid preparation may aid in dampening the inflammatory response that accompanies glaucoma.

Endophthalmitis describes an intra-ocular inflammation usually caused by infection affecting the aqueous or vitreous humour and may occur as a result of direct inoculation of infectious agent to the eye (e.g. foreign body penetration) or endogenously via spread from a pre-existing primary focus. Systemic antibiotics are usually indicated for infectious causes and may be treated adjuvantly by administration of antibiotic and steroid directly into the eye. Involvement of an ophthalmologist is always indicated and should be performed immediately once the diagnosis is suspected. Retinitis pigmentosa is a complex inherited disorder of the retinal photoreceptors and pigment epithelium. There is a slight male predominance in affliction due to the more frequent X-linked varieties. Loss of night vision and peripheral vision are the most common complaints in those affected. Treatment modalities have been shown to have modest benefit and are mainly involved in symptom control. These include massive vitamin A dosing, the use of acetazolamide along with experimental procedures such as retinal prosthesis or transplantation. Retinal detachment may occur as a result of traction from retinal neovascularisation with attachment to the vitreous humour, a tear in the surface with mechanical detachment by subretinal vitreous humour invasion or as a result of vascular changes in the retina (e.g. hypertension or vasculitis). The sensation of flashing lights and floaters associated with patches of lost vision (scotomata) are the most commonly described phenomenon. Retinal artery occlusion usually presents with painless sudden loss of vision in one eye and is caused by emboli. The pathophysiology is similar to that of cerebral stroke. There may be a role for thrombolysis if an embolus is detected within the first 4–6 hours but the mainstay of treatment is expectant management with investigation of the underlying cause.

52 **e.** Hyperglycaemia and diabetes has been linked to the development of posterior subcapsular cataract by a mechanism thought to be due to chronic osmotic changes, modification of lens protein and oxidative damage in the lens. A distortion in vision can often be experienced with accumulation of high blood glucose levels and is often complained of in patients who present with hyperosmolar hyperglycaemic and diabetic ketoacidotic states and who experience large and often rapid shifts in the osmotic content of the lens whilst on treatment. Steroids, hypertriglyceridaemia, obesity and hypertension have all been demonstrated to be associated with this type of senile cataract at a young age. Posterior subcapsular cataracts tend to present with more florid and disabling visual disturbance than cortical, nuclear or mixed cataracts (the other subclassifications of senile cataracts). Glare, especially in sunlight or with bright headlights at night, reduction in visual acuity and sometimes a reduction in accommodation. Treatment is primarily surgical with lens extraction and replacement providing great improvement in vision. Cataract operations have become almost standard procedures in day surgery units and can be performed with complete removal of the lens (intracapsular cataract extraction, ICCE) or with removal of the lens nucleus only with retention of the posterior capsule (extracapsular cataract extraction, ECCE). ECCE is the currently preferred method of extraction, however, the choice of procedure depends on the surgeon, patient and the type of cataract present.

53 **d.** Amiodarone is a drug notorious for its detrimental effect on the lungs, thyroid and liver and is best remembered for these derangements by the mnemonic 'PFTs, LFTs and TFTs.' Amiodarone can cause a picture of hyperthyroidism as it is structurally similar to thyroxine and thus thyroid function tests must be monitored on a regular basis with a low threshold to stop or reduce dosing if thyroid derangement is detected. Pulmonary fibrosis and skin manifestations such as photosensitivity reactions have also been reported. Atorvastatin has been linked to myositis (like all the statin drugs) and attention to the development of muscle pain and weakness should prompt assessment of dosing and or consideration of changing to another statin or other class of lipid-regulating drug. Statins must be used with caution in hypothyroidism due to the increased risk of myositis with untreated hypothyroidism and correction of thyroid dysfunction may itself lead to an amelioration of lipid profile. Amlodipine is associated with many diffuse symptoms including gastrointestinal upset but the main problem with use is the development of ankle swelling, which may only partially respond to diuresis. Atenolol and other beta-blocking medication may exacerbate asthma and other bronchospastic diseases, however, this effect may be minimised by the use of cardio-selective beta-blockers such as bisoprolol. Acarbose is an inhibitor of intestinal glucosidases (acting at the brush border) and may cause diarrhoea and loose stools due to the osmotic effect of a higher glucose load in the stool. Flatulence is also a side-effect reported by those taking acarbose due to the amount of glucose present in the colon available for metabolism by lower gastrointestinal organisms.

54 b. Lid retraction is a sign of sympathetic overactivity and can be seen in normal individuals who ingest large amounts of thyroxine with normal thyroid function. It can be used as a fairly reliable measure of the degree of treatment with thyroid-blocking medication. Hyperthyroidism is assessed clinically and confirmed biochemically with high levels of thyroid hormones (T4 and T3) and low levels of thyroid-stimulating hormone (TSH) due to negative feedback. The normal thyroid produces T4 and T3 as driven by TSH from the pituitary, which in turn is driven by hypothalamic thyroid-releasing hormone (TRH). T4 is produced in abundance relative to T3, however, T3 is 4 times more metabolically active than T4 and is converted from T4 in peripheral tissues. Symptomatic control of hyperthyroidism is achieved acutely with beta-blockade such as propranolol until thyroid-blocking agents such as propylthiouracil or carbimazole have taken effect. This usually occurs over a period of weeks and therapy must be monitored in this period with regular tests of thyroid activity until a stable dosage regime has been established.

Beta-blockade is not usually required as long-term therapy if control of overactivity can be managed medically or surgically with subtotal or total thyroidectomy (if refractory to medical treatment).

55 e. In this gentleman with a history of peripheral vascular disease an exercise tolerance test would provide inadequate information. A thallium cardiac scan can assess the heart without putting pressure on the peripheral vasculature. The results of an ETT can be influenced by pain from intermittent claudication and therefore the thallium scan is a better alternative for risk stratification in this patient. The gold standard for investigation in this case is a coronary angiogram. It allows the vasculature of the heart to be visualised with ease and any obvious lesions may be managed at the same time, providing a relief from symptoms.

56 a. Both verapamil and diltiazem are calcium channel blockers. They block calcium entry into the cell and its utilisation within the cell. They relax the coronary arteries and reduce the force of left ventricular contraction, which in turn reduces oxygen demand. Diltiazem has a negative chronotropic effect which helps alleviate the symptoms of angina as will regular long-acting nitrates.

57 b. Warfarin is not indicated in the immediate management of myocardial infraction (MI). The anti-platelet effect of aspirin and clopidogrel has been shown to be beneficial in the treatment of MI.

58 e. New-onset atrial fibrillation should ideally be converted to sinus rhythm by DC cardioversion. DC cardioversion may precipitate systemic emboli from intracardiac thrombus. To avoid thromboembolic events, formal anticoagulation is required for a month before and after the cardioversion, unless:
- The arrhythmia is of less than 72 hours standing.
- No intracardiac thrombus is apparent on trans-oesophageal echocardiography.

Co-ordinated atrial activity may not resume for 2 weeks following cardioversion even if sinus rhythm is apparent on the ECG, for this reason anticoagulation should continue for 1 month usually in the form of warfarin. In this case it is inappropriate to start conservative medical management since the atrial fibrillation is of new onset (past 72 hours is cut off for cardioversion).

59 c. PTCA is the most appropriate management option for this gentleman. PTCA restores artery patency in more than 90% of patients. PTCA has fewer bleeding complications and recurrent ischaemia when compared to thrombolysis, however, a major drawback of PTCA is the need for 24-hour availability of an angioplasty suite and staff. The time for treatment is longer for patients receiving primary PTCA as compared to those receiving thrombolysis but if the facilities are available it is the preferred treatment option. None of the other options listed above are appropriate in the management of this case.

60 b. Contraindications to thrombolysis include:
- Known active bleeding source (e.g. peptic ulcer, active dyspepsia).
- Active menstruation.
- Cerebrovascular accident within 3 months.
- Surgery or head injury within last 3 months.
- Severe hypertension:
  - Systolic more than 200 mmHG or diastolic more than 100 mmHg.
  - Must be sustained (e.g. not responding to i.v. nitrates).
- Hypotension:
  - Systolic less than 90 mmHg and not corrected by atropine (if bradycardia) or other rhythm correction.
- Chest trauma due to prolonged cardiac massage – if CPR more than 5 minutes assess risks with senior staff.
- On warfarin.
- Known or suspected aortic aneurysm.
- Known sensitivity to streptokinase or prior administration within last 24 months (for streptokinase administration only).

Extended matching questions

61 h. HSP is usually seen between the ages of 2 and 11 but approximately a quarter of cases may present in adulthood. HSP commonly presents with a diffuse purpuric rash over the lower limbs and buttocks that can often be mistaken for non-accidental injury in a young child (hence the incorrect and improper involvement of social services on admission to hospital) associated with abdominal pain, vomiting and oedema. Joint pain is also a common presenting feature and bloody stool indicated gastrointestinal involvement. The pathology is one of a small-vessel vasculitis with immune complex deposition in the vessels thus predictably leading to glomerular inflammation and signs of glomerulonephritis. About half of those presenting with HSP describe a preceding upper respiratory infection although many other putative triggers have been postulated.

Treatment is supportive and usually requires admission to hospital for monitoring of renal and gastrointestinal complications. Resolution is the rule but corticosteroids have been trialled to ameliorate symptoms.

62 b. IgA nephropathy (Berger's disease) is the commonest cause of glomerulonephritis worldwide – it is seen much more prevalently in Asian as compared to other populations. Berger's disease typically affects males more commonly than females and those in their twenties and thirties. The usual clinical presentation is with haematuria, which may be recurrent, usually following an upper respiratory tract infection. Less than 1 in 20 cases will present with acute renal failure and the nephrotic syndrome but spontaneous resolution does occur. An association with conditions such as gluten enteropathy and respiratory tract infections has led to the hypothesis that mucosal dysfunction is likely to play an important part in the development of the disease. Renal biopsy is the only modality to reliably diagnose IgA nephropathy and mesangial deposition of IgA and C3 seen on immunofluorescence is pathognomonic of the condition. Prognostically between 20% and 40% of all patients will eventually progress to end-stage renal failure (ESRF) requiring renal replacement therapy or transplantation.

63 a. Minimal change disease is the commonest cause of glomerulonephritis in children and can be difficult to distinguish from post-streptococcal glomerulonephritis as both can be brought on by preceding upper respiratory tract infections. An association in adults is with Hodgkin's lymphoma and this should be considered in adult patients presenting with signs of hypertension, proteinuria and oedema in whom a diagnosis of minimal change disease is considered. Renal biopsy should only be considered in children when tissue diagnosis is likely to alter management strategies and most renal physicians favour a therapeutic trial with corticosteroids with renal biopsy in more resistant cases. Histology by definition under light microscopy demonstrates little or no change thus electron microscopy is relied upon to look for subtle changes in foot process (podocyte) anatomy with podocyte fusion and retraction being the most common pathology.

64 i. Systemic lupus erythematosus is a systemic autoimmune condition with multi-organ involvement. Vasculitis is the underlying component that ties much of the organ dysfunction together with renal involvement predicting a poorer prognosis. Characteristically exhibiting the malar rash (butterfly rash

– so-called because of the double-winged appearance on either side of the nose) with a spectrum of symptoms ranging from neuropsychiatric to pulmonary, SLE can be difficult to diagnose unless it is borne in mind. Immune complex deposition of immunoglobulins directed against nuclear elements causes a glomerulonephritis often referred to as lupus nephritis with features on light microscopy graded by the WHO from I to VI. Wire-loop lesions are seen in Grade IV microscopic appearances and are due to hyaline deposits. Treatment is directed at medically stabilising the patient until such time that they may require more definitive treatment of renal compromise such as replacement therapy or transplantation. Corticosteroids are the first-line therapy for all but severe renal disease at which point immunosuppressive agents such as azathioprine and cyclophosphamide improve renal function more significantly.

65 e. RPGN can manifest with a variety of conditions such as the systemic vasculitides, other systemic autoimmune conditions such as SLE, Goodpasture's disease, rheumatoid arthritis and glomerulonephritides of unknown or infectious aetiology. Malignancy and drug therapy such as penicillamine and anti-tuberculous drugs can also cause a florid glomerulonephritis. As the name suggests the decline in renal function to a level where intervention is required can be very rapid occurring anywhere from days/weeks at most aggressive to a few months. Therefore early medical therapy is key in trying to influence the course of disease. Pathological correlates on renal histology are primarily of fibrinoid necrosis with crescent formation seen in over half the specimens biopsied.

66 c. Multi-infarct dementia (vascular dementia) usually presents in patients who have suffered multiple cerebrovascular events such as transient ischaemic attacks or strokes. Typically there is a step-wise deterioration of cerebral function with each event and relatives will often remark that the patient never recovered to the level he/she was before the stroke. Multi-infarct dementia accounts for about 25% of all strokes and should be considered in those with a history of cerebrovascular disease with global impairment of cognition.

67 g. Lewy-body dementia, as the name suggests, is characterised by the presence of Lewy bodies in the brainstem and cortex with a myriad of features of dementia and Parkinsonism. The difficulty in treating patients with this dementia is that using traditional anti-parkinsonian drugs may lead to delusions, which themselves are a common finding in dementia, and using neuroleptic drugs to counter delusions will worsen features of parkinsonism.

68 a. Alzheimer's dementia should be suspected in adults who demonstrate long-lasting problems with spatial navigation and visual awareness usually manifest as wandering or becoming lost. The mini-mental state examination is a relatively sensitive tool for screening for dementia but an ideal diagnosis requires exclusion of other reversible causes of dementia along with neuroimaging and histology. Found more commonly with increasing age there is evidence that 20% of those over 80 years old have dementia with many people with Down's syndrome manifesting signs of dementia earlier than 40 years of age.

69 h. Pseudo-dementia is a psychiatric illness that can mimic the apparent cognitive decline of true dementia. It is linked to depression and will characteristically ameliorate once the depression has been treated. The mini-mental state examination is not as sensitive a test for dementia in these cases as motivation plays a large part in determining a representative score. Clues to the diagnosis tend to come from the patient's affect and mood, however, as with any apparent dementia, it is important never to ascribe a reduction in cognition to pseudo-dementia without ruling out any organic cause of pathology.

70 e. This patient is too young to fit into the typical patterns of dementia and thus it is important that all organic causes for his behaviour be explored. The patient's nationality has an important bearing on narrowing down possible diagnoses and in a patient from Sub-Saharan Africa it is important to consider whether the patient's HIV status is a factor. More importantly, however, is to consider whether knowledge of HIV status is likely to alter the management strategy.

71 i. Haemophilia A and B and von Willebrand's disease may manifest as bleeding from the gastrointestinal tract, mucous membranes, into joints and from any wounds (including surgical wounds). von Willebrand's disease is the most common inherited coagulopathy and results from either a reduction or lack of von Willebrand factor (vWF) or abnormally functioning vWF. vWF is involved in platelet function thus manifests in laboratory studies as an increase in bleeding time, high APTT with a normal INR. Haemophiliacs are much more likely to exhibit major bleeding than von Willebrand's disease sufferers and bleeding into joints after trauma or exercise and into muscle after intramuscular injections are more commonly seen. The haemophilias are caused by a deficiency of factor VIII (haemophilia A) and factor IX (Christmas disease, haemophilia B) and behave clinically similarly. It should always be borne in mind when considering the differential diagnosis of any cause of bleeding that general bleeding diatheses may be responsible.

72 **d.** Haemorrhoids (or piles) are congested vascular cushions that aid the anal sphincter mechanism in maintaining continence. It is postulated that poor dietary fibre and straining at stool may contribute to the increase in rectal venous pressure that may precipitate haemorrhoid formation but mechanical factors such as rectal carcinoma, pelvic tumours and pregnancy all predispose to haemorrhoids. Typically bleeding is bright red and painless unless a prolapsed haemorrhoid becomes trapped in the sphincter or thrombosed. Sometimes patients have a sensation that something is descending in the rectum and may actually be able to feel prolapsed haemorrhoids. These are termed second-degree when they reduce spontaneously (first-degree haemorrhoids do not prolapse) and third-degree when they remain prolapsed. Sclerotherapy, banding or surgical removal form the mainstay of treatment measures.

73 **a.** Angiodysplasia may be clinically asymptomatic or present with rectal bleeding; either occult in nature or associated with life-threatening haemorrhage. Due to their frequency in the elderly as opposed to young population the diagnosis is often only made at colonoscopy or mesenteric angiography. Angiodysplasia refers to vascular abnormalities, usually of veins, and are most commonly found in the caecum or ascending colon. Treatment is restricted to hemicolectomy if bleeding is severe or recurrent or if lesions are small or solitary then a trial of electrocoagulation during colonoscopy may be of benefit.

74 **b.** Osler–Weber–Rendu syndrome (hereditary haemorrhagic telangiectasia) is an autosomal-dominant disease involving dilatation of small arterioles and capillaries causing an increased tendency to bleed. Anticoagulation and anti-platelet agents should be avoided if the syndrome is diagnosed. At one end of the spectrum small red blanching lesions are found on skin, mucous membranes and the gastrointestinal tract but at the other end the syndrome has been associated with the development of hepatic and pulmonary arteriovenous fistulas leading to high-output heart failure, cerebral embolism and cerebral abscesses. Recurrent epistaxis and gastrointestinal bleeds are the

most common presentation of Osler–Weber–Rendu syndrome although stroke and cerebral abscess in young patients should always alert the clinician to the possibility of this disease.

75 f. Mesenteric embolus is a difficult diagnosis to make due to the myriad of insidious causes of rectal bleeding. The presentation of shock may be a feature of both hypovolaemia and infarction of bowel leading rapidly to faecal peritonitis and overwhelming sepsis if not caught early. Atrial fibrillation, bruit or other risk factors for thromboembolism may aid in pointing the surgeon to the right diagnosis. A careful history may reveal preceding symptoms of intermittent pain on eating and resultant weight loss due to reduction in blood flow through the mesenteric system, however, this is often uncommon in acute-on-chronic cases with the development of good collateral supply in the gastrointestinal tract even in the face of marked blockage. Resection of the necrotic bowel with either primary anastomosis or secondary closure of colostomy depending on site, age and co-morbidities is often the only treatment available at emergency presentation.

76 a. In the post-operative patient there are several potential causes of fever and shortness of breath. In this situation the answer is atelectasis. In the first 24 hours post-operatively this is most likely to be the cause of any shortness of breath or fever. In the first 2–3 days pneumonia is more likely to be the cause. In either case it is important to confirm the diagnosis by sending off blood tests, blood cultures and requesting a chest X-ray.

77 f. This gentleman has suffered a massive pulmonary embolus, which culminated in cardiac arrest. With his history of being treated for an embolus during the resuscitation streptokinase was administered although unfortunately, despite 3 cycles of resuscitation, this gentleman showed no signs of improving. As advised on the advanced life support course during a cardiac arrest reversible causes should be sought including:

- Hypokalaemia/hyperkalaemia.
- Hypothermia.
- Hypoxia.
- Hypovolaemia.
- Tension pneumothorax.
- Toxicity (drugs).
- Thromboembolism.
- Tamponade.

By working through these potential causes of cardiac arrest it is possible to treat those reversible causes effectively. During every cardiac arrest call that you attend you should always be thinking about the cause for each particular case as that quick thinking can be lifesaving.

78 **c.** This gentleman has suffered an aspiration pneumonia secondary to a stroke. If patients are not carefully monitored by the nursing staff they may continue to eat and drink despite having altered neurological status. If a patient's ability to swallow is impaired then they can develop aspiration pneumonia. The commonest part of the lung to be affected by an aspiration pneumonia is the right lower lobe, this is due to the angulation of the right main bronchus meaning that food or any aspirate will preferentially end up there. Presentation of an aspiration pneumonia is identical to that of a normal pneumonia although the history may vary, the key difference is in the management. Aspiration pneumonia will require coverage for organisms normally found in the gastrointestinal tract, usually cefuroxime and metronidazole.

79 **b.** Given the details in the history it is sensible to be suspicious of a malignancy. Although this lady is young it is not uncommon for malignancies to present in this age group. She is complaining of a gradually worsening shortness of breath with a long history of cigarette smoking. The clinical findings of an effusion fit with the diagnosis of a lung cancer and analysis of the fluid would show an exudate with greater than 30g/L of protein and presence of malignant cells. Whilst other causes of pleural effusions should be considered the presence of malignant cells confirms the diagnosis and further imaging tests should be carried out to confirm the location and subgroup of the cancer.

80 **e.** This scenario is clearly describing an exacerbation of COPD. These are commonly caused by concurrent infection. In this case it appears that omission of her inhalers has resulted in reduced lung function and an opportunist infection has exacerbated the problem. With this subgroup of patients it is important to ensure that the infection is treated and that they are back on their usual bronchodilators and steroids before discharge in order to optimise their chances of coping once discharged. It is always important that appropriate follow-up arrangements are made to prevent similar episodes occurring in the future.

81 **a.** Appendicitis is both one of the easiest surgical conditions to diagnose and simultaneously one of the most difficult. The classical presentation of a young male or female with central colicky

abdominal pain associated with nausea and vomiting, which subsequently localises to the right iliac fossa (with local peritoneal involvement) causing rebound tenderness and guarding leaves little else on the list of differentials. However, the variable position of the appendix and often relatively uncharacteristic presentation can often cause diagnostic conundrums. It must be heeded that torsion of the testis may present with the same clinical findings as appendicitis and there are cases of missed necrotic testes that were only discovered on the table when preparing the patient for appendicectomy. The abdominal examination must always include examination of the external genitalia, hernial orifices and consideration of digital rectal examination.

82 c. Diverticulitis is often colloquially referred to as the 'left-sided appendicitis'. It presents with many of the features of appendicitis: nausea, vomiting, rebound tenderness and guarding and localised pain in the left iliac fossa. The sigmoid colon is the unhappy recipient of the brunt of gastrointestinal disease for reasons still unknown and diverticulitis is most commonly found here. Terminology in diverticular disease is precise and should be used correctly:

- *Diverticulosis*: diverticula that are present and asymptomatic.
- *Diverticular disease*: refers to symptomatic diverticula.
- *Diverticulitis*: active inflammation of diverticula.
- *Complicated diverticulitis*: the presence of complications of diverticulitis, e.g. fistula, abscess or perforation.

The Hinchey classification grades perforated diverticulitis from Stage 1 to 4 depending on the extent of peritoneal contamination and forms a useful guide to the severity of diverticulitis complication.

83 i. Rectosigmoid carcinoma may present with local, general or metastatic features. A change in bowel habit, large bowel obstruction, perforation, stricture or fistula associated with fresh rectal bleeding may all occur. General features associated with cancer are malaise, weight loss, a pyrexia of unknown origin (PUO) caused by activation or inflammatory cytokines and anaemia. As a rough guide right-sided tumours are more inclined to cause large bowel obstruction whilst those presenting on the left side (e.g. caecal carcinoma may present purely with an anaemia). Any unexplained anaemia or episode of rectal bleeding in older patients merits outpatient investigation such as colonoscopy if there is any suspicion of malignancy. More recently there has been a national initiative to introduce a colon cancer screening programme similar to that already in place for breast and cervical cancer screening and is planning to employ home faecal occult blood testing as part of the process.

84 f. Epigastric pain, vomiting and features of peritonism should alert the clinician to the possibility of a perforated peptic ulcer. Risk factors for ulceration include drug therapy especially NSAIDs and steroids, smoking, excess alcohol intake, presence of *Helicobacter pylori* organism, severe burns (Curling's ulcer), acute stress reaction (Cushing's ulcer) and Zollinger–Ellison syndrome. Perforation is investigated by both clinical examination and erect chest radiograph. Air under the diaphragm can help to confirm clinical suspicion and is present in more than 70% of cases of perforation.

85 b. Pancreatitis can be a complication of a myriad of causes. These are best summarised by the mnemonic 'GET SMASHED' standing for **G**allstones, **E**thanol, **T**rauma, **S**teroids, **M**umps, **A**utoimmune disease, **S**corpion venom, **H**yperlipidaemia (also hypertension, hypercalcaemia, and hypothermia), **E**RCP and **D**rugs (rarely but significantly HMG-CoA reductase inhibitors ('statins') and anti-epileptic medication). Surgical signs associated with pancreatitis are the oft-quoted but rarely seen Grey-Turner's sign (bruising discolouration in the flanks) and Cullen's sign (bruising discolouration around the umbilicus). Reactive pleural effusions can occur secondary to systemic inflammatory response evoked by severe pancreatitis and can be significant enough to affect the respiratory system.

86 g. It is important to remember that children are not simply small adults. There are a range of conditions that are specific to children and as a result their baseline observations vary.

Age (years)	Respiratory rate (breaths per minute)	Heart rate (bpm)	Systolic BP (mmHg)
<1	30–40	110–160	70–90
1–2	25–35	100–150	80–95
2–5	25–30	95–140	80–100
5–12	20–25	80–120	90–110
>12	15–20	60–100	100–120

87 c. By the age of 9 months it is expected that a child will be able to sit up unaided. In all of these cases gestational age needs to be taken into account and any pre-term births need to have allowances made when assessing for normal development. Between the ages of 13 and 18 months it is expected that a child will be able to walk unaided.

88 a. The vaccination schedule in the United Kingdom starts at the age of 2 months. At 2, 3 and 4 months infants are immunised against diphtheria, tetanus, pertussis, polio, *Haemophilus influenza B* and meningitis C. At the age of 12–15 months children are immunised against measles, mumps and rubella (MMR). Between the ages of 3 and 5 years booster doses of diptheria, tetanus, pertussis, polio and MMR are administered. The next step in the schedule is the BCG aged 10–14 which provides approximately 75% protection against tuberculosis and the final step is a booster dose of diptheria, tetanus and polio aged approximately 18 years old.

89 a. This is a presentation of acute bronchiolitis. It is most commonly seen in those children under the age of 6 weeks or in those with chronic respiratory, cardiac or neurological deficits. The commonest causative organism is the respiratory syncitial virus which accounts for 75% of cases. Those infants in respiratory distress may require non-invasive ventilation in the acute phase in addition to inhaled bronchodilators and there is some evidence for the use of ribavirin; a nucleoside analogue. Long-term consequences may include an obstructive bronchiolitis.

90 a. By 6–8 weeks it is believed that babies are able to follow movements with their eyes. At this age experts belies that their eyesight is developing and their vision extends up to a distance of approximately 30 cm. This is one of the reasons that babies are believed to form a strong bond with their mother as they can focus their gaze on them whilst feeding.

PAPER 4

Answers and notes

Multiple choice questions (single best answer)

1 d. Decreased oesophageal sphincter is reduced, which results in the patient developing symptoms of heartburn. Other common findings include reduced gut motility, which can lead to constipation and raised platelets, erythrocyte sedimentation rate, cholesterol and fibrinogen. With the physiological changes taking place in the vascular compartment a systolic flow murmur is common whilst water retention occurs leading to ankle oedema and carpal tunnel syndrome.

2 e. Risk factors for developing an ectopic pregnancy include:
- Pelvic inflammatory disease.
- Pelvic surgery/adhesions.
- Previous ectopic pregnancy.
- Endometriosis.
- Assisted fertilisation.
- IUCD.
- Progesterone-only pill.
- Congenital anatomical variants.
- Ovarian/uterine cysts and tumours.

Although previous Caesarean section may result in development of adhesions it is not in itself responsible for future progression onto an ectopic pregnancy.

3 d. Tetralogy of Fallot is the most common congenital cyanotic heart abnormality. This abnormality is characterised by variable obstruction to the right ventricular outflow due to pulmonary stenosis, dextroposition of the aorta overriding the ventricular septum, ventricular septal defect (VSD) and right ventricular hypertrophy. Due to the VSD there is a shunt of blood from the left to the right side of the heart. Children have learned that squatting decreases the cyanosis and the hypoxaemia. This increases the left ventricular afterload and decreases the left to right shunt. Other mechanisms listed in the question do not have any effect on the left to right shunting of the blood flow in the heart.

4 c. The most likely diagnosis given the history and clinical findings is of pyloric stenosis. This condition is usually seen in newborn males and results in forceful vomiting immediately after meals. The condition is most likely to occur in the first-born males. The most cost-effective and useful investigation to make this diagnosis is an abdominal ultrasound. It will reveal hypertrophy of the pylorus. Management of this condition is surgery to make an incision in the hypertrophied muscle to relieve the pressure.

5 b. This patient has two main problems: as he is drowsy he is not likely to protect his airway and thus is risk of aspiration, and on clinical examination he has evidence of a right-sided tension pneumothorax. Most clinicians would consider needle thoracocentesis to drain a tension pneumothorax before attempting to intubate additionally as intubation in situations of lung compromise carries significant risk. A nasopharyngeal airway is contraindicated due to the complex facial fractures as the risk of basal skull fracture is high. An emergency cricothyroidotomy is a last resort attempt to secure an airway and can be avoided by early intubation if airway management is likely to become difficult. Chest drain insertion is not the recommended procedure for releasing a tension pneumothorax.

6 a. Jaundice is a feature of acute pancreatitis due to inflammation of the pancreatic head obstructing bilious outflow. Pseudocyst formation is a late complication of pancreatitis and usually takes about a week to develop thus not seen in the acute inflammation. Hypocalcaemia as opposed to hypercalcaemia is often seen and is useful as one of the Glasgow criterion for predicting severity of pancreatitis along with a low albumin. Bowel necrosis is not associated classically with pancreatitis.

7 a. These signs are characteristic of arterial occlusion. The '6 P's' are:
- **P**ale.
- **P**ulseless.
- **P**arasthesiae.
- **P**ainful.
- **P**aralysed.
- **P**erishingly cold.

The popliteal artery is the most susceptible artery to acute occlusion, being small in calibre. Cellulitis would cause pain in the leg, erythema and warmth, which is not seen in this case. Reduced circulating volume would provide more generalised symptoms. Distal pulses may be weakened but will be present, although the limbs may be cold there should be no pain. Venous insufficiency would lead to oedema in the limbs and in the longer-term trophic skin changes including venous eczema and lipodermatosclerosis. Vasculitis would provide a different clinical picture with vasculitic lesions on the skin, presence of pulses and blood tests that typically reveal increased inflammatory markers.

8 d. Taking the patient to CT scan in the first place was a huge risk – the notoriously named 'doughnut of death' should only be considered in the management of trauma patients when the patient is stabilised. The presence of free fluid in the abdomen or pelvis is a warning sign as this could signify bleeding. Exsanguination into the abdomen and pelvis can occur rapidly and internal bleeding should be considered in any patient who sustains blunt trauma to the chest, abdomen or pelvis. Noradrenaline would indeed be the inotrope of choice for maintaining blood pressure but is only used in a critical care setting and never to correct a surgical cause of hypotension. A GCS of 11/15 suggests a significant degree of deterioration, however, intubation is not necessary at this stage unless airway compromise is suspected. Fluid resuscitation is absolutely needed before, during and after surgery, however, a repeat CT scan of the abdomen is not only unnecessary in making the diagnosis but may in fact endanger the patient by delaying surgery.

9 a. Complex abdominal trauma requiring emergency surgery may require massive transfusion in the peri-operative period. Packed red cells are the most commonly used blood product for transfusion, however, are relatively platelet and clotting factor deplete. Transfusion of as little as 4 units can predispose a shocked patient to coagulopathy manifest by oozing from all wound sites and bleeding from mucous membranes that cannot be easily controlled. Replacement of clotting factors and platelets forms the mainstay of therapy acutely. Vitamin K is a useful agent in cases of warfarin overdose, however, is not beneficial in this situation.

10 d. The cause of the obstruction is at the level of the ureteric orifices as suggested by the dilated ureters and kidney with small bladder volume. Insertion of a suprapubic catheter will be of no use in this situation as there is no evidence of bladder outflow obstruction. Intravenous antibiotics are useful for treating a suspected urinary tract infection as evidenced from the urine dipstick but are not the modality that will ultimately aid in recovery. Intravenous fluids are useful in the management of urinary tract infection and sepsis, however, without surgical decompression of the renal tracts is likely to overload the cardiovascular system. The indications for renal dialysis include: (1) metabolic derangement refractory to medical treatment, e.g. hyperkalaemia, severe metabolic acidosis, (2) advanced symptomatic uraemia, (3) signs of volume overload and (4) end-stage renal failure.

11 **b.** Acute pulmonary emboli is normally present with type I respiratory failure, e.g. low PaO_2 and normal or low PCO_2. This option represents type II respiratory failure which is seen in the context of chronic pulmonary emboli. The diagnosis of a pulmonary embolus should be considered in patients with hypoxia and tachypnoea in the absence of any clinical signs, e.g. pneumonia. Occasionally on chest X-ray a pulmonary embolus can cause a wedge-shaped infarct (due to loss of blood supply to an area of lung), more commonly the chest X-ray is clear. In cases of large pulmonary embolus the characteristic $S_I Q_{III} T_{III}$ pattern may be seen on ECG, more commonly a tachycardia and right axis deviation are seen. Calf swelling unilaterally virtually confirms the diagnosis in a patient who has become acutely short of breath – in fact, guidelines state that in patients with a confirmed deep vein thrombosis with acute onset shortness of breath the diagnosis of a pulmonary embolism should be assumed and treatment continued for the appropriate length of time, usually 6 months.

12 **d.** Patients with underlying lung conditions are more likely to develop pneumothoraces than those without. Young, tall men are at risk of developing pneumothoraces spontaneously simply due to their body shape. This diagnosis should always be considered in a young patient with acute onset shortness of breath – although most small pneumothoraces will be reabsorbed, larger ones will require treatment with a chest drain and underwater seal whilst tension pneumothoraces require emergency treatment.

Pulmonary emboli do not predispose to pneumothoraces as they are not predominately a condition of the lung parenchyma but the associated vasculature.

13 **e.** Charcot's triad describes the clinical findings of right upper quadrant pain, jaundice and fever/chills. It is associated with acute (ascending) cholangitis most often due to Gram-negative bacterial infection such as *Escherichia coli*, *Enterobacter* and *Pseudomonas*. Reynold's pentad simply adds features of shock

and altered mental state to Charcot's triad and occurs in acute cholangitis. Fitz–Hugh–Curtis syndrome occurs in young women who have been exposed to chlamydia and manifests as perihepatic adhesions involving the diaphragm and nearby structures. The pain experienced may mimic that of biliary obstruction and may spread transcoelomically to involve other abdominal viscera causing generalised peritonitis. Leriche's syndrome is found in arteriopathic patients who exhibit absence of femoral pulses with buttock pain and claudication and impotence. The syndrome occurs because of occlusion of the aortic bifurcation by atherosclerosis or thromboembolism. Wernicke–Korsakoff's syndrome is comprised of the triad of Wernicke's encephalopathy; nystagmus, ophthalmoplegia and ataxia and Korsakoff's psychosis, which is manifest as the inability to acquire new memories with confabulation of missing information. The latter is irreversible but may be prevented by parenteral administration of thiamine.

14 d. The clinical picture shows many of the characteristic hallmarks of hereditary haemochromatosis (HHC). This autosomal recessive disease is common in older males of Northern European descent and has been genetically linked to the C282Y mutation on the short arm of chromosome 6. Abnormal iron metabolism leads to deposition of iron and haemosiderin in liver, heart, pancreas, pituitary, joints, adrenals, testes and kidneys. This in turn leads to a spectrum of cirrhosis, pancreatic dysfunction and diabetes mellitus, skin pigmentation, cardiac dysfunction and dilated cardiomyopathy and hypogonadism. Diagnostic investigations include radiography of joints for chondrocalcinosis, fasting transferrin saturation (a level $>45\%$ is very sensitive for HHC), liver biopsy to assay the degree of hepatic iron loading, MRI scan if liver biopsy is contraindicated and genetic mutational analysis. Management of HHC is by twice-weekly venesection to render the patient mildly iron-deficient, then maintenance venesection every 2 months. The iron-chelating agent desferrioxamine has some clinical benefit in reducing iron levels.

15 d. This woman most likely has Wilson's disease (hepatolenticular degeneration), a rare inborn error of metabolism that leads to a failure to excrete copper. The build-up of copper can sometimes be seen as a green-brown pigmented ring at the junction of cornea and sclera known as a Kayser–Fleischer ring. Four-vessel neck angiography would be a useful discriminative test in cases of suspected arteriovenous malformations or vessel occlusion. Hyperthyroidism can lead to a slender frame and an anxious disposition but this is not the clinical picture of thyroid dysfunction. Serum bilirubin and liver enzymes would be a useful test to do if there were any clinical signs of jaundice or any liver disease, which is associated with Wilson's disease, however, it would not be the most discriminative test to do. Peripheral blood films and vitamin B_{12} levels are useful in cases of suspected subacute combined degeneration of the spinal cord secondary to vitamin B_{12} deficiency.

16 c. The patient is showing a response to a placebo. Normal saline is not known to have any pain-reducing qualities, and this amount of normal saline is unlikely to alter any electrolyte abnormality this gentleman may have. His pain could be psychogenic in origin although he does have a slightly raised white cell count, which may suggest some pathology. There is no evidence in the question that he is suffering with a personality disorder of any kind. His pain may be somatic in origin, this is unlikely to be directly affected by a bolus dose of normal saline and is likely to be improving with rest and conservative measures.

17 c. Antihypertensive medications are known to cause a depressed mood in susceptible individuals. Other drugs that are strongly associated with depression are steroids and hypnotic medications. Digoxin, calcium supplements and oral hypoglycaemics are not usually associated with depression.

18 e. An increase in adipose tissue in the elderly resulting in a reduction in number of insulin receptors available for glucose leads to a mild glucose intolerance. Bone changes and degenerative arthritis are responsible for an increase in alkaline phosphatase, whilst creatinine clearance reduces with age due to a reduction in the glomerular filtration rate. With age a reduction in the level of testosterone, the stimulation of erythropoietin falls resulting in a mild anaemia in the elderly.

19 c. The median nerve innervates most of the flexor compartments of the forearm. It does not pass around the lateral epicondyle – in fact this is the course of the ulnar nerve which is often damaged following injuries to the elbow or distal humerus fractures. The median nerve does provide sensation to the lateral 3½ digits of the hand on the palmar aspect of the hand and may become trapped in the carpal tunnel as it passes deep to the flexor retinaculum at the wrist which may result in pain, paraesthesiae and weakness in the distribution of the nerve.

20 e. Chronic alcohol abuse lowers the seizure threshold and can put drinkers at risk of withdrawal fits. Hypoglycaemia is the most common metabolic cause of seizures and may be seen in poorly controlled diabetics or alcoholics who are prone to dropping their blood sugars. Any form of cerebral mass can result in seizures depending on its location, the mass itself may be responsible as can the surrounding oedema and raised intracranial pressures. Overdosing on antidepressants is known to result in seizures. Benzodiazepine overdose is not associated with seizures; in fact they form the mainstay of the treatment of seizure disorders initially.

21 e. Whilst in approximately 50% of cases no cause is found, many people can improve the severity and number of attacks that they experience by avoiding certain risk factors. Risk factors can be remembered by the mnemonic 'CHOCOLATE'.
CH: CHeese
O: Oral contraceptive
C: Caffeine (or its withdrawal)
OL: AlcohOL
A: Anxiety
T: Travel
E: Exercise
Depression is not a risk factor although it is documented that migraines may lead to depression.

22 e. In cases such as this one, investigations are not always necessary. If you are happy that it is purely a syncopal attack after appropriate examinations have been carried out then no further tests need to be done. In this case there is a clear and obvious role for an ECG and blood tests are self-explanatory looking for any undiagnosed hypoglycaemia or anaemia. An echocardiogram may have a role if a murmur is heard on auscultation or if there is any concern on cardiovascular examination. A CT scan of the head is unlikely to yield any information in this case and should be reserved for cases when no cause can be found on other simple tests.

23 d. Causes of proximal myopathy are varied. Patients will notice that they have difficulty in climbing up stairs or difficulty in standing from a low chair. Causes include metabolic problems including hyper or hypocalcaemia, alcoholism, steroid use, thyroid disease, inflammatory myositis and myasthenia gravis. Syphilis infection is known to cause a sensory deficit resulting in a high-stepping gait but not a proximal weakness and waddling gait.

24 e. This case is describing a right-sided homonymous hemianopia (homonymous – same side, hemianopia – loss of half a field of vision) with macular sparing. The macular sparing suggests that the lesion is not in the occipital cortex. The bilateral symptoms suggest that the lesion is at a place in the pathway where fibres for both eyes will be affected (posterior to the optic chiasm). Causes for this gentleman's symptoms may be an infarct, a haemorrhage or a tumour producing a mass effect. Isolated lesions of the upper or lower optic radiation provide a quadrantaniopia and lesions of the optic nerve alone will affect only one eye.

25 d. This man has developed a rare complication of renal cell carcinoma – a left-sided varicocoele manifest due to venous congestion of the left testicle. In 1% of cases of renal cell carcinoma (also called Grawitz tumour) advancement of the tumour along the left renal vein can cause occlusion at the inlet of the left testicular vein. This complication is not seen on the right hand side due to the differential anatomy of the venous drainage on the right hand side. To respect laterality the left testicular vein drains into the left renal vein, which then crosses the midline to drain into the inferior vena cava. On the right hand side the right testicular vein drains directly into the inferior vena cava thus a right-sided varicocoele is 'never' seen in right renal vein tumours.

26 e. Haematuria is seen in nephritic conditions such as glomerulonephritis and is not associated with nephrotic syndrome by definition. Components of the nephrotic syndrome are proteinuria defined as protein loss in the urine at a rate of greater than 3g in a 24-hour period, hypoalbuminaemia defined as an albumin level less than 30g/L and oedema. Fourth and fifth elements are sometimes described as part of the syndrome and are hypercholesterolaemia and normal renal function respectively. Nephrotic syndrome can occur as a primary event or a secondary phenomenon but this definition is not clinically of great benefit in the management of cases of nephrotic syndrome as treatment is supportive in the first instance whilst the underlying cause is sought. Management focuses on use of diuretics to reduce oedema along with fluid and salt restriction, adequate nutrition to replace protein loss (approximately 1–2g/kg/day) and venous thromboembolism prophylaxis unless contraindicated. This is due to the loss of clotting factors with heavy proteinuria and predisposes those with the nephrotic syndrome to thromboembolism. Hypercholesterolaemia usually requires no active treatment and will resolve alongside the nephrotic syndrome, however, if persistent, a role for statins may be indicated.

27 c. Treatment of acute severe hyperkalaemia (potassium level above 6.5 mmol/L or electrocardiogram changes) is managed firstly by intravenous injection of 10 mL of 10% calcium gluconate as cardioprotection. Secondly infusion of, e.g. 10 units of short-acting insulin with 50 mL of 50% dextrose over 30 minutes will shift potassium intracellularly. Correcting the underlying cause, e.g. hypovolaemia may stabilise the potassium level, however, depletion of total body stores of potassium may be indicated and can be achieved by using calcium resonium (although this may take up to 6 hours or more to take effect). Other modalities used are beta-agonists such as salbutamol but this is less commonly employed. Haemodialysis is indicated in conditions of uraemic complications, e.g. pericarditis, metabolic acidosis or hyperkalaemia refractory to drug treatment and fluid overload refractory to drug treatment. Patients may exhibit few signs or symptoms but may complain of fatigue, weakness and parasthesias. ECG changes seen in hyperkalaemia depend on the level and duration of hyperkalaemia and in summary can be broken down into peaked T waves, shortened QT interval and ST depression initially progressing to bundle branch blocks with associated widening of the QRS complex with PR shortening and P wave flattening. Eventual irreversible changes occur leading to sinusoidal character of the ECG and eventual ventricular fibrillation and asystole.

28 a. The history given from the patient is of a young man with recurrent aerodigestive tract bleeding and haemoptysis and non-specific symptoms that would be consistent with renal failure. A clinical impression (confirmed with biochemical tests of renal function) would be of a process affecting both the kidneys and lungs. Pulmonary–renal syndromes must be excluded as a matter of some urgency as therapy is dependent upon early diagnosis and treatment. This clinical scenario lies at the more extreme end of the presentation spectrum. Autoantibody screen comprising anti-neutrophil cytoplasmic antibodies (ANCA), anti-glomerular basement membranes (anti-GBM), complement, lupus anticoagulant and cardiolipin antibodies as well as double-stranded DNA (ds-DNA) antibodies is an easily performed screening tool for vasculitic and autoimmune processes. Goodpasture's syndrome (to which the clinical vignette alludes) comprises the triad of glomerulonephritis/renal impairment, pulmonary haemorrhage and anti-GBM antibodies. Renal biopsy will definitively provide histological confirmation of the disease with immunofluorescent staining demonstrating linear deposition of antibody (usually IgG) along the glomerular basement membrane, however, should not be undertaken until after simple screening blood tests. CT chest aids definition of the extent of pulmonary involvement but again can be pursued at a later date. High-dose immunosuppression plus plasmapheresis forms the mainstay of medical treatment for Goodpasture's syndrome.

29 c. Urine analysis is a cheap, simple and non-invasive screening tool for a variety of conditions and should be performed as standard in the investigation of suspected renal or urinary tract disease. Red-cell casts are simply impressions of the renal tubules that have been formed by compaction of red cells. These are almost always pathological and are associated with glomerulonephritis and vasculitic processes and occasionally seen in malignant hypertension with renal involvement. Glucose can be detected on urine dipstick analysis once the renal threshold for glucose reabsorption has been surpassed and occurs in conditions such as pregnancy, renal tubular damage, diabetes and in conditions of altered reabsorption of solutes such as chronic renal failure. Bilirubin can be seen in the urine with obstructive jaundice (post-hepatic jaundice) as water-soluble bilirubin, conjugated in the liver, overflows into the systemic circulation and is excreted by the kidneys. Nitrites are commonly seen in urinalysis with conditions such as urinary tract infection and high-protein meals (as nitrites are breakdown products of protein metabolism). Cystine crystals are diagnostic of the rare condition cystinuria.

30 c. Chronic renal failure is associated with small, shrunken kidneys and ultrasound is in fact a useful guide in determining whether renal impairment found clinically or on blood tests is an acute phenomenon or whether it has been persistent for some time. Amyloidosis is an unusual and rare disease of extracellular deposition of an abnormal protein that is particularly resistant to breakdown (amyloid). Classified as primary or secondary (reactive) or localised versus systemic there are various inherited forms of amyloid that are associated with organ failure with renal, cardiac and liver being the most commonly affected. Deposition in the kidneys causes bilateral enlargement of the kidneys detectable ultrasonographically and leads to renal failure by a mechanism that is thought to be mechanical disruption of tissue architecture in the main. Compensatory hypertrophy of a single kidney allows maintenance of normal renal function and manifests as a larger and thicker remaining kidney. Polycystic kidney disease results in an irregularly enlarged kidney filled with cysts easily detectable and reliably diagnosed on ultrasound scan. Renal cell carcinoma is the most common primary tumour of the kidney representing over 90% of all renal cancers. Presentation is frequently as an abdominal mass palpable on clinical examination associated with loin pain and haematuria.

31 b. In this sort scenario we should consider the possibility of a posterior shoulder dislocation. On a single antero-posterior X-ray it is not possible to exclude a posterior dislocation of the shoulder as on a single AP view this can look normal. This injury is caused by an epileptic fit, electric shock or fall from a motorbike usually due to a forced internal rotation of the abducted arm or a direct blow to the front of the shoulder. This injury can usually be reduced in the accident and emergency department. Anterior dislocations of the shoulder are visible on AP views and are commonly caused by falls backwards onto an outstretched hand or by forced abduction and external rotation of the shoulder. This causes the head of the humerus to be driven forwards tearing the capsule or avulsing the glenoid labrum, associated fractures are occasionally seen.

32 c. Fractures in children can be difficult to assess particularly in areas such as the elbow where there are several growth plates involved. The history in this case is of a minor injury with very limited clinical findings, which suggests that the X-ray is unlikely to show anything significant. The mnemonic for remembering which of the growth plates fuse around the elbow is 'CRITOL' and the ages at which they close are roughly two, four, six, eight, ten and twelve;
C: Capitulum.
R: Radial head.
I: Internal epicondyle.
T: Trochlear.
O: Olecranon.
L: Lateral epicondyle.
Variations do occur among children and if there is any doubt or difficulty in interpreting the X-rays comparison views of the unaffected side should be taken and compared.

33 b. Macule is a descriptive term for a flat but well-defined area of skin change. Papule refers to a raised macule that is less than 0.5 cm in diameter, i.e. a circumscribed area of skin that is elevated. A nodule is the counterpart to a papule that is greater than 0.5 cm in diameter. Plaques refer to more discoid elevations of the skin that can be small when less than 2 cm in diameter or large when greater than 2 cm. A vesicle describes a localised collection of fluid less than 0.5 cm in diameter such as found typically in herpes zoster. A bulla describes the counterpart that is greater than 0.5 cm in diameter. A pustule is simply a collection of pus in the skin. A weal is usually associated with allergic reactions such as seen in urticarial disorders and represents a localised area of oedema within the skin.

34 d. Seborrhoeic keratoses are encountered universally in medicine in whichever specialty one trains in as they are frequently an incidental finding in the elderly population. Most often found on the back and chest the lesions may take on an oily appearance due to the sebaceous nature of the growth and resemble segmented discrete flat brown abnormalities that arise from the skin surface. Malignant melanoma may be suspected in seborrhoeic keratoses that have a darker, more atypical appearance; however, the melanomas occur in a younger population that other skin cancers and are predisposed by frequent sun exposure, typically in a pale-skinned patient with a history of repeated sunburning episodes. Malignant melanomas are aggressive once spread past the superficial layers of the skin has occurred and must be caught early if effective curative resection is to be achieved. Keratoacanthoma is often classified as a benign tumour although histologically it closely resembles a squamous cell carcinoma. However, excision and further histological analysis is usually recommended if the diagnosis is not clear. It often presents as a round discrete nodule with a central darker area filled with keratin. Campbell de Morgan spots are seen often again in the elderly population and are essentially abnormal vascular regions developing within the deeper layers of the skin. They present as cherry red round lesions in the skin and are harmless. Basal cell carcinoma (BCC) is the commonest malignant skin tumour seen in dermatological practice and is locally invasive with metastasis being extremely rare. BCC is classically described as having a pearly appearance with areas of superficial telangiectasia and a rolled edge surrounding a sunken central area. Treatment is with excision and biopsy with or without radiotherapy.

35 c. Causes of testicular swelling can be divided into the following categories:

Painful	Hard and painless	Soft
Torsion of testis	Tumour	Varicoele
Torsion of hydatid of Morgagni	Syphilis	Epididymal cyst
Epididymitis	Tuberculosis	Hydrocele
Orchitis: viral or bacterial	Haematoma	

Other causes of scrotal swelling include an inguinal hernia, which extends above the scrotum and sebaceous cysts, which sit superficially on the scrotum.

36 b. This history is classical of bladder cancer. The one major clue is PAINLESS haematuria, a classical feature of bladder cancer. Predisposing factors to bladder cancer include working in the rubber injury with exposure to carcinogens, smoking and schistosomiasis. Other risk factors include chronic bladder stones and a congenital abnormality of the urinary tract. Most bladder cancers are transitional cell histologically and spread by direct invasion initially but by lymphatic spread to the peri-aortic nodes and haematogenous spread to the liver and lungs eventually; 95% of cases present with painless haematuria. Benign prostatic hyperplasia (BPH) presents with urgency and difficulty in initiating urination and terminal dribbling with an incomplete sense of emptying. Prostatism is an acutely painful condition.

37 c. The biggest clue to this question is in the patient's age, as is true of many examination questions, and real life! The symptoms are not unlike those experienced by patients with colon cancer, but the infrequency of cancer in this age group makes this one of the most unlikely possibilities. Ulcerative colitis is bimodally distributed, peaking between ages of 15 and 30 years and then again in later life. The patient's ethnic background is also suggestive of the diagnosis with a slightly increased prevalence among the Jewish population. Pseudomembranous colitis is typically due to antibiotic-associated overgrowth of *Clostridium difficile* and both angiodysplasia and haemorrhoids are usually present with fresh rectal bleeding in the absence of abdominal symptoms.

38 a. Digoxin is the first-line agent in treating atrial fibrillation with fast ventricular rate. (Note the concept of 'fast' atrial fibrillation is a misnomer as atrial fibrillation is, by definition, fast. It is the rate of conduction to the ventricles that should be described.) Loading is given as 500 µg oral (there is no evidence that intravenous digoxin works better) once in every 12 hours for two doses then conversion to digoxin maintenance, usually at a dose of 62.5 µg. Patients should be placed on a cardiac monitor in a ward setting where this can be adequately observed. Digoxin will act over a 24–48-hour period and care must be taken not to over digitalise patients leading to bradycardia. If the rate is not adequately controlled with digoxin in the first instance then beta-blockade may be added if left ventricular function is adequate. Finally, although still somewhat controversial, anticoagulation should be considered in patients who present with atrial fibrillation. If there is documented evidence of either known atrial fibrillation or structural heart disease the evidence weighs heavily in favour of long-term anticoagulation with an agent such as warfarin. In cases where patients are younger than 65 years with echocardiographically normal hearts and a potentially reversible reason for atrial fibrillation then the decision to anticoagulate over the long term becomes more subjective.

39 b. Schizotypal personality disorders form part of Cluster A of the Diagnostic and Statistical Manual of Mental Disorders (DSM-IV), which groups personality disorders by similarly matched characteristics. The definition of a personality disorder is an enduring pattern of inner experience and behaviour that differs markedly from the expectations of the individual's culture, is pervasive and inflexible, has an onset in adolescence or early adulthood, is stable over time, and leads to distress or impairment. Schizotypal personality disorders manifest with behaviour or thinking that is odd, often associated with excessive social anxiety, an inability to form close confiding relationships with other individuals and often paranoid ideation. It can be difficult to distinguish from schizoid personality disorders, which typically exhibit an emotionally flat affect with a lack of enjoyment for activities, close relationships and sexual activity.

Antisocial personality disorders are usually over 18 years but many have evidence of early conduct disorder in early adolescence. A lack of respect for authority and lawmaking characterise this disorder that is one of the only psychiatric conditions that one may be put in prison for. A lack of remorse for aggressive and often dangerous behaviour is a common feature.

Dependent personality disorders refer to a cluster of character traits that include dependence on other individuals, an inability to be alone or not in a close relationship with excessive demands on those around them for support and reassurance. Similarly clustered with the avoidant personality disorder, which differs slightly in a lack of a close relationship unless acceptance is guaranteed. Avoidant personalities tend to shun social situations and activities that bring attention to themselves for fear of criticism and exhibit anxiety in social contexts.

40 a. A fluctuating level of consciousness suggests a diagnosis of delirium rather than dementia the latter of which can be defined as the deterioration of cognitive functions, such as memory, concentration and judgement, and personality and behavioural changes resulting most commonly from an intrinsic disorder of the brain but infrequently from a reversible organic cause. Dementia typically presents with features of cognitive impairment manifests as forgetfulness, inability to recognise familiar objects, persons and places, and behavioural manifestations that may range from wandering behaviours to aggression or emotional lability and inappropriateness. Dementia encompasses a wide range of disease pathologies such as vascular dementia, neurodegenerative aetiologies such as Pick's disease and Alzheimer's disease, infectious processes and metabolic, endocrine and traumatic derangements, some of which may ameliorate with correction of the abnormality.

Sundowning is a phenomenon that is common to both dementia and delirium and describes the worsening of symptoms that occurs towards the end of the day. It has been postulated that the reduction in ambient light levels and external cues causes an increase in disorientation and this forms the basis of simple nursing strategies for orientating demented patients. Strict adherence to routines such as medication timing, bright lighting and set sleep–wake patterns and reinforcement of external cues such as the time, date and place are important nursing tasks that can make a significant difference in the care for this often difficult but vulnerable population.

41 e. Myelodysplasia is a clonal disorder of the bone marrow in which morphologically and structurally abnormal blood cells are produced. Patients tend to have a macrocytic anaemia, leukopaenia and thrombocytopaenia. In most cases no cause is identified but occasionally radiotherapy or cytotoxic drugs are found to be the cause. Clinical features include recurrent infections, pallor and easy bruising and bleeding. Management involves symptomatic relief – treating infections and blood transfusions in addition to platelet transfusions to help in haemorrhage resulting from thrombocytopaenia. Allogenic bone marrow transplant is an option in younger patients if donors can be found. After 2–3 years this condition may progress onto acute myeloid leukaemia, which is refractory to treatment.

42 e. Polycythaemia is an increase in haemoglobin by >2g/dL. Increased haemoglobin occurs in myeloproliferative diseases. Most commonly polycythaemia is secondary to chronic hypoxaemia from chronic lung disease and heavy cigarette smoking with systemic hypertension (Gaisbock's syndrome). Other causes include cyanotic heart disease and dehydration and rarer causes include excess erythropoietin from erythropoietin-secreting tumours in the kidneys. Polycythaemia may be asymptomatic or produce a hyperviscosity syndrome. Most polycythaemia is secondary to other causes and therefore investigations should include arterial blood gases and lung function tests. Venesection is occasionally used to provide symptomatic relief.

43 c. This child is suffering from acute otitis media. It is a common complaint in children between the ages of 3–6 years and often follows an upper respiratory tract infection. The commonest pathogens implicated are *Haemophilus influenzae* and *Streptococcus pneumoniae*. The presentation may be accompanied by fever and irritability in the child and typically hearing loss precedes pain. Examination of the ear canal shows an inflamed tympanic membrane with loss of the light reflex and bulging of the eardrum. It is important to feel the mastoid bone to look for any associated pain implying a secondary mastoiditis. Treatment of otitis media involves analgesia and antibiotics are the subject of debate. Those commonly prescribed are amoxicillin or erythromycin. This presentation differs from otitis externa, which is commonly seen in swimmers and pain precedes hearing loss. Cholesteatoma is an erosive condition of the middle ear and has an associated offensive smelling discharge from the ear canal.

44 a. This patient is suffering with tonsillitis. Acute tonsillitis may be caused by a variety of organisms including: *Epstein-Barr virus herpes simplex virus, group A β-haemolytic Streptococcus* and *Mycoplasma*. The most common presenting features include a sore throat headache, fever and mild odynophagia. Examination of the tonsils reveals an inflammation, presence of pus suggests a bacterial infection whilst generalised lymphadenopathy is indicative of infectious mononucleosis. Any concern regarding presence of pus or abscess should be followed up by referral to ENT surgeons for further evaluation.

45 e. Prednisolone is used as a treatment option in systemic lupus erythematosus and has not been reported to be associated with drug-induced lupus in the literature. A useful mnemonic for remembering four drugs commonly associated with drug-induced lupus is 'It's not HIPP to have Lupus' (**H**ydralazine, **I**soniazid, **P**rocainamide, **P**henytoin). The associated lung and skin manifestations usually resolve on cessation of drug therapy.

46 a. Anticardiolipin and lupus anticoagulant antibodies are most strongly associated with antiphospholipid syndrome. Antireticulin antibodies are commonly found in coeliac disease and other enteropathies, antinuclear antibodies are raised in a variety of conditions such as systemic lupus erythematosus (SLE), Sjögren's syndrome, systemic sclerosis, chronic active hepatitis and rheumatoid arthritis. Anti-Ro antibodies are found in Sjögren's syndrome and SLE and antineutrophil cytoplasmic antibodies (ANCA) are raised in systemic vasculitides such as Wegener's granulomatosis, microscopic polyangiitis and Churg–Strauss disease.

47 a. Ductal carcinoma *in situ* (DCIS) is a pre-malignant condition. Approximately 40% of DCIS lesions will progress to become invasive breast cancers. As carcinomas *in situ* they are unable to metastasise. They present in the same way as invasive breast cancers but are more readily picked up on mammography – they account for approximately 25% of all cancers picked up in that way. Management normally involves a wide local excision with possible radiotherapy depending on the clinical decision made at the time of surgery. If the lesion is large axillary node clearance may also be required.

48 d. Indications for performing a mastectomy in lieu of any other procedure include:
- A lump of 4 cm or greater.
- A multi-focal cancer.
- Centrally located cancer.
- Patient choice (in the presence of a breast lump).

Fibroadenomas are often managed conservatively and 1/3 regress and disappear in their own time. If they cause significant discomfort or are greater than 4 cm they may be considered for removal.

49 a. Proliferation of new blood vessels on the retina is associated with the development of vitreous haemorrhage and retinal detachment (usually by attachment of new vessels into the vitreous humour with traction detachment of the retina) as the most clinically significant sequelae of retinal neovascularisation (= new blood vessel formation). Treatment modalities include laser photocoagulation of peripheral parts of the retina with theoretical reduction of retinal oxygen requirements. Another rational for laser therapy is that photocoagulation is thought to supplement the oxygenation of the retina by increasing the supply from the choroid layer and thus reducing the ischaemic burden shouldered by the retinal vessels.

Aqueous haemorrhages are not seen due to the lens capsule separating the posterior (vitreous) compartment of the eye from the anterior (aqueous compartment). The pathogenesis of retinal neovascularisation is thought to be a direct consequence of retinal ischaemia with resultant compensation in blood flow through the rapid formation of new but friable blood vessels. Rupture and haemorrhage of these delicate vessels can cause acute changes in vision due to clouding of the vitreous humour with blood and patients may experience floaters and progressive deterioration in visual acuity.

Optic neuritis is a condition most often occurring in association with demyelinating conditions such as multiple sclerosis and is due to inflammation of the optic nerve. Typically presenting as pain on eye movement with distortion of central vision it may be associated with a relative afferent papillary defect detectable upon examination of pupillary reflexes to light. A bitemporal hemianopia is sometimes referred to colloquially as tunnel vision and is seen in conditions of central compression of the optic chiasm such as an enlarging pituitary tumour. Often a focused history will lead to a diagnosis of pituitary disease such as acromegaly presenting with symptoms of coarse skin, thick heavyset features and other manifestations of soft tissue overgrowth.

50 c. Retinoblastoma is the most common ocular malignancy of childhood and exhibits a peak in incidence at between 10 and 20 months. There is no significant difference in sex and both unilateral and bilateral disease has been described with bilateral disease presenting an average of 7 months before unilateral disease. The aetiology of retinoblastoma has been linked to a mutation in the *retinoblastoma* gene located on the long arm of chromosome 13. A deletion or non-functional mutation cause inactivation of this gene, which actually suppresses the formation of retinoblastoma and when both loci are inactivated the tumour occurs. Treatment is directed at preservation of as much visual function as possible and can be delivered through external beam radiotherapy (however, with a very unfavourable side-effect of facial hypoplasia due to cessation of bony growth with radiotherapy), chemotherapy to achieve local control or radionuclide plaque treatment. Surgical treatment, however, still remains the most definitive option in retinoblastoma and involves enucleation for very poor prognosis tumours with photocoagulation and cryotherapy additional options in very selected cases.

Endophthalmitis is an inflammation of the internal cavities of the eye and can occur after trauma to the eye with inoculation of bacteria, after retained lens material during cataract operations or by metastatic spread to the eye from a distant focus. It presents with pain in the eye, redness, swelling and a decrease in visual acuity. Antibiotic therapy both systemic and occasionally into the ocular cavities is merited and the choice of antibiotic will depend upon the putative organism responsible, e.g. skin flora inoculation during eye surgery and any patient allergy to antibiotic therapy. Congenital cataract presents with opacity of the lens, which may be very subtle, and irregularity of the red reflex. If the cataract is in the visual axis then reduction in vision may occur and this must be corrected as soon as possible to minimise long-term deficits in vision. Congenital cataract may be associated with infection, genetic diseases such as Down syndrome and prematurity. ROP is a disease that is related to the degree of prematurity of a newborn and is a serious disorder of vascular proliferation due to underlying retinal ischaemia from untimely birth. Laser therapy, cryotherapy and even ablative therapy are the main modes of treatment.

51 c. Pituitary adenoma accounts for over 95% of all causes of acromegaly and results in a plethora of clinical features; often noticed by those around the patient rather than the patient themselves. Headache and visual disturbance are common complaints due to the enlarging adenoma causing compression of the neighbouring optic chiasm usually in the central portion leading to the classical pattern of visual loss, bitemporal hemianopia (tunnel vision). Adenomas are almost always benign and can be classified as secretory or non-secretory (null-cell tumours); 25% of the secretory adenomas produce prolactin, 20% produce growth hormone and 10% produce ACTH accounting for the endocrine disturbance in addition to the mass effect of the adenoma. Craniopharyngioma is a squamous, calcified cystic tumour arising from the remnant of the craniopharyngeal duct or Rathke's pouch and manifests with similar signs and symptoms as acromegaly. Headache due to mass effect is a predominant complaint but over 50% present with signs of endocrinopathy such as hypothyroidism, adrenal failure or diabetes insipidus and around 75% may present with visual disturbance.

Craniopharyngioma exhibits a bimodal distribution in children aged around 6–10 years and then again in adults in their mid-to-late 50s. Hypothalamic glioma is typically a disease of children and young adults and tends to be aggressive in nature. Subtle endocrine disturbance may occur related to the area of hypothalamus affected and range from disturbance in temperature regulation and appetite to syndrome of inappropriate ADH production (SIADH) and cranial diabetes insipidus. Parasella meningioma usually causes local compression effects and causes a local osteoblastic reaction to the surrounding bone that is usually depicted on plain radiographs and CT scan. MRI is the definitive imaging modality and may help to assess surgical resectability by defining involvement of the cavernous sinus and carotid artery. Metastases can also been seen to the pituitary and are usually clinically silent unless large in size. Lymphoma, breast and bone marrow tumours are the most commonly seen metastases at this rare site and most diagnoses of pituitary metastases at this are made only at autopsy. Diabetes insipidus may sometimes be a consequence of large secondary deposits.

52 e. Long-term use of steroids (greater than 2 weeks) with abrupt withdrawal causes the clinical state of hypoadrenalism similar to Addison's disease due to exogenous suppression of the endogenous production of corticosteroids. Patients who are on steroid medications should carry a 'steroid card' with information regarding dosing and length of dosing and side-effects of abrupt cessation of steroids. High-dose regimens for acute flares of autoimmune diseases are usually tapered over a matter of weeks usually with fixed increment reduction in dose (e.g. 5 mg/week) to prevent a hypoadrenal crisis by slow regaining of endogenous adrenal axis function. Intravascular depletion is often a cause of hypotension in the elderly and is usually seen in the context of an infective process such as a urinary tract infection or pneumonia with good response to intravenous fluids. In this case there were abnormal requirements for parenteral fluids to maintain a barely adequate blood pressure indicating an underlying process more complex than intravascular depletion. Septic shock (especially with Gram-negative organisms) can cause a profound hypotension that is refractory to fluid resuscitation and may in fact lead to fluid overload and pulmonary oedema. The pathophysiology is one of a decreased systemic vascular resistance due to bacterial endotoxins and intravascular depletion and hypotension. Inotropic support in a critical care setting with an agent such as noradrenaline may be required. Haemorrhagic stroke usually presents acutely with neurological signs and symptoms, and hypertension due to a reflex response to cerebral injury and loss of autoregulation in order to ensure adequate cerebral perfusion pressure (CPP). As cerebral perfusion is a function of mean arterial pressure (MAP) minus the intracerebral pressure (ICP), in the face of increased ICP e.g. cerebral insult, adequate CPP is achieved by an increase in the MAP manifest as hypertension. It is vital not to treat this primary hypertension acutely. Vasovagal syncope is unlikely to cause such a lasting hypotension and would be responsive to fluid resuscitation.

53 b. If the causative organism is not known empirical therapy is as follows:
- Intravenous benzylpenicillin and gentamycin unless staphylococcal infection is suspected when vancomycin is substituted for penicillin.
- Vancomycin and gentamycin if patient is allergic to penicillin.

54 e. Cullen's sign is periumbilical bruising or yellow-blue discolouration. Originally it was described in ruptured ectopic pregnancy but is more commonly associated with severe, acute pancreatitis. The cause of the discolouration is pancreatic enzymes having tracked along the falciform ligament and digested subcutaneous tissues around the umbilicus. Aortic regurgitation is associated with De Musset's sign (head-bobbing) and Quinke's sign (visible nail bed pulsations). Kussmaul's sign is a rising jugular venous pressure (JVP) on inspiration associated with a diagnosis of constrictive pericarditis and cardiac tamponade. Corrigan's sign is associated with aortic valve incompetence.

55 a. The scenario is describing a classic history of pericarditis. This is often associated with a history of a recent URTI. The history of chest pain that is exacerbated by lying flat and inspiration is characteristic of pericarditis. Classical ECG findings are described including concave upwards ST segment elevation. Management of pericarditis includes non-steroidal anti-inflammatories for pain control and rest. Accident and emergency referral would be appropriate management if there was uncertainty about the diagnosis. No further useful information would be gleaned from a chest X-ray or an echocardiogram.

56 a. Identification of cardiac tamponade relies upon 'Beck's triad': hypotension, jugular vein distention and muffled heart sounds. This results from fluid accumulation in the pericardial sac that dampens the transmission of sounds through the chest wall. Identification of the quiet heart sounds can be difficult just using a stethoscope, which is why a hospital setting is useful for further investigations. Bradycardia is not associated with cardiac tamponade, in fact, tachycardia is often seen as there is reduced filling time in the cardiac cycle due to reduced capacity of the chambers.

57 b. A PDA is a defect between the pulmonary artery and the aorta. The ductus arteriosus normally closes within the first 48 hours of life. In premature babies it may remain open for longer, sometimes up to 3 months. If it remains patent longer than this it is unlikely to close spontaneously. A persistently patent ductus is a common congenital heart lesion, occurring either singly or in combination with other defects. Girls are more likely to be affected by PDA, and those affected by congenital rubella syndrome are more likely to suffer a PDA.

All other options are correct.

58 d. Hypothyroidism is associated with bradycardia. It often has an insidious onset with symptoms such as fatigue, weight gain and cold intolerance. Cardiovascular symptoms include angina, cardiac failure, pericardial and pleural effusions. Ehlers–Danlos syndrome is associated with joint laxity and hypermobility and mitral valve prolapse. Whilst superficially Turner's syndrome is associated with a webbed neck, cardiovascular complications can include coarctation of the aorta, which can be how the syndrome is discovered in young girls. Noonan's syndrome is similar to Turner's but it has a normal phenotype. Cardiovascular lesions affect the right side of the heart in this condition.

59 b. The ideal anticoagulation regime for management of a pulmonary embolus is commencement of warfarin (with a loading dose) and administration of low molecular weight heparin in addition until the dose of warfarin becomes therapeutic.

Dalteparin is a low molecular weight heparin. It exerts its effect on factor Xa in the clotting cascade and requires no monitoring; once administered it becomes effective immediately and its effects last for approximately 24 hours. Warfarin is a vitamin K antagonist and its effects need to be monitored. When commencing a patient on warfarin it is important to remember that it is procoagulative for the first 24 hours and it takes up to 3 days for its effect to be exerted. For patients being treated for a pulmonary embolus the target INR (International Normalising Ratio) range is 2–3, meaning that their blood will be 2 to 3 times thinner than a patient who is not being anti-coagulated. To maintain this, regular blood tests are required as over-anti-coagulation can be dangerous and under-anticoagulation may result in development of further clots.

Both aspirin and clopidogrel have anti-platelet action and therefore are not useful in the management of pulmonary emboli. Whilst unfractionated heparin is an adequate choice, its effects require monitoring up to 4 hourly and it requires the patient to be hooked up to an infusion pump and is therefore less desirable than low molecular weight heparin. The benefits of unfractionated heparin is that once stopped its effects will be reversed 4–6 hours after this whereas with low molecular weight heparin it takes 24 hours after administration for the effects to normalise and roughly 3 days for the effects of warfarin to be reversed.

60 d. The analysis of the pleural fluid shows that the effusion is an exudate (due to the protein content <30 g/L = transudate, >30 g/L = exudate). Causes of transudates can be considered as failures (e.g. heart failure, renal failure, liver failure, etc.).

The following cause transudates:
- Congestive heart failure.
- Cirrhosis.
- Atelectasis (which may be due to malignancy or pulmonary embolism).
- Nephrotic syndrome.
- Myxoedema.
- Constrictive pericarditis.

In contrast, exudates are produced by a variety of inflammatory conditions and often require more extensive evaluation and treatment.

The more common causes of exudates include the following:
- Parapneumonic.
- Malignancy (carcinoma, lymphoma and mesothelioma).
- Pulmonary embolism.
- Tuberculosis.
- Asbestos related.
- Pancreatitis.
- Trauma.

- Drug induced.
- Sarcoidosis.

Extended matching questions

61 a. Combined oral contraceptives should be started with caution in patients. Questions should be asked about past or family history of venous thrombosis. Other factors that should be discussed include obesity, immobility and varicose veins. Two or more of these risk factors should urge you to think again about contraceptive solutions. In this case, she is a young healthy girl who wants to control excessive bleeding and the combined oral contraceptive should help reduce the proliferation of the uterine endometrium and in turn the associated pain and bleeding.

62 d. This lady has too many risk factors or contraindications for the standard option of the combined oral contraceptive pill. The remaining options for regular contraceptives include progesterone-only solutions including a pill or an intramuscular injection. Since she is known to be scatty the option of a daily progesterone-only pill is less than ideal. Standard progesterone-only pills require to be taken at the same time every day and the window is shorter than your average combined oral contraceptive. The other option is the progesterone-only injection; it is a 3 monthly preparation that is injected intramuscularly that avoids the need to remember a daily pill.

63 g. This girl has sought advice at the correct time. Although, when a patient commences on any contraceptive solutions they should be advised that in the presence of any inter-current illness either abstinence or a barrier method of contraception should be sought. In this case, this girl has essentially had unprotected sexual intercourse and therefore the most appropriate contraception is the emergency contraception (or 'morning after pill'), which can be used up to 72 hours after the event.

64 b. Any oral contraceptives require regular checks on simple observations including blood pressure. For those patients whose blood pressure is found to be outside of the upper range of normal on a combined oral contraceptive, there are a few options. A progesterone-only option should be considered, in addition to a low oestrogen combined pill or a period without hormonal treatment. In this case since the patient is a medical student with a regular schedule it is assumed that she could be trusted to take the pills at the same time each day. This is a good alternative for those patients with blood pressure problems.

65 c. This lady is a great candidate for an intra-uterine contraceptive device. There are two options either hormonally based devices or a copper device. These are rarely used in nulliparous ladies. The hormonal device is impregnated with progesterone and works in a similar way to the progesterone-only pills. The copper device is well known to have side-effects of heavy bleeding, but can be used as emergency contraception up to 5 days after unprotected sexual intercourse or up to 5 days prior to the next predicted ovulation.

66 j. Oesophageal carcinoma usually presents with progressive dysphagia initially for solids then progressing to liquids. There is usually associated marked weight loss due to both the anorexic effects of cancer and the inability to tolerate food. In the main oesophageal carcinoma is squamous in histology but may be adenocarcinoma in the distal oesophagus. Risk factors include Barrett's oesophagus, Plummer–Vinson (Patterson–Kelly) syndrome, achalsia of the cardia, caustic stricture, excessive alcohol intake, coeliac disease, smoking and tylosis.

67 a. Mallory–Weiss tear is characteristically described following a large meal and alcohol ingestion with subsequent severe retching and vomiting causing a tear in the oesophageal mucosa leading to fresh haematemesis that usually resolves spontaneously. This is a relatively benign type of oesophageal tear when compared to the catastrophic transection of the oesophagus that is seen in Boerhaave's syndrome. This can also occur precipitated by vomiting after a large meal and causes severe chest pain with a collapsed patient. Chest radiography aids in the diagnosis with air seen in the mediastinum usually leading to acute mediastinitis and the clinical sign of surgical emphysema in the neck.

68 h. Aorto-enteric fistula is a rare but devastating complication of previous aortic surgery. Adhesion and erosion of the repair line into the adjacent small bowel can cause massive gastrointestinal haemorrhage that may be fatal if not diagnosed and treated early. Patients have been described as experiencing a 'warning' bleed preceding massive and life-threatening haematemesis. The presentation of the patient described is one of florid hypovolaemic shock. Tachypnoea, signs of sympathetic activation and a markedly reduced GCS are important signs of shock as blood pressure may be maintained until approximately 30% of the blood volume has been lost.

69 e. Gastric ulceration can occur for a variety of reasons; postoperatively it is usually a combination of poor oral intake, acute stress reaction and the addition of non-steroidal anti-inflammatory drugs as pain relief. It is more likely to occur in patients with a history of dyspepsia and presents acutely with coffee ground vomiting due to altered blood by stomach contents, with occasional melaena (black tarry stools again due to altered blood) if the bleeding is significant. Treatment is in the first instance by stopping any gastric irritant drugs, starting either high-dose proton pump inhibitor, e.g. omeprazole or a 72-hour infusion at a rate of 8 mg/h depending on the severity of haematemesis/melaena. Fluid and/or blood resuscitation may be required if the patient is in hypovolaemic shock and uncontrolled bleeding may require urgent endoscopic therapy or emergency laparotomy.

70 g. Gastric carcinoma carries a very poor prognosis, mainly due to the relatively late presentation of disease in which the carcinoma is already established and may well have invaded local organs or metastasised to liver, lungs and bones. A feature of gastric carcinoma that is not seen in many other tumours is transcoelomic spread of tumour to peritoneal structures such as the ovaries causing bilateral Krukenburg tumours. Tumours near the pylorus (as in this example) can lead to pyloric obstruction leading to projectile vomiting following meals and may require endoscopic dilatation or surgical palliation. Risk factors for the development of gastric cancer include pernicious anaemia, partial gastrectomy, *Helicobacter pylori* infection (tentatively thought to be the cause behind the high rates of gastric cancer in the Japanese population), chronic peptic ulceration, blood group A and genetic predisposition such as hereditary non-polyposis colon cancer syndrome (HNPCC).

71 g. The most useful test in this case is a PEFR. It will give instant results and allow the status of her asthma to be quickly assessed. By using results charts we can tell whether her PEFR values are optimal and this helps in deciding on her management. Although this girl claims to be using her inhalers regularly in a person of her age, noncompliance must be considered as an important cause for deterioration in her normally well-controlled asthma.

72 c. In any patient with reducing saturations it is very import-ant to get an arterial blood gas. Although sats machines on the ward give fairly accurate readings, in those patients where the readings are very important it can be useful to get an arter-ial sample that gives more accurate readings. In deteriorating patients it will give an idea of respiratory function and any associated metabolic function and is a quick and easy test to both perform and interpret.

73 b. This patient has suffered a pneumothorax. The most appro-priate investigation is a chest X-ray to confirm the diagnosis. Pneumothoraces are common in tall people, those with pre-existing lung disorders and those with connective tissue dis-eases. Treatment depends on the size of the pneumothorax. If it is small it can be left to be reabsorbed although larger ones require insertion of a chest drain.

74 e. This lady requires a V/Q scan to investigate for a pulmonary embolus. She has clinical symptoms consistent with a diagnosis of a pulmonary embolus and associated risk factors. Since her chest X-ray is clear a V/Q scan is the investigation of choice. Should her chest X-ray show anything either the diagnosis should be reconsidered or computed tomography with pulmo-nary angiography (CTPA) should be requested.

75 d. This patient requires a high-resolution CT of his chest. The diagnosis under consideration is of pulmonary fibrosis which may be confirmed on CT. The characteristic appearance on chest X-ray is a ground-glass appearance whilst on CT scan it is linear opacities and honeycombing. Although arterial blood gas studies will show a change from the norm these will not be diagnostic, neither will lung function tests.

76 b. Riedel's lobe is a congenital anatomical variant that is benign and often found incidentally on physical examination. It is found as an enlargement of the right lobe of the liver below the costal margin and is usually completely asymptomatic unless it is hugely enlarged. Patients should be reassured that it is nor-mal and that no further action needs to be taken.

77 h. This woman has the clinical features of reactive systemic amyloidosis (AA amyloid). Amyloidosis can be subdivided into three main categories: (1) plasma cell dyscrasia (AL amyloid) associated with abnormal production of amyloidogenic immu-noglobulins, (2) reactive amyloid (AA amyloid) associated with an increase in the production of an acute phase protein called serum amyloid A and is highly associated with chronic inflammatory and infective conditions and (3) familial amyloidoses. Rheumatoid arthritis is especially linked to the development of AA amyloid due to the chronic nature of the inflammation and may present with multi-organ involvement and even failure. Renal disease is very common in amyloid and manifests as nephrotic syndrome. Hepatomegaly may be found on examination but does not usually present with the acute nature of renal disease. Histological diagnosis (80% pick-up rate from rectal tissue) is preferable with staining either with Congo red or under polarised light, where the fibrillar protein deposits exhibit an apple-green birefringence.

78 e. Colorectal and breast cancer are the two most common metastatic deposits in the liver and a derangement in liver enzymes may be one of the only red-flag signs that an undiagnosed malignancy has disseminated. The liver is richly supplied with venous blood from the gastrointestinal tract via the portal vein and thus is the first organ encountered when haematogenous seeding of primary gastrointestinal malignancy metastasises. Unlike the other more benign or reversible causes of hepatomegaly the liver edge is often non-tender, craggy and nodular. Recent advances in hepatobiliary surgery have now allowed restricted case-by-case resection of liver segments in an attempt to provide curative therapy for early metastasised malignancy, however, lesions are usually only considered when single and anatomically accessible. A staging CT scan of the chest, abdomen and pelvis should be performed if there is a high index of suspicion of malignancy with discussion at a multidisciplinary meeting (MDM) involving oncologists, palliative care clinicians, surgeons, gastroenterologists and radiologists.

79 a. Right heart failure can occur secondary to many causes but in the main due to pulmonary hypertension and left heart failure leading to the clinical syndrome of congestive cardiac failure. Commonly after large myocardial infarctions a part of the left ventricular muscle becomes non-functional and reorganises to become scarred fibrotic tissue leaving the rest of the viable tissue to take on the burden of systolic output. With time the remaining left ventricle will start to fail causing backpressure through the pulmonary system and eventual pulmonary vascular changes, which may manifest as pulmonary hypertension. This in turn increases the work of the right heart due to increased afterload and the resultant pressure overload will cause hypertrophy and eventual failure. Functional regurgitation may occur through any of the valves involved in the failing heart and tricuspid regurgitation, although rare, may be a mechanical consequence of changes in the right myocardium. A pulsatile liver is a sign that there is an open communication between the right ventricle and the inferior vena cava (as a patent tricuspid valve will direct pressure waves up through the pulmonary valve during systole). Other causes of tricuspid regurgitation such as endocarditis caused by intravenous drug use may give the same clinical picture of right-sided heart failure without the co-existent left-sided signs and may aid the diagnosis.

80 **i.** Falls are a common presenting complaint in those who abuse alcohol. Right upper quadrant pain may also be complained of and suggests the development of alcoholic hepatitis. Signs may vary from florid signs of chronic liver disease, i.e. ascites, spider naevi, oesophageal, rectal and umbilical varices but may be as mild as an unwell patient with a faint jaundice. Typically there is a tender smoothly enlarged liver edge, however, if the patient has progressed to alcoholic cirrhosis (with a shrunken impalpable and fibrotic liver) there is an increased risk of the development of hepatocellular carcinoma, which may present with nodular hepatomegaly and raised alpha-feto protein. Alcoholic hepatitis is usually treated with adequate pain relief, alcohol withdrawal programmes and intravenous or high-dose oral vitamins and thiamine to prevent complications such as Wernicke–Korsakoff syndrome and neurological sequelae of vitamin B_{12} deficiency such as peripheral neuropathy and subacute combined degeneration of the cord.

81 **b.** Systemic lupus erythematosus fits with the clinical scenario of multi-organ involvement that appears clinically fairly mild from the history and a simple autoantibody screen will aid the diagnosis in the first instance. Haematuria with slightly elevated urea and creatinine along with positive urinalysis are signs that there may be an element of renal glomerulonephritis, but the rise in renal markers may be due to dehydration and thus renal biopsy may be indicated at some point in the future to indicate prognosis if the renal function has not ameliorated with steroids and rehydration. Daily urea and creatinine should be considered for this patient as it is important to see the trend in renal function, but the diagnosis needs to be established first to allow future management and follow-up to be planned.

82 **c.** A renal tract ultrasound should be considered a first-line imaging investigation in renal disease as a lot of information

can be reliably gained easily and quickly. The history is consistent with that of autosomal dominant polycystic kidney disease (ADPKD) suggested by the previous stroke and renal failure in such a young woman. Renal ultrasonography has a high sensitivity and specificity for diagnosing polycystic kidney disease in addition to picking up other renal masses, size of kidneys, obstruction to outflow, collections and bladder volumes. Other rare causes of 'enlarged' kidney include renal tumours, benign cysts, single kidney hypertrophy, amyloidosis and renal contusion and trauma. The association of polycystic kidney disease with subarachnoid haemorrhage due to rupture of a berry aneurysm should be noted as well as the association with cardiac valvular lesions (especially mitral valve prolapse) and diverticulitis.

83 f. Bence–Jones protein is an easily performed assay for multiple myeloma and should be considered in a patient who presents in the above fashion with new-onset renal failure. Myeloma causes a monoclonal gammopathy of mainly immunoglobulin G (60%) and sometimes immunoglobulin A (25%) and is the most common primary malignancy of the skeletal system. Light-chain fragments are found in abundance due to overexpression of a plasma cell clone and are nephrotoxic causing renal failure. Lytic lesions are sometimes seen on radiography and are associated with the development of hypercalcaemia causing abdominal pain, psychiatric disturbance, renal stones and bony pain – famously described as 'stones, bones, abdominal groans and psychic moans'. Interestingly although one immunoglobulin line is overexpressed, patients are susceptible to infection especially from encapsulated organisms and this is due to the resultant suppression of the other immunoglobulin lines. A pancytopaenia may be seen additionally due to the suppression of other blood cell lines.

84 a. Although daily urea and creatinine is important to monitor in a young man with rapidly deteriorating renal function it is vital to making the diagnosis that a renal biopsy is considered. In this case the diagnosis appears to be one of rapidly progressive glomerulonephritis and diagnosis of any remediable cause is key to prognosis and survival. Autoantibodies are a useful screen to perform, however, for extent and tissue diagnosis a biopsy is key. Twenty-four hour urine protein collection would quantify the amount of proteinuria associated with glomerulonephritis and the nephrotic syndrome, and could be done as an inpatient, however, it is unlikely to alter the management.

85 h. Renal artery stenosis (RAS) is often diagnosed on commencement of an ACE-I and can lead to flash pulmonary oedema, a sharp rise in urea and creatinine associated with a sharp decline in renal function. Reduced renal perfusion with bilateral RAS leads to a reliance on the intrinsic tone of the glomerular efferent arteriole to maintain glomerular filtration pressure. Reducing this efferent tone markedly drops the filtration pressure and thus an acute deterioration in renal function can occur. The investigation of choice is the renal artery Doppler and has replaced the invasive renal arteriography as the first line in diagnosis. Doppler flow studies are very sensitive for stenosis and are able to quantify the degree of stenotic lesion. A form of renal artery stenosis may be seen in young women (fibromuscular dysplasia) and may present in a similar fashion. Radiographically definable via renal artery angiography this manifests as a string-of-beads appearance.

86 e. This history is of cavernous sinus thrombosis. Although the symptoms seem vague, a high index of suspicion is required to make the diagnosis. Clinical features include:
- Fevers and rigors.
- Pain in the eye and forehead – ophthalmic division of trigeminal nerve.
- Exophthalmos and occasionally papilloedema.
- Cranial nerve palsies – III, IV, VI.
- Oedema of the peri-orbital structures and forehead due to blockage of venous drainage.
- Symptoms are most usually unilateral, but can extend via the circular sinus to become bilateral.

87 c. The history describes a subdural haemorrhage. It is most commonly seen in people with pre-existing cerebral disease or in the elderly due to atrophy of the brain or in alcoholics. Subdural haemorrhages result from rupture of cortical bridging veins. These connect the venous system of the brain to the large intradural venous sinuses and lie relatively unprotected in the subdural space. Acute subdural haemorrhage is usually associated with severe brain injury following trauma. It can occur at any age.

88 a. This is a case of a tension headache. It is believed that four out of every five people suffer with these over the course of their lifetime and approximately 40% of the population will suffer with them each year. Characteristically they are bilateral and the pain is band-like and exerts a pressure over the head.

There is no neurological deficit associated with these episodes and patients should be reassured and given adequate analgesia.

89 b. This case is describing a subarachnoid haemorrhage. The headache is sudden in its onset and described by the patient as feeling like being kicked in the head. The severity of the symptoms will depend on the extent of the bleed. It is bleeding from the intracranial vessels that is accrued in the subarachnoid space. Its incidence is approximately 1 in 10,000.
- 80% due to 'congenital'/berry aneurysm that rupture resulting in a bleed.
- 10–15% due to other aneurysms:
  - Arteriosclerotic/fusiform.
  - Inflammatory/mycotic.
  - Traumatic.
- 5% due to arteriovenous malformations – more common in younger patients.
- Less than 5% due to:
  - Bleeding diatheses, anticoagulants e.g. warfarin.
  - Tumours.

90 g. This patient is suffering from sinusitis. This can often cause the symptom of headache and often follows close after an upper respiratory tract infection. On further questioning patients may occasionally complain of feeling congested with increased amounts of nasal secretions. Sinusitis is the inflammation of the mucous membranes of the paranasal sinuses. It usually results from inadequate drainage of the sinuses secondary to physical obstruction, infection or allergy.

PAPER 5

Answers and notes

Multiple choice questions (single best answer)

1 **b.** Hypertrophic cardiomyopathy is defined as the unexplained, asymmetrical or concentric hypertrophy of the undilated left ventricle. There is also hypertrophy of the right ventricle. It may be inherited as an autosomal-dominant condition, but at least half of cases may be the result of sporadic mutation and therefore the patient may be unaware of the condition.

Symptoms may include:
- Angina
- Dyspnoea
- Palpitations
- Syncope
- Sudden death

Clinical signs include:
- Jerky pulse
- JVP: large a waves, indicating right ventricular flow obstruction
- Double impulse at apex
- Loud fourth heart sound due to the left ventricular hypertrophy
- Third heart sound
- Late systolic murmur

It is unlikely that this episode has been caused by a pulmonary embolus as she is a fit and well lady with no obvious risk factors. A pneumonia or pneumothorax would have caused some symptoms and are unlikely to have resulted in a cardiac arrest.

2 **c.** Warfarin acts as a vitamin K antagonist and so affects the synthesis of active factors II, VII, IX, X, protein C and protein S. The therapeutic goal is to cause a partial inhibition of clotting factor synthesis, to prolong prothrombin time 2-to 4-fold. Once administered warfarin does not exert its effect for 2–3 days and therefore during this lag period alternative anticoagulation should be used. This anticoagulation is usually in the form of a

low molecular weight heparin, its anticoagulation action is via factor Xa and is much more rapid in its onset.

3 a. Inhibition of (HMG Co-A) in the liver, which is the rate limiting step in cholesterol synthesis, is the mechanism of action of statins. They are appropriately prescribed in the evening since the synthesis of cholesterol appears most active overnight.

The cytochrome p450 is a group of enzymes that control concentrations of drugs and endogenous substances. Succinate Co-A is involved in the Krebs cycle.

4 c. Adenosine is a naturally occurring purine nucleoside with a pharmacological half-life of less than 2 seconds. Its principal role is in the diagnosis and management of paroxysmal supraventricular tachycardia. Cautions include atrial fibrillation or flutter caused by accessory pathways and contraindications include second- or third-degree heart block and sick sinus syndrome. Before administering adenosine to a patient it is important to tell them that they may experience a strange sensation that may lead them to feel like they are about to die. This sensation may last for a few seconds.

Atenolol is a beta-blocker and has limited use in an acute setting whilst atorvastatin has a role in reduction of cholesterol in a chronic capacity. Amlodipine is a calcium channel blocker and amiodarone has a role in refractory ventricular fibrillation or atrial flutter.

5 b. Simvastatin has been linked to inflammation of muscle tissue (myositis) causing a rise in creatinine kinase associated with muscle aches, malaise and abdominal pain. Also reported is a derangement of liver enzymes especially of aspartate transaminase and alanine aminotransferase. A rare but serious side-effect of simvastatin in particular is the development of rhabdomyolysis leading to acute renal damage. Diclofenac may be associated with abdominal pain but the mechanism of pain is usually due to gastric ulceration caused by the inhibition of protective prostaglandins in the gastric mucosa. Metformin is a diabetic medication that unlike the sulphonylureas does not cause hypoglycaemia due to a mechanism of action that increases insulin sensitivity in tissues rather than increase insulin levels. Metformin can cause a metabolic acidosis and renal impairment when given in conjunction with contrast agents such as those used in radiographic investigations. It should be stopped on the day of the investigation and the patient should be encouraged to drink fluids for the next 24–48 hours post contrast.

6 b. Ventricular fibrillation is uncoordinated ventricular activity which can be corrected by unsynchronised DC shock. Pulseless ventricular tachycardia can also be managed by unsynchronised DC shock. Atrial fibrillation, provided it is new in origin, can be managed by electrical current but this requires synchronised current. Asystole and pulseless electrical activity do not benefit from treatment with electrical current.

7 c. Phentolamine and other alpha-blockers are the agents of choice in the rapid treatment of hypertension caused by phaeochromocytoma. Beta-blockade can be added to control dangerously high blood pressure but only after institution of an alpha-blocker otherwise there is a significant risk of exacerbating hypertension. Surgical intervention in patients with phaeochromocytoma must only be performed once the patient has been medically treated and blocked from the effects of excess circulating catecholamines. Catecholamine-induced cardiomyopathy and life-threatening hypertensive crisis due to uncontrolled release of catecholamines intra-operatively are a significant cause of mortality and morbidity.

Imaging modalities such as a CT scan of the abdomen and renal artery Dopplers are useful studies in the investigation of any patient with uncontrolled newly diagnosed hypertension; however, these are not urgent and CT scan would be contraindicated in an unstable patient (the 'doughnut of death'). Renal artery Dopplers are used commonly to detect clinically significant arterial stenosis, which can lead to hypertension and flash pulmonary oedema.

Surgical management of phaeochromocytoma is usually performed transabdominally with identification and ligation of the adrenal veins to isolate the tumour from releasing a surge of catecholamine into the systemic circulation. Laparoscopic approaches have been favoured recently but prove more difficult to assess for extra-adrenal sites of catecholamine production, e.g. elsewhere in the sympathetic chain.

8 e. Extra-ocular muscles are supplied by three main cranial nerves: the oculomotor nerve (III), trochlear nerve (IV) and abducens nerve (VI). The abducens nerve supplies motor innervation to the lateral rectus muscle, the trochlear nerve supplies motor innervation to the superior oblique muscle and medial rectus, inferior oblique, superior and inferior rectus are all motor innervated by the oculomotor (III) nerve. A useful way of remembering this information is the 'chemical formula' – $LR_6SO_4AL_3$ (**L**ateral **R**ectus **6**, **S**uperior **O**blique **4**, **AL**l the rest **3**).

The innervation to levator palpebrae superioris (the muscle responsible for eyelid opening) is dual, involving both the sympathetic nervous system and the third cranial nerve (oculomotor nerve). This dual supply is evidence by the degree of ptosis (drooping of the eyelid) seen in oculomotor palsy and in conditions affecting the sympathetic supply to the head and neck, e.g. Horner's syndrome. Partial ptosis is seen in Horner's syndrome due to sparing of the oculomotor innervation to levator palpebrae superioris, whilst complete ptosis occurs in oculomotor palsies due to loss of both oculomotor *and* sympathetic tone (as sympathetic fibres run along the course of the oculomotor nerve). Supply to the lacrimal glands is from the parasympathetic nervous system and is delivered via the greater petrosal nerve, the deep petrosal nerve, and zygomatic and lacrimal nerves.

9 **c.** All of the signs above are suggestive of a locally invasive breast cancer. A growing mass with overlying skin ulceration is highly suggestive of malignancy. Other signs to look out for include peau d'orange skin changes and axillary lymphadenopathy, which are not mentioned in the case. A breast abscess or mastitis are unlikely to be the case in this lady as she reports no pain from the lump and is not strictly in the right age range for those conditions. Although ductal carcinoma *in situ* may present in a similar manner to an invasive breast lump the extent of the spread of this lump suggests that a more sinister cause is responsible.

10 **d.** Thalassaemia major is a life-threatening illness. Most well-treated thalassaemic patients survive into their 30s and 40s. Thalassaemia is associated with a microcytic anaemia. The other associations are correct.

11 **c.** Upper gastrointestinal bleeds (UGIB) manifest themselves both as haematemesis, typically with coffee ground vomiting from the alteration of blood by digestive enzymes and stomach acid, or with the presence of melaena (dark, offensive, altered blood per rectum). Evidence of an actively bleeding source in the upper GI tract can often be difficult to objectively assess as the subjective description of passing melaena stools may vary greatly. Clinical and laboratory indices of bleeding are often relied upon as a proxy measure and include pulse rate, lying versus standing (or sitting if patients are not able to stand) blood pressures looking for significant postural hypotension (arbitrarily described as a drop in systolic of > 20mmHg) and a systolic pressure lower

than 90 mmHg, a drop in haemoglobin (which will only occur after a period of bleeding lasting longer than about 24 hours due to the acute effect of haemoconcentration during an acute bleed leading a falsely normal haemoglobin reading) and a rise in urea due to break down of blood into nitrogenous products. Once the diagnosis of UGIB has been made then patients should be commenced on proton pump inhibitors and any non-steroidal drugs should be stopped (as these increase the risk of GI bleeds by inhibiting the protective effect of prostaglandins in the GI tract. Decisions as to the urgency of endoscopy should then be made. Indications for urgent endoscopy depend on the clinical risk prediction for active bleeding and in this case are fulfilled. A postural drop and tachycardia approximate a 20% blood loss and with biochemical evidence of a clinically significant bleed endoscopy may identify and treat any actively bleeding source. Surgical referral is not merited at this time as the patient may be adequately and safely treated endoscopically. Persistent bleeding in an unstable patient who may not be treatable endoscopically and in whom urgent control of bleeding is required are candidates for laparotomy and direct surgical intervention although the mortality is high in cases of emergency surgery for UGIB. Coeliac arteriography is an option to consider in a patient in whom no readily identifiable lesion has been demonstrated but who continues to bleed and a small bowel source of bleeding is suspected. Colonoscopy is only useful for assessing sources of bleeding in the lower GI tract and is mostly often applied in the investigation of colonic malignancy.

12 **c.** The history of colicky pain radiating from the loin to groin and occasionally down to the testis is classical of ureteric stones. He is within the right age group for this problem and microscopic haematuria is seen with calculi. Calculi may develop or be the cause of associated urinary tract infections although most stones pass without any surgical intervention. Investigation should include a full set of bloods and a plain abdominal X-ray since 90% of urinary calculi are radio-opaque. Other useful investigations include urine culture and intravenous urogram, which can identify the level of the stone if indeed one is present.

13 **e.** Pyoderma gangrenosum is associated with inflammatory bowel disease such as ulcerative colitis and Crohn's disease. It presents as wet sloughly ulcers with heaped edges and scattered areas of black necrotic tissue. Pyoderma gangrenosum may also be associated with haematological malignancy and rheumatoid arthritis. The cutaneous manifestations of diabetes mellitus are

legion and range from diabetic foot ulcers to atrophy of the fat layers in the skin causing thinning and an abnormal appearance to the area (lipoatrophy). Necrobiosis lipoidica diabeticorum are usually found on the shins and present as shiny, yellow-brown heterogenous areas of skin discolouration with associated skin thinning and predisposition to break down. Xanthomas and xanthelasma are seen in condition of hypercholesterolaemia and are not discrete to diabetes; however, endocrine disturbance, as seen in diabetes mellitus, is frequently associated with derangement in other biochemical profiles such as lipid homeostasis. Acanthosis nigricans (the presenting complaint of this gentleman) manifests as a result of insulin resistance, although it may be seen in association with gastrointestinal malignancy. Granuloma annulare often present in association with diabetes when generalised rather than discrete and are characteristically described as crops of hard raised areas of skin in a ring-like arrangement occurring on the back of the hands and soles of the feet. A conservative approach is adopted in most cases as spontaneous resolution tends to be the rule.

14 b. The case in question is describing a Weber C fracture (a fracture arising above the syndesmosis). Ankle fractures were described by Weber and his simple classification is still used in orthopaedics today:
- Weber A – fibular fracture below the syndesmosis.
- Weber B – fibular fracture through the syndesmosis.
- Weber C – fibular fracture above the syndesmosis.

Management of these fractures depends on the classification. Weber A are always managed conservatively, Weber B fractures are sometimes managed surgically and sometimes managed conservatively, and Weber C fractures as a rule are always managed operatively. These rules apply for isolated fibular fractures, when other injuries co-exist management may change.

15 a. Primary post-partum haemorrhage is defined as vaginal blood loss in the first 24 hours after delivery of the baby. The bleeding is often related to gestational products and blood loss.

16 e. This patient is suffering from ischaemia of the bowel or mesenteric ischaemia. This condition is most commonly seen in elderly men, particularly known arteriopaths. Commonly the disease involves the superior mesenteric artery, which provides blood supply to both the small and large bowel. It is characteristically identified by severe abdominal pain approximately 30 minutes after eating, which results in anorexia to avoid the pain and subsequent weight loss. Angiography would be useful to confirm this diagnosis. A congenital cause of a bowel abnormality would more than likely have presented itself before the age of 67 years and a psychogenic cause can be ruled out due to physical signs being present. Imaging, including barium enema and colonoscopy, would identify the large majority of colonic neoplasms and therefore these can be ruled out although they are important differentials in an elderly patient with weight loss.

17 c. The Glasgow criteria for predicting the severity of pancreatitis can be used for pancreatitis due to any cause, though the Ranson criteria are reserved for pancreatitis due to alcoholism. The mnemonic 'PANCREAS' is useful for remembering the Glasgow criteria, especially on surgical ward rounds!

P: $PO_2 < 8\,kPa$
A: Age > 55 years
N: Neutrophils $> 15 \times 10^9/L$
C: Calcium $< 2\,mmol/L$
R: Raised enzymes – LDH/AST
E: Elevated urea $> 16\,mmol/L$
A: Albumin $< 32\,g/L$
S: Sugar $> 10\,mmol/L$

18 a. Femoral hernias are more common in women. The small bowel herniates through the femoral canal underneath the inguinal ligament, medial to the femoral artery. (Use 'NAVEL' to remember from lateral to medial in the femoral canal – **N**erve, **A**rtery, **V**ein, **E**mpty space, **L**ymphatics.) The neck of femoral hernias is narrow and therefore strangulation ensues. Indirect hernias pass through both the deep and superficial inguinal rings, ventral hernias, also known as incisional hernias, are most commonly seen in those patients with particular risk factors including obesity, old age, wound infection postoperatively and violent coughing. Direct hernias do not protrude into the scrotal sac although inguinal hernias cannot be classified adequately until surgery is performed.

19 b. This patient has acute infection of the parotid gland or acute parotitis. Patients with poor dental hygiene and those who have been intubated are most at risk. *Staphylococcus aureus* is the organism most commonly responsible for this. Most often the treatment for this condition would require surgical drainage and antibiotics. Mumps is a common cause of parotitis although now only seen in outbreaks usually among children and young adults that have failed to be immunised. Haemorrhage into the gland is incredibly rare and trauma during this surgery is unlikely due to its position. Sialolithiasis or stones in the salivary glands could be the cause of this presentation, although there is no relationship between stone development and surgery.

20 b. A ruptured spleen must be considered with blunt trauma to the chest or upper abdomen particularly if rib fractures are involved. Splenic trauma can be diagnosed by peritoneal lavage, CT scan or radionucleotide scanning; however, in this situation surgery is necessary immediately, due to the development of shock, in order to assess the level of damage to the spleen and potentially prevent its removal. The location of the injury and the associated hypovolaemia argue against both transection of the abdominal aorta and injury to the liver capsule. Trauma to the lungs is unlikely to lead to normal breath sounds on examination.

21 b. Paraphimosis is frequently seen as a result of urethral catheterisation. This unfortunate complication can be avoided by careful attention to replacing the foreskin after catheterisation and by regular inspection of the penis whilst a catheter is *in situ*. Phimosis is usually picked up in childhood by a concerned parent that the child has problems passing urine or that his foreskin balloons up on passing urine. The condition is due to a narrowing of the preputial orifice and will usually require correction by circumcision. Epispadias is a defect in penile development where the urethra opens on the ventral aspect of the penis. More commonly found is the 'opposite' defect; hypospadias, where the urethra opens on the dorsal aspect of the penis in an abnormal position anywhere from base of the shaft to the glans penis. Peyronie's disease manifests as an angulation of the erect penis due to fibrosis. It is associated with Dupuytren's contracture and atheroma.

22 c. The results of the ABG can be broken down into components:
1. pH 7.40 – this is within the normal range (7.35–7.45).
2. PO_2 7.3 kPa – this is clearly suboptimal. Even in patients suffering from COPD the PO_2 should be greater than 8.0 kPa.
3. PO_2 4.8 kPa – this is also within the normal range. Some patients with COPD retain CO_2 which can suppress their respiratory drive.

On balance, this patient is hypoxic with a normal PCO_2, therefore the main problem is hypoxia, which can be improved by administering oxygen. In these patients it is always important to be on the look out for the signs of CO_2 narcosis particularly when increasing concentrations of oxygen.

23 a. Sarcoidosis is a multi-system inflammatory disease of unknown aetiology that mainly affects the lungs and intrathoracic lymph nodes. Sarcoidosis is manifested by the presence of non-caseating granulomas in affected organ tissues. It is more common in men than women (2:1) and peak incidence occurs from ages 25 to 35 years with a second peak in women aged 45 to 65 years. Characteristic appearance on chest X-ray is bilateral hilar lymphadenopathy.

Pulmonary fibrosis presents with a ground-glass appearance on chest X-ray and rarely has symptoms manifest outside of the chest. In a person of this age it is unlikely that this would be malignancy. In lung cancer unilateral hilar lymphadenopathy is seen but rarely is this bilateral.

24 d. Cystic fibrosis is not a disorder that is seen very often. On examination of the chest in a patient suffering from cystic fibrosis you would expect to hear coarse inspiratory crackles due to the production of thick secretions and difficulty of the mucociliary system in clearing these. The result is coarse crepitations heard on auscultation.

25 e. Causes of fibrosing alveolitis are vast and varied. When all causes have been excluded and the diagnosis is certain it can be said that the patient is suffering with cryptogenic fibrosing alveolitis, e.g. of unknown cause. Rheumatoid arthritis, Sjögren's syndrome and ulcerative colitis are all systemic conditions that are known to cause fibrosing alveolitis. *Aspergillus* is associated with extrinsic allergic alveolitis as it causes an immune response by which it medicates its effects.

26 e. Malignant mesothelioma is associated with a history of asbestos exposure. In most cases the exposure is approximately 40 years prior to onset of the symptoms and discovery of the cancer. It is believed that some women suffer with mesothelioma after exposure via their husband's work overalls, others became exposed by living down-wind from the asbestos factory. Men usually have a good history of occupational exposure to asbestos. Pleural mesothelioma is 1.6 times more common on the right side than on the left and the prognosis of the condition from diagnosis is poor. Males are usually more commonly affected than females.

27 a. Sleep apnoea is a problem of overweight middle-aged men. It is believed that the weight of the additional fat surrounding their necks places pressure on their trachea during sleep and subsequently they have apnoeic episodes. Due to this interruption to their sleep daytime somnolence is a common feature as is morning headache. Reduced libido and cognitive function are associated with sleep apnoea although rarely considered to be part of the same condition as sleep apnoea is commonly overlooked. Cough is not a feature of this condition.

28 e. Acute asthma does not cause cor pulmonale. It is caused by chronic conditions that result in high pressures in the lungs resulting in high backpressure being transmitted to the heart which ultimately has a remodelling effect on the right-sided heart chambers. Chronic asthma has been associated with the development of cor pulmonale but acute lung diseases do not cause this problem. The main symptom is shortness of breath and occasionally chest pain, if the condition is prolonged both sides of the heart become involved, symptoms such as bipedal oedema will develop.

29 c. The history is describing a respiratory emergency. It is a case of a tension pneumothorax. With every additional breath that the patient takes his pleural cavity is filling up with air and his lung is being pushed over to the opposite side of the chest. Not only is the pleural pressure causing the lung to deflate, but is also reducing venous return to the heart. In this situation urgent action is required.

Clinical symptoms include:
- Tracheal deviation away from the affected side.
- Increased resonance to percussion on the affected side.
- Reduced breath sounds on the affected side.
- Reduced chest expansion on the affected side.

In this clinical picture insertion of a large bore cannula into the second intercostal space as soon as possible is lifesaving (always remember to remove the needle once inserted!!). A hissing sound should be heard if your diagnosis is correct and gradually the patient should find it easier to breathe as the lung re-inflates. You should always seek senior support in this scenario.

30 c. There are few clues to the diagnosis in the question; however, the clinical picture suggests an episode of acute pancreatitis with classical radiological features. The best discriminatory investigation is the serum amylase, which, if raised 4-fold above the upper limit of normal (90u/L), is highly suggestive of pancreatitis. Diabetic ketoacidosis should also be ruled out and a simple bedside blood glucose and urine dipstick is a quick and easy screen whilst serum levels are awaited. A pleural tap is unlikely to be useful in the diagnosis of this patient's abdominal pain and trans-oesophageal echo is usually employed in the visualisation of the heart and cardiac function. Endoscopy is a useful option if amylase levels are normal and an upper gastrointestinal cause of pain is suggested.

31 **a.** *Candida albicans* is a fungal infection responsible for causing thrush in women and balanitis in males. Although it is common in normal healthy women it is relatively uncommon in males and thus any male presenting with signs of candidal infection should have blood glucose levels checked. Diabetes mellitus predisposes to infection and the clinical history of polyuria, polydipsia and a candidal infection in the absence of genitourinary tract infection in a young male is almost enough to make the diagnosis itself. Full blood count might be useful if a sexually transmitted infection with systemic involvement was suspected. Erythrocyte sedimentation rate (ESR) is a non-specific index of disease, e.g. inflammatory conditions, disseminated malignancy and infection but would not be beneficial in this case. ESR rises with age and anaemia and an easy guide to interpreting ESR with respect to age is by using the Westergren formula:

Males: (Age in years)/2
Females: (Age in years + 10)/2

HTLV-1 and-2 (human T cell leukaemia virus) are oncogenic retroviruses that are of the same family as HIV. HTLV-1 has been linked to the development of T cell leukaemia and lymphoma and neurological diseases such as tropical spastic paraparesis and the Brown-Séquard syndrome. Urine analysis would be useful in determining the clinical probability of urinary tract infection and on the basis of dipstick positive findings would be evidence enough to start empirical antibiotics. Urine specimen for microscopy, culture and sensitivities should be considered if there is a negative urine dipstick or suspicion of a more resistant or atypical organism.

32 **b.** Benign oesophageal strictures are associated with gastro-oesophageal reflux disease (GORD) and are caused by backwash of acid through an incompetent lower oesophageal sphincter with resultant scarring, fibrosis and stenosis of the lower oesophagus. The history of taking antacid remedies points the clinician to

a diagnosis by proxy of GORD and the patient's body habitus makes acid reflux a likely problem. GORD can be treated medically with antacids, proton pump inhibition or H_2 antagonism and surgical therapy (Nissen fundoplication) may be necessary for those refractory to medical treatment. Systemic sclerosis would likely manifest with clinical obvious features such as peri-orbital or digital skin changes or lung, cardiac or renal involvement. Autoantibody screen especially for Scl-70 and RNA polymerases will aid in diagnosis if any doubt is present. Oesophageal carcinoma is very unlikely given the patients' age; however, if there were any sinister features to the history or examination an outpatient barium swallow study would aid in making the diagnosis. The typical radiological finding suggestive of oesophageal carcinoma is of an apple-core appearance as the tumour encircles a portion of oesophageal lumen causing dilatation of the proximal segment. Oesophageal candidiasis would again unlikely in an immunocompetent individual but if retrosternal pain on swallowing persists in the face of effective proton pump or H_2 receptor inhibition for GORD then further investigation may be warranted. There is no history of radiotherapy to the chest or mediastinum that may raise the suspicion of a radiation stricture.

33 c. Drug therapy is one of the causes of gynaecomastia but must not attributed as a cause without exclusion of the aggressive male breast cancer. Spironolactone, digoxin, cimetidine, alcohol and ketoconazole have been linked to the development of gynaecomastia and the mnemonic 'some drugs cause awesome knockers' aids in remembering these. Other causes of bilateral benign breast swellings include liver cirrhosis, testicular and adrenal tumours, hypogonadism and renal failure with the pathogenetic link being an abnormality in the normal ratio of oestrogens to androgens (either due to failure of production in liver cirrhosis, testicular and adrenal tumours or a failure to clear hormones from the body as in renal failure).

34 e. Rectal bleeding is a distressing symptom for patients and every effort should be taken to reassure the patient. An accurate history can be more useful than investigation and should always be undertaken as the difficulty in finding an occult source of bleeding should never be underestimated. Classifying rectal bleeding into fresh red and altered dark bleeding can help to differentiate between upper and lower gastrointestinal causes. The presence of melaena, i.e. altered changed blood almost exclusively locates the source of bleeding to the upper gastro-intestinal tract as blood is altered by digestive enzymes and acid found in the stomach and proximal small intestine. Fresh red blood suggests lower tract bleeding. Further classifying lower tract bleeding into painful versus painless helps to exclude conditions such as anal fissure, which causes excruciating pain on passing stool. Angiodysplasia is a cause of fresh rectal bleeding from an arteriovenous malformation often in the elderly. It can be seen at colonoscopy as a luminal vascular abnormality that may bleed on pressure over it. Rectosigmoid carcinoma typically presents with obstruction and may only bleed when advanced. Inflammatory bowel disorders tend to present with altered bowel habit and bloody diarrhoea mixed in with mucus rather than bright red blood.

35 a. Microcytic anaemia with weight loss in an elderly patient is colorectal carcinoma until proven otherwise. Right-sided tumours, e.g. caecum and ascending colon, tend to cause occult bleeding and a microcytic anaemia whilst left-sided tumours, e.g. rectosigmoid, tend to cause obstruction and sometimes fresh red rectal bleeding. The derangement of liver enzymes is a sinister sign of potential hepatic metastases and a coagulation profile should be requested in case of liver dysfunction. In the first instance an OGD and colonoscopy ('top and tail') should be performed as this will both identify any suspicious masses and allow tissue harvest for histological analysis. A staging CT scan of the chest, abdomen and pelvis should then be performed if endoscopy results demonstrate a lesion. The images and case details should ideally be discussed in a multidisciplinary meeting (MDM) involving surgeons, oncologists, palliative care physicians and radiologists so active decisions regarding management can be made. A simple chest radiograph is a useful screening tool if a colorectal cancer is suspected and will be done more quickly than a staging CT. Liver biopsy is rarely necessary unless disseminated malignancy is found with no apparent primary focus *and* histological diagnosis will influence management strategy.

36 b. Meig's syndrome describes the association of an ovarian thecoma or fibroma with ascites and pleural effusion. Usually occurring to women of childbearing age the benign ovarian thecoma is one of the commonest sex-cord stromal tumours. The Jarisch–Herxheimer reaction occurs secondary to penicillin use in syphilis and is caused by a release of TNF-α, IL-6 and IL-8. As it is not a dose-related phenomenon penicillin should not be withheld or reduced in dose. Fitz–Hugh–Curtis syndrome is seen in chlamydial infection of young women leading to perihepatic adhesions through transcoelomic spread of chlamydia from the genitourinary tract. Peyronie's disease is seen in males leading to angulation of the penis due to fibrosis of soft tissue. It is associated with Dupuytren's contracture and atheroma. Raynaud's syndrome describes intermittent digital ischaemia with colour changes in the hands often precipitated by cold weather or emotion. It has been linked with the use of vibrating machinery, CREST syndrome and smoking.

37 c. The presentation of abdominal pain, new-onset neuropsychiatric symptoms in a young woman should always alert the clinician to the possibility of acute intermittent porphyria (AIP) as the diagnosis. The porphyrias are a set of genetic disorders of haem biosynthesis resulting in increased levels of porphyrin precursors such as porphobilinogen and 5-δ-aminolaevulinic acid. Skin involvement is a feature of some varieties of porphyria and may be the presenting feature. Other clinical features can be summed up by 'the four H's, P's and S's':
- **H**ypotonia, **H**ypotension, **H**yponatraemia, **H**ypokalaemia
- **P**roteinuria, **P**sychosis, **P**aralysis, **P**eripheral neuritis
- **S**eizures, **S**hock, **S**ensory impairment, vi**S**ual abnormalities

The urine may appear dark or deep red especially on standing and testing for urinary porphobilinogen and 5-δ-aminolaevulinic acid levels aids in diagnosis. Thyroid function tests may be helpful in patients with features of thyroid dysfunction and confusion or psychiatric symptoms; however, the clinical picture is not typical for thyroid dysfunction. Phaeochromocytoma may cause symptoms of anxiety, depression and a sense of impending doom. Levels of adrenaline metabolites can be assayed in a 24-hour urine collection; however, a phaeochromocytoma crisis manifests with sympathetic overactivity, which can help to differentiate organic from functional causes of psychosis. CT scan of the abdomen is a reasonable line of investigation to proceed with once simple causes of abdominal pain and psychiatric disturbance have been ruled out as malignancy and especially hormone-secreting tumours may cause the above picture.

38 a. Faecal impaction with overflow diarrhoea is a common cause of spurious diarrhoea in an elderly poorly mobile patient. Radiological and clinical features show a ground-glass appearance throughout the gastrointestinal tract with hard faecal matter per rectum and a lumpy abdomen. Treatment involves the use of phosphate enemas once obstruction has been ruled out or aperients such as senna, lactulose or sodium docusate. Faecal stool softeners such as glycerine suppositories can additionally be used if constipation is not relieved by the above measures. Sigmoid volvulus is a cause of large bowel obstruction and a surgical emergency if absolute constipation (obstipation) has set in. It is commoner in men than women and presents acutely with sudden onset colicky abdominal pain with radiographic appearance of a 'bent inner tube' if the two segments of sigmoid lie adjacent to each other. Cholesterol embolus can occur from the mobilisation of cholesterol atheromatous plaques from the aorta or renal arteries causing back and abdominal pain with evidence of end-artery ischaemia, e.g. retina/digits. Usually occurring after arterial catheterisation, especially renal artery angioplasty, it may lead to gastrointestinal bleeding, purpura, progressive renal failure and a net-like rash (livedo reticularis). Cauda equina syndrome is a neurosurgical emergency due to compression of the spinal cord at the level of the cauda equina. It manifests typically with perineal numbness (saddle anaesthesia), loss of anal sphincter tone, incontinence and paraparesis of both legs. *Clostridium difficile* infection is usually associated with the use of antibiotics, in particular clindamycin and the cephalosporins. Diarrhoea is profuse, watery and offensive, and direct imaging of the colon demonstrates a pseudomembranous colitis appearance. Oral metronidazole and fluid rehydration are the first line in treatment along with stopping other antibiotic therapy.

39 b. Total parenteral nutrition (TPN) has been linked with derangement of liver enzymes, sepsis, thrombosis and hyponatraemia. Cholestasis has been shown to occur after commencement of TPN and frank liver damage can occur. It is extremely common for patients to exhibit a rise in liver enzymes after starting TPN and these must be monitored 3 times weekly for acute rises. Enteral nutrition is the preferred route of administration of nutrition even in the face of gastrointestinal disease and recent advances in the management of pancreatitis aim to re-establish enteral feeding slowly once vomiting and abdominal pain allow. Blood transfusion reactions are usually acute events occurring within minutes to an hour of the transfusion with pyrexia, flushing and in severe cases anaphylaxis. Biliary leak usually occurs after hepatobiliary surgery and manifests in the days post-operatively with pain, peritonitis and a rise in liver enzymes. Hepatitis in a very rare complication of blood transfusion and although a theoretical risk nowadays, would be low down on the differential diagnosis of a rise in liver enzymes in this case. Sedation on the ICU is usually maintained with infusion of benzodiazepine and opioid such as midazolam and morphine. Both agents have not been linked with hepatic damage in doses used for sedation although use in pre-existing severe hepatic dysfunction may prolong the sedative effects and is recommended with caution.

40 d. Multiple sclerosis is one of the most common of a group of inflammatory conditions affecting the CNS. It leads to a relapsing and remitting course for the disease but ultimately most patients develop progressive permanent neurological symptoms. It is a fairly common disease and normally presents in young patients. Its effects are wide reaching, in addition to the physical disability that develops, psychological problems often accompany the physical symptoms. At present there is no proven treatment, β-interferon has been shown to reduce the relapse rate of exacerbations but not alter the disease progression. Patients are plagued with a combination of eye problems, motor weakness, sensory loss, cerebellar and brainstem lesions in addition to spinal cord damage. Its investigation remains challenging due to the intermittent course that the disease initially undertakes.

41 a. In a patient with a confirmed diagnosis of bacterial meningitis we would expect to see a raised opening CSF pressure. Normal pressure is seen in cases of viral infection and sometimes encephalitis but not in bacterial meningitis. Protein levels are elevated and glucose is low due to the active bacteria affecting the fluid and greater than 50 polymorphs should be seen. Confirmed cases are public health issues and the appropriate departments should be contacted.

42 b. The condition that this case is alluding to is an acute cord compression. The history of niggling pain is a red herring. Whilst that may be significant, in the acute setting the worry is that he is unable to pass urine and complaining of saddle anaesthesia. Whilst in a scenario such as this one spinal X-rays may provide some information and clues the diagnosis will be made on MRI scan. Any evidence of acute cord compression regardless of cause should be discussed with a neurosurgical centre for potential surgery to decompress. There is no evidence that these symptoms are caused by a cerebral lesion and blood tests are unlikely to be of diagnostic value alone.

43 d. Tight control of blood sugars in diabetic patients is essential to reduce the risk of developing later complications. Bilateral pupillary abnormalities are caused by an autonomic neuropathy. The pupils have a poor reaction to light, but better to accommodation. The third nerve palsy results from a microvascular lesion to the nerve trunk, often the pupil is spared in this condition.

Hemiparesis may occur transiently due to hypoglycaemia or due to transient ischaemic attacks. There is no evidence that headaches are associated with diabetes.

44 a. This case is describing trigeminal neuralgia. It commonly affects the maxillary and mandibular divisions of the trigeminal nerve and occasionally affects the ophthalmic division. It can be an intensely painful condition and may result in the face completely screwing up as a result. The symptoms may be precipitated by washing, brushing or simply touching the overlying skin. It has a number of causes including idiopathic, cerebello-pontine angle tumour, multiple sclerosis or a vascular malformation. Although the condition may resolve spontaneously drugs directed at the nerve ganglion may provide relief. These include carbamazepine and phenytoin.

45 d. Patients suffering from Parkinson's disease develop a typical gait. It is normally a shuffling gait with difficulty both initiating and stopping movements. As the condition progresses the posture becomes increasingly flexed.

Other characteristic gait findings include:
• Spastic – circumduction of legs.
• Frontal – difficulty getting feet off floor.
• Cerebellar – wide-based gait.
• Myopathic – waddle, difficulty climbing stairs.

46 b. This is a classical history of an extradural haemorrhage. They commonly follow head injuries, particularly those causing fractures of the temporal or parietal bones resulting in damage to the middle meningeal artery and vein. Damage to the dural venous sinus will also result in an extradural haemorrhage. Important signs to look out for include a deterioration in the patients level of consciousness and a lucid interval that may be mistaken for an uncomplicated recovery. This lucid interval may last for anything from a duration of hours to days as the blood accumulates between the bone and dura. The bleed finally declares itself by a reducing level of consciousness with rising intracranial pressure and increasingly severe headaches. Vomiting and confusion may also be features and hemiparesis and upgoing plantars may be seen as the deterioration progresses.

Management of this bleed is by the neurosurgeons releasing the pressure through burr holes in the skull.

Subdural haemorrhages are most common in the elderly or amongst alcoholics. A subarachnoid haemorrhage is often described as being kicked in the back of the head whilst a stroke would provide neurological evidence at presentation.

47 b. This lady is most likely to be suffering from delirium, otherwise known as an acute confusional state. It is a fairly common condition in hospitalised patients and occurs in approximately 5–15% of inpatients on general medical or surgical wards.

Symptoms and signs include:
- Impaired consciousness with acute onset over hours to days. It will fluctuate throughout the day often being worse in the late afternoon to evening.
- Disorientation in time, place and person.
- Altered behaviour, including quietness and reduced speech to agitation and aggression.
- Thinking may be slow and muddled and occasionally paranoid.
- Their mood is likely to be labile and depressed.
- Memory is often impaired.

All presentations similar to this one should have a full screen of tests carried out to discover the underlying cause. Dementia is much slower in its onset and more chronic in its course. Whilst it is easy to assume that this presentation could be due to a psychiatric illness, other organic causes should be excluded first.

48 e. The causes of peripheral neuropathy may be remembered by the mnemonic 'DANG THERAPIST':
D: Diabetes
A: Amyloid
N: Nutritional (e.g. B1, B6 or B12 deficiency)
G: Guillain–Barre syndrome (GBS)
T: Toxic (e.g. amiodarone, arsenic)
H: Hereditary
E: Endocrine e.g. diabetes
R: Recurring (10% of GBS)
A: Alcohol
P: Pb (lead) or Porphyria
I: Idiopathic
S: Sarcoid
T: Tumours

49 a. Causes of pin-point pupils include both an opioid overdose and a pontine event including a haemorrhage. Remember this as:
'**P**in-**P**oint **P**upils are due to o**P**ioids and **P**ontine **P**athology'.

50 b. The most common cause of acute renal failure post-surgery is dehydration and hypovolaemia. In this particular case acute renal failure can be deduced by the normal renal function pre-operatively and acute onset of biochemical derangement post-operatively. Remaining nil by mouth prior to surgery with inadequate fluid maintenance on top of any pre-existing dehydration in addition to increased losses such as vomiting in this case all contribute to dehydration and reduction of blood flow to the kidneys if volume loss is significant. Acute rather than chronic renal failure can also be reasoned if there is a disproportionate rise in urea relative to creatinine. Analgesic nephropathy typically causes an interstitial nephritis but would be unlikely to manifest with therapeutic doses of analgesia used over a short period of time. Renal metastases would be unlikely to present acutely post-surgery with no stigmata pre-operatively and is an uncommon site for metastases from an isolated colonic carcinoma. Post-surgical rhabdomyolysis is not the cause of renal failure in this case; muscle injury is usually significant in cases of rhabdomyolysis and is usually associated with crush injuries, acute drug reactions or elderly patients immobile on a hard surface over a period of time. If rhabdomyolysis is suspected as a cause of renal failure, creatinine kinase levels and urinary myoglobin assay will usually aid diagnostic uncertainty. Urinary retention post-surgery is very common in the elderly population especially males with pre-existing prostatic hypertrophy, however, is a less likely cause in this case. Urinary catheterisation with replacement fluids if a palpable bladder or significant bladder residual volume is usually all that is required.

51 e. Reversal of renal failure once the end stage has been reached is extremely unlikely and usually represents a misdiagnosis of the initial cause or an acute event that required supportive therapy until intrinsic renal function was restored. Dialysis has been implicated in the development of cardiovascular disease and incidence of such disease related to the process of dialysis itself has been shown to be higher in dialysed patients. Complications associated with β_2-microglobulin amyloidosis associated with dialysis for periods greater than 5 years have been well described and include bony fractures due to bone weakening by formation of amyloid-related bony cysts, carpal tunnel syndrome due to accumulation of amyloid in tendon sheaths and arthralgia. Aluminium toxicity with the associated risk of dementia and cognitive impairment is a phenomenon seen less frequently with current dialysis methods but has been described in patient dialysed using non-aluminium-depleted dialysate. Bleeding tendency may occur with long-term dialysis and is due to platelet dysfunction that may be exacerbated by anticoagulants used to prevent clotting whilst on the dialysis machine.

52 **a.** Staging CT scan of the chest, abdomen and pelvis will be of most help in assessing the extent of any presumed metastatic spread and may provide information regarding a primary focus in malignancy is strongly suspected. However, CT is only of diagnostic use when contrast medium is used and this is contraindicated in renal failure as a potential side-effect of contrast use is contrast-induced nephropathy. Around 5% of the population will experience this side-effect with those already exhibiting renal failure at a 5–10 times increased risk above this baseline. Ultrasonography of the liver is a useful, non-invasive and safe tool if liver enzymes are elevated and should be considered in patients in whom metastatic cancer (especially breast and colon) is suspected. Thoracic radiography requires no contrast and may demonstrate bony metastases in this woman who is experiencing mid-back pain. Breast examination should be carried out possibly with mammography or breast ultrasound depending on age and breast characteristics if clinically indicated. Bony metastases are an extremely common presentation of cancer and may manifest as bony pain, pathological fractures, hypercalcaemia and a raised alkaline phosphatase. Thyroid, breast, lung, kidney, colon and prostate are the most common sites of primary neoplasm metastasising to bone.

53 **b.** Metformin is primarily excreted by the kidneys and dosing is dependent on the intrinsic renal function. Although the biguanides are not directly nephrotoxic when used at therapeutic doses, in the face of renal failure and oliguria or anuria metformin levels may build up to toxic levels in peripheral tissues. This in turn may rarely lead to an increase in lactate production and lactic acidosis. Metformin therefore should not be continued in cases where contract injection (such as CT scanning) is necessary. It should be withheld on the day of the planned study (occasionally the day before if renal failure is significant) and for at least 48 hours post-contrast with documentation of the renal function on a daily basis. Once normal renal function has been shown metformin can be instituted with adequate hydration. This is especially important in the elderly and those not able to take in adequate oral hydration, e.g. surgical patients and these patients should be well hydrated prior to undergoing any contrast procedures with diligent monitoring

of renal function. Shortness of breath in this case is related to a degree of acidosis caused by both renal failure and the build-up of lactic acid due to metformin use and thus respiratory compensation in the form of hyperventilation. An arterial blood gas possibly with a plasma lactate will help to confirm the diagnosis and assess the extent of the acidosis.

54 d. Renal vein thrombosis typically presents in association with nephrotic syndrome or sometimes in cases of thrombophilic states such as malignancy. Loss of clotting factors in the nephrotic syndrome causes an increase in venous thrombosis, particularly seen in association with membranous glomerulonephritis causing the nephrotic syndrome. Pain over the affected kidney with haematuria in addition to the stigmata of nephrotic syndrome coupled with occasionally palpable renal enlargement and progressive renal failure provides a clue to the diagnosis. Pyelonephritis is a reasonable differential for the clinical presentation but the absence of temperature, lack of sensitive indicators in the urine dipstick (leucocytes and nitrites) and markedly raised D-dimer are less likely. Diagnosis is by renal vein Doppler ultrasound, CT scan or rarely with renal angiography. Treatment is similar to that for pulmonary embolus with oral anticoagulation for up to 6 months. Pancreatitis does present with abdominal pain and can cause deterioration in renal function when severe, however the clinical picture is one of renal pathology. Addisonian crisis can occur when patients are taken off long-term steroids abruptly due to suppression of the normal hypothalamo-pituitary-adrenal axis and manifests clinically with hypotension, lethargy, hyperkalaemia, hyponatraemia and hypoglycaemia. Pulmonary embolus may indeed mimic abdominal pain if thrombosis involves the lower lobe blood supply; however, usually signs of hypoxia, tachypnoea and tachycardia prevail. D-dimer findings are raised in any venous thrombosis but may be raised in a variety of disorders and is only of clinical value in ruling out venous thrombosis. Arterial blood gases aid the diagnosis and should be considered in any patient with signs of respiratory compromise.

55 d. Non-steroidal anti-inflammatory drugs act on cyclo-oxygenase to reduce formation of prostaglandins thereby dampening the inflammatory response as well as reducing pain sensation. Prostaglandins play an important role in vasodilatation of renal vasculature. Inhibiting the production of prostaglandins adversely affects the flow of blood to the kidney. This can cause huge changes in glomerular filtration rate (GFR, and hence renal function and urine output) in patients with already compromised renal function and thus should be avoided in cases of moderate to severe renal impairment. Simply stopping the offending medication and rehydrating the patient should bring the renal function back to pre-existing baseline. Analgesia is often difficult in patients with severe renal failure as doses, e.g. morphine, may need to be much reduced to prevent the build-up of drug and toxic metabolites, however the reduced dose may not always provide effective pain relief. Amoxicillin should be given at a reduced dose and has an increased tendency to cause crystalluria and rashes in severe renal failure but it itself is not strongly associated with intrinsic renal damage. Clarithromycin should be used at half the normal dose if the GFR is less than 30 mL/minute. Paracetamol and sodium docusate are safe to use at normal doses in renal failure.

56 a. Severe psychiatric illness is an absolute contraindication to renal transplantation except in very exceptional cases where a patient has been assessed by a psychiatrist and deemed fit to comply under very rigorous criteria. An ability to attend regularly for follow-up appointments, total compliance with post-transplantation medical care and a high level of motivation and understanding of the drastic lifestyle implementation required with a transplanted kidney are crucial factors in selecting candidates for receipt of organs. Relative contraindications, which may be considered on an individual basis, include cardiac disease assessed by a cardiologist to be compatible with the demands of immunosuppression and transplantation, chronic non-active hepatitis, minor treatable infections (excluding active tuberculosis and HIV) and quiescent or well-treated cancer. Renal transplantation is the modality of choice for diabetic nephropathy and paediatric patients with ESRF but due to a worldwide shortage of suitable donors the wait for an available organ may be on average in excess of 2 years. The life expectancy at 3 years for a first renal transplant is approximately 90% with between 2% and 6% of those on the waiting list for a transplant dying before transplantation.

57 d. Rifampicin is known for causing a reddish/orange discolouration to the urine among other non-therapeutic effects that include liver enzyme induction and resistance when used not in combination with other anti-tuberculous medications. These effects are helpfully summed up by 'the three R's of Rifampicin' (**R**evs up liver enzymes, **R**ed/orange discolouration and **R**esistance when used alone). True causes of haematuria are best described anatomically from the kidney downwards and include glomerulonephritic processes, polycystic kidney disease, trauma and urinary tract stone. Infectious processes include TB, cystitis of the bladder and schistosomiasis (especially if the patient has a positive travel history) and prostatic carcinoma, urethral trauma, urethritis or neoplasm. General causes of abnormal coagulation must always be excluded in any case of bleeding and inherited bleeding disorders such as haemophilia and any derangement in coagulation profile must be excluded. Malaria can cause haematuria and a full history of recent travel must be elicited. Investigation of this often benign but occasionally life-threatening parasitic disease must be undertaken swiftly but should not delay empirical treatment if laboratory turn around times of thick and thin films looking for malarial parasites is slow. Treatment of *Plasmodium falciparum* malaria is of vital importance due to the association with cerebral malaria and should depend on local sensitivities to anti-malarial drugs; however, a week's course of quinine followed by fansidar (with glucose-6-phosphatase deficiency, G6PD, investigation) is usually an adequate treatment regime. G6PD deficiency poses a risk of haemolytic anaemia with certain medications notably antimalarials and G6PD status is usually taken as soon as possible to but not delaying the start of treatment.

58 b. The history of a crush injury with radiographic confirmation of extensive soft tissue swelling with deranged renal function makes the diagnosis of rhabdomyolysis the most likely explanation. When interpreting renal biochemical tests it is important to have an idea about a patient's baseline creatinine as the investigation and treatment strategy of acute renal failure are very different to that of chronic renal failure. Muscle injury from trauma, ischaemia, cold or toxins releases myoglobin and protein fragments that are nephrotoxic and cause tubular damage. Urine myoglobin levels (where available) or creatinine kinase levels are useful tests to aid the diagnosis. Renal contusions may present with varying degrees of haematuria but usually there is a history of damage to the renal angle and for acute renal impairment to occur usually bilateral involvement (or rarely a lone damaged kidney!) is required. Cholesterol embolus should be suspected if a net-like rash (livedo reticularis) is associated with renal failure in association with invasive procedures such as cardiac catheterisation or multiple trauma but usually occur on a background of atherosclerosis. Acute interstitial nephritis is well associated with certain medications most notably the penicillins and non-steroidal anti-inflammatory drugs but a typical history usually includes haematuria, proteinuria, eosinophiluria and raised eosinophil count due to the type IV hypersensitivity reaction. Urethral rupture should be considered in any case of trauma with pelvic injury and a failure to pass urine and digital rectal examination may reveal a free-floating prostate. Urinary catheterisation should not be attempted until this diagnosis has been excluded due to the risks of creating a false passage or in fact exacerbating any pre-existing anatomical disruption.

59 a. Creatinine kinase and myoglobin urinalysis are two useful screens for assessing the likelihood of rhabdomyolysis causing renal failure. Often the diagnosis is self-evident from the history; however, in the elderly and unconscious there may be a lack of clinical information regarding possible muscular damage. A typical scenario for rhabdomyolysis outside of the sphere of trauma is an elderly patient who is brought to hospital with a fall who has been lying on a cold hard floor for hours to days. A renal ultrasound scan is a useful and non-invasive investigation of renal failure without a readily identifiable cause and may show obstruction, renal masses and kidney size that may guide further investigation. Twenty-four-hour urine protein collection is a useful test for quantifying proteinuria, which in the nephrotic syndrome is found in the urine at a rate of 3g/24 hours. Normal range of proteinuria is up to 150mg/24 hours but can be elevated above this level (but below 3g/24 hours) in times of stress, heavy exercise, infection and in children. Bence–Jones protein is an assay for the light-chain breakdown products of monoclonal immunoglobulins that are excreted by the kidney in excess in myeloma. It is commonly encountered in elderly patients who may present with bone pain, signs of hypercalcaemia and even pathological fractures associated with signs of renal failure. Renal artery Dopplers would be a useful investigation of suspected renal artery stenosis (RAS) and allow waveform morphology and flow velocity in the renal and perirenal aorta to be assessed. A reduction in flow below a threshold velocity indicates a significant degree of stenosis. Bilateral RAS is a contraindication to using angiotensin-converting enzyme inhibitors (ACE-I) and renal function must be watched when starting ACE-I in case this condition is present.

60 e. Acute pyelonephritis itself usually does not cause hypertension and blood pressure is usually within the normal range. However, hypotension may in fact be seen due to systemic sepsis and the systemic inflammatory response syndrome causing systemic release of inflammatory mediators, which in turn causes peripheral vasodilatation and a drop in blood pressure. Recurrent urinary tract infections, especially in childhood when associated with abnormalities of the urinary tract (most commonly vesicoureteric reflux), can lead to renal scarring seen on renal ultrasonography. This in turn predisposes to hypertension by a mechanism thought to be due to the abnormal blood flow through scarred regions. Interestingly only reflux of infected urine has been linked to renal scarring; sterile refluxing urine requires only low-dose prophylactic antibiotic to prevent infection that will lead to scarring. RAS is often diagnosed after an angiotensin-converting enzyme inhibitor (ACE-I) has been started with a sharp rise in urea and creatinine shortly after commencement. This is due to the decrease in glomerular efferent arteriole tone being lost when levels of angiotensin II (the end-product of ACE) fall secondary to ACE-I use. As those with RAS have a reduced flow through the glomerular afferent arteriole they require an intrinsically high tone at the efferent arteriole to maintain an adequate glomerular filtration pressure. Once the efferent tone is reduced then the glomerular filtration rate tails off rapidly and renal failure ensues. The intrinsic reduction in blood flow to the kidney in RAS is detected by the juxtaglomerular apparatus, which is responsible for upregulating renin–angiotensin levels to increase blood pressure to maintain adequate perfusion and thus these patients often present with hypertension.

Extended matching questions

61 e. A diagnostic coronary angiogram is indicated in this case. The mildly positive troponin and associated ECG changes increase the likelihood that this lady is suffering from cardiac chest pain. Whilst she has no cardiovascular history it is not inconceivable that this could be the first presentation of underlying problems. Information could be gleaned from echocardiogram but the most appropriate diagnostic investigation is a coronary angiogram.

Risk factors for cardiovascular disease include:
- Male sex
- Hypertension
- Hypercholesterolaemia
- Diabetes
- Smoking
- Family history
- Homocysteine levels

62 b. An ECG is the most sensible place to start in investigation of this lady's symptoms. The most likely cause for her symptoms is either sinus pauses or arrhythmias. Should she have been taking vast numbers of medications this would have been a sensible place to start. If an ECG does not yield a diagnosis it may then be sensible to proceed onto a 24-hour tape to hunt for further answers.

63 c. An echocardiogram would provide useful information about the necessity for anticoagulation in this case. In cardiovascular disease anticoagulation may be divided into two levels, warfarinisation or antiplatelet therapy. Antiplatelet therapy includes both aspirin and clopidogrel. In the absence of a dilated left atrium warfarinisation is unnecessary as the likelihood of a thrombus forming in a normal atrium is slim. Should an echocardiogram reveal a dilated left atrium warfarinisation should be discussed with the patient, since there are serious implications to warfarin particularly in elderly patients.

64 d. An ETT is the next logical step in risk stratification of this patient. He has ECG changes, a history of chest pain but negative troponin. Any changes on ETT will help to identify risk to this patient of developing cardiovascular disease or symptoms. Depending on the findings, it may be necessary to proceed onto a coronary angiogram.

65 f. These findings are suggestive of some form of arrhythmia. With rate variations such as this, in excess of 40 beats per minute, a cause should be sought. A 24-hour tape should provide adequate information about the cause of these rate variations. Based on this information treatment may be commenced. An ECG alone is unlikely to show any cause for this rate variation as it captures a period of 6 seconds only.

66 a. Pneumococcal pneumonia is the commonest bacterial pneumonia affecting all ages but is especially common in the elderly. Other groups commonly affected are alcoholics, patients after splenectomy, immunosuppressed patients and patients with chronic heart failure or those with pre-existing lung disease. Patients usually complain of fever and pleurisy. A classical chest X-ray appearance is one of a lobar pneumonia.

67 d. *Psuedomonas* is a common pathogen in those patients suffering with cystic fibrosis and bronchiectasis. It is often associated with an increasing mortality and a general deterioration in their clinical condition. The treatment is usually with anti-pseudomonal penicillins, e.g. piperacillin.

68 e. Mycoplasma pneumonia affects young, well people. It presents with general features that often precede the chest signs and symptoms by 4–5 days. Often physical signs in the chest are scanty and don't fit the clinical picture. The chest X-ray does not frequently correlate with the clinical state of the patient. Following diagnosis treatment is usually with erythromycin. Occasionally extrapulmonary features take over the clinical picture.

69 b. Usually follows a viral illness, especially seen in i.v. drug abusers or in those patients with indwelling central venous catheters. Chest X-ray appearances are normally of patchy consolidation, which can break down to form abscesses, forming a cystic appearance on chest X-ray. Other complications include pneumothoraces, effusions and empyemas. The mortality with this form of pneumonia is approximately 25% and treatment with i.v. antibiotics (flucloxacillin) is usually advised.

70 f. This is most likely to be due to infection with *Legionella pneumophila*, which infects water supplies to hospitals, hotels and workplaces. It characteristically follows a prodrome of a viral illness with a high temperature and associated extrapulmonary features including diarrhoea, hyponatraemia and confusion. Once diagnosed either by sputum, bronchial washings or urine analysis treatment is simple with clarithromycin, ciprofloxacin or rifampicin for 2–3 weeks.

71 a. Viral hepatitis presents with a patient who is unwell with lethargy and malaise and who may present with jaundice and abdominal pain. There is often hepatomegaly, which is smooth and tender (unlike the non-tender craggy hepatomegaly of carcinoma or metastasis) and the patient may feel nauseated, anorexic and have experienced some weight loss. Intrahepatic cholestasis causes a deepening jaundice and derangement of liver enzymes, notably the aminotransferases indicate hepatic inflammation. Groups at risk from hepatitis infection include haemophiliacs prior to the 1980s (when routine screening for blood-borne viruses was not undertaken in donated blood products), intravenous drug users, those engaging in risky sexual practice, health care workers and from vertical transmission.

72 d. Lower lobe pneumonia may present with abdominal signs and indeed may occasionally be investigated from the general surgical standpoint. In a confused patient from a nursing home, infection should always be at the top of the differential and a septic screen should be performed. This involves a urine dipstick, chest radiography, blood cultures, urine, sputum and faeces culture as well as routine blood tests. If this does not reveal any source of infection then other causes of confusion must be rule out and CT scan of the head, thyroid function tests, syphilis serology and haematinics may be considered as clinically indicated. In this particular case there is strong suspicion that the patient may have aspirated, as she is PEG fed and was observed to have regurgitated her feed. Starting antibiotics for an aspiration pneumonia such as cefuroxime and metronidazole would be appropriate if clinical and/or radiographic findings confirmed the diagnosis.

73 **f.** DKA is almost exclusively seen in type I diabetics requiring insulin injection. DKA can be precipitated by acute disease such as surgery, infection and even a myocardial infarction. Insulin requirements increase in time of homeostatic stress and a failure to increase or even take insulin during a period of illness may cause blood glucose levels to become very high. This causes a lack of glucose metabolism and an increase in ketone formation due to the increased availability of circulating free fatty acids. Ketone bodies are acidic in nature and cause a metabolic acidosis, which is compensated by an increase in ventilation rate to blow off carbon dioxide. The treatment of DKA hinges around adequate fluid rehydration (up to 5 L in an 18-hour period) and reduction of blood glucose with suppression of ketogenesis. The latter two are achieved by insulin infusion at a rate of 3–6 units of short-acting insulin an hour. Potassium replacement is almost always required in addition as insulin will drive potassium intracellularly and an apparently 'normal' level may quickly become low once therapy is instituted.

74 **b.** Cholecystitis is often depicted as a disease affecting a population described as 'Fat, Female, Forty and Fertile'. Whilst slightly outdated in approach this aide memoire does provide some useful guidelines when considering those at risk for gallstone disease. Only 10% of gallstones contain calcium and thus are radio-opaque on plain abdominal radiographs (in stark contrast to over 90% of renal stones) and thus the first-line investigation for suspected cholecystitis is ultrasound. This patient additionally exhibits a sonographic positive Murphy's sign – the patient will typically 'catch their breath' on inspiration with the ultrasound probe placed at the right upper quadrant as the inflamed gallbladder descends on inspiration and impinges on the probe. The presence of pericholecystic fluid and a thickened gallbladder wall as well as the presence of gallstones aids in the diagnosis of cholecystitis. Intrahepatic duct

dilatation suggests common bile duct obstruction and many centres suggest further imaging of the biliary tree with magnetic resonance cholangiopancreatography.

75 **h.** Subphrenic abscess is a recognised complication of liver and biliary tree surgery. Seen at around 2–5 days post-surgery the patient typically presents with a swinging fever, pain in the right (or left) upper quadrant and raised inflammatory markers. Septic screen results may return normal and the surgical aphorism, 'pus somewhere, pus nowhere, pus under the diaphragm', reminds the clinician to consider subphrenic abscess as the cause of a patient's pyrexia. Small abscesses may respond to a conservative approach with antibiotic therapy and may resolve. Larger or loculated (organising) abscesses merit drainage and/or surgical evacuation.

76 **d.** This woman is suffering an attack of inflammatory bowel disease and has a history consistent with a moderate to severe exacerbation. She should be managed initially medically unless any complications such as perforation, uncontrolled bleeding or toxic megacolon should occur, and should be started on oral prednisolone and a 5-aminosalicylate such as mesalazine for symptom relief initially. The history of conjunctivitis and arthritis in a young person with bloody diarrhoea and mucous in the absence of foreign travel or sexually transmitted infection is likely to be an extra-gastrointestinal manifestation of either Crohn's disease or ulcerative colitis.

77 **a.** *Clostridium difficile* is the most likely agent to have caused this man's diarrhoea. Treatment with antibiotics has been linked to selection of drug-resistant strains of *C. difficile* with resultant overgrowth and the development of pseudomembranous colitis. Particularly linked with the development of pseudomembranous colitis is clindamycin; however, the cephalosporins have also been demonstrated to cause this and few antibiotics are free from this rare but serious side-effect. The colonoscopic appearance is one of an erythematous colonic mucosa with a faint cream or grey pseudomembrane. A stool sample for parasites, bacterium and *C. difficile* toxin should be taken and it is important that antidiarrhoeal therapy is not instituted unless the sample is clear for fear of prolonging and exacerbating the infection. Treatment is either with oral metronidazole or oral vancomycin and rationalisation of antibiotic therapy.

78 **b.** This man is showing the clinical signs and symptoms of diabetic ketoacidosis (DKA) with a low pH and metabolic acidosis,

ketonuria and hyperglycaemia. Precipitants of DKA can range from infection to myocardial infarction and typically a history is given of an acute illness with a failure to increase insulin requirements appropriately. Travel and erratic eating pattern can disrupt the normal rhythm of blood glucose regulation and a superimposed infection can quickly cause even the most disease-aware individuals to become unwell. The diarrhoea is due to osmotic sequestration of fluid in the gut due to high glucose and electrolyte levels and will cause massive dehydration of up to 5 L quite easily along with polyuria. The treatment strategy includes fast fluid rehydration and high level of insulin infusion to reduce glucose level and suppress ketogenesis. Conversion to sliding scale of insulin can be undertaken after a few days once the initial hyperglycaemia and ketogenesis (as monitored effectively by simple urine dipsticks) have settled.

79 **e.** These are the classical signs and symptoms of hyperthyroidism with heat intolerance, diarrhoea, mood changes especially anxiety and mania and weight loss. Physical signs include increased sweating, tachycardia that does not abate at night or at rest, proptosis, lid lag and exophthalmos if Grave's disease is causative and a fine tremor. The exact opposite is true for those suffering from hypothyroidism and represent one of the starkest physiological correlates of biochemical disturbance with neurokinetic manifestations. Treatment is aimed to cure and to palliate symptoms and employs both a beta-blocker such as propranolol (in the absence of contraindication) to control symptoms of tremor, tachycardia and excess sympathetic over-activation and a thioureylene such as carbimazole is used to inhibit the iodination of thyroglobulin thereby reducing the synthesis of the end-products T3 and T4. A rare but serious side-effect of carbimazole is the development of agranulocytosis and repeat full blood counts must be undertaken. Patients are told to report immediately to hospital or their GP if they develop symptoms such as a sore throat as this may signify the development of agranulocytosis.

80 **i.** Bulimia nervosa can manifest in many different ways but the core symptoms that allow a diagnosis to be made are prevalent in all. Typically the patient is a young female with characteristic episodes of binge eating, particularly of sugar-rich foods and snack. The period of overeating is then countered with a period of self-induced vomiting, food avoidance or restriction or even laxative abuse and may present to hospital with diarrhoea. Patients are often aware that their behaviour is

detrimental to their health and may be ashamed and disgusted with it. Rapid weight losses can lead to a cessation of periods (secondary amenorrhoea) and usually occurs when total body weight falls below 45 kg. Biochemical disturbances due to vomiting and diarrhoea are common and low levels of potassium may be seen. Treatment strategies may involve psychiatrists when symptoms are severe especially in cases of self-harm or suicidal behaviour and is focused on changing the behaviour that drives the impulses behind binge eating.

81 a. Benign prostatic hyperplasia (BPH) and prostate cancer can cause haematuria although this is a rarer clinical finding in BPH due to prostatic vein congestion. BPH most commonly presents with lower urinary tract symptoms (LUTS), which can be neatly summed up by the mnemonic 'WISE FUN' standing for **W**aiting to pass urine, **I**ntermittency, **S**training to pass urine, **E**ffortless passing (incontinence), **F**requency, **U**rgency and **N**octuria. Conversely prostatic carcinoma tends not to cause these symptoms until it is very advanced due to neoplastic growth of the peripheral rim of prostatic tissue rather than the central enlargement of the prostatic core seen in BPH. A digital rectal examination is vital in the assessment of prostatic enlargement due to hyperplasia or neoplasm and prostate-specific antigen levels may help monitor treatment for confirmed malignancy. Typically the enlargement of the prostate gland felt in BPH is smooth whilst that of prostatic carcinoma is craggy and nodular. Surgical therapy to ameliorate BPH is usually performed via the urethra (transurethral resection of the prostate) and consists of coring out the enlarged periurethral prostate to relieve the symptoms of bladder outflow obstruction.

82 d. Bladder carcinomas in Western populations are overwhelmingly transitional cell carcinoma (TCC) with a very small number showing histology of other cell types such as squamous cell or adenocarcinoma. Although TCC of the bladder is often of unknown aetiology associations between chemical exposure (in particular aniline dyes, hair dye and smoking – nitrosamines present in carcinogenic quantities in cigarette smoke) have been described. Chronic infection with organisms such as schistosomiasis and bladder stone disease has been linked to an increased incidence of squamous cell carcinoma. Embryological abnormalities such as a persistent urachal remnant (communicating between umbilicus and bladder) have also been shown to predispose to bladder carcinoma. Seen more commonly in men than females and in the latter during the later decades of life, bladder carcinomas are the second most common urological cancer (after cancer of the prostate) and the most frequent malignant tumour of the urinary tract. Painless haematuria is the most common presenting complaint but may be complicated by clot retention, i.e. where the build-up of clotted blood inside the bladder obstructs the bladder outflow tract causing urinary retention. Treatment of clot retention is by insertion of a three-way urinary catheter into the bladder and constant irrigation until the urine runs clear.

83 c. Schistosomiasis affects over 200 million people in the tropics and is found commonly in those from the Middle East and Africa. Three main strains of *Schistosoma* cause disease in humans: *Schistosoma mansoni, S. japonicum and S. haematobium* of which *S. japonicum* is most commonly linked to severe disease. The life-cycle of *Schistosoma* revolves around carriage in the water snail – an intermediate host, before being released into water where they attempt to penetrate the mucous membrane and skin of the human host. Each strain of *Schistosoma* presents slightly differently and *S. mansoni* primarily affects large bowel with migration to the liver with diarrhoea, hepatitis and portal hypertension. *S. japonicum* affects both large and small bowel as well as the liver but may cause neurological and respiratory symptoms if migration to the brain and lung occur. *S. haematobium* (bilharzia), as the name suggests, usually affects the bladder causing painless haematuria with progressive obstructive symptoms as bladder inflammation increases in severity and hydronephrosis, renal failure and loin pain may develop. The treatment for trematode disease in the main is praziquantel tablets at a dose of 40 mg/kg taken with food with the aim of treatment not necessarily being to eradicate the disease but to reduce the effect of chronic infection of which a serious complication is squamous cell carcinoma of the bladder.

84 f. UTI is a common cause of transient haematuria (which is often only discovered on urine dipstick as microscopic haematuria) and one of the commonest causes of confusion in the elderly. Any patient who presents with confusion should have a urine dipstick and sample sent for microscopy, culture and sensitivity as this is an easily treatable and thus reversible cause of confusion and should never be missed. The signs of pyrexia accompanying suprapubic tenderness point strongly to a diagnosis of UTI and the clinician must be quick to treat empirically on the basis of clinical suspicion whilst sensitivities and organisms are awaited to prevent the development of the more serious pyelonephritis, which in compromised patients may be life threatening. A choice of a cephalosporin such as cefuroxime or alternatively trimethoprim if a 'simple' UTI is suspected for a period of 3–7 days depending on severity is usually enough to resolve the infection. A single UTI in a young male prompts investigation of at least blood glucose (for diabetes) and occasionally a renal tract ultrasound to assess for renal tract abnormalities as this type of infection is uncommon in this population and may point to an underlying hitherto undiscovered cause.

85 **h.** Renal trauma can be divided up into categories based upon type of injury to the kidney, i.e. laceration, vascular disruption or contusion (bruising) and the mode of injury causing the damage, i.e. blunt or penetrating injury. When assessing a patient with suspected renal trauma it is of paramount importance that a systematic method is adopted, such as the 'ABCDE' approach to trauma. Assessing the airway and cervical spine should be the first priority with any immediate intervention, e.g. airway adjuncts performed before moving to assess other systems. A quick assessment of breathing starting with the presence or absence of breath sound, symmetry of lung expansion and any abnormal findings should be performed with any appropriate intervention carried out as necessary. Circulation should then be assessed starting with examination of pulses and vital signs (blood pressure, capillary refill, etc.). Disability refers to any deficit in function that may have occurred as a result of trauma, e.g. neurological upset and musculoskeletal system for fractures and dislocations. A more complete examination may be performed once the clinician is satisfied that the airway, breathing and circulation are stable and abdominopelvic examination should always be considered as exsanguination (catastrophic and fatal blood loss) can quickly and insidiously occur with abdominal and pelvic visceral or bony injury. Exposure forms the last part of the primary survey with assessment of areas previously not examined such as the spine (normally accessed by log-rolling patients until the cervical spine has been radiologically and clinically cleared from injury) and the level of exposure to the environment, e.g. temperature, soft tissue injury and wound assessment

86 **a.** This gentleman has injured his common peroneal nerve. It is a branch of the sciatic nerve and may be damaged following trauma, application of a plaster cast or by repeated kneeling. It provides the motor supply to the muscles of the anterior and lateral compartments of the leg. It is the most commonly

damaged nerve in the lower limb and is relatively unprotected as it traverses the lateral aspect of the head of the fibula.

Clinical features include:
- Foot drop.
- Weakness of dorsiflexion and eversion of the foot.
- Weakness of extensor hallucis longus.
- Loss of sensation over the lower lateral part of the leg and dorsum of the foot.

87 h. The axillary nerve winds around the head of the humerus. It is this tortuous course that puts it at risk from damage from trauma, e.g. from cast application or during rotator cuff surgery. It supplies the deltoid muscle and teres minor and therefore results in problems with shoulder elevation and abduction. It also provides sensation to the skin on the lateral aspect of the arm over the body of deltoid muscle.

88 b. This lady is describing symptoms of median nerve palsy. In addition to these symptoms she may note a weakness in the muscles of her thenar eminence with associated wasting. This is likely to be caused by carpal tunnel syndrome, which results in compression being applied to the median nerve as it passes under the flexor retinaculum on the palmar aspect of the wrist. If this is the cause it can be treated with a carpal tunnel decompression, although since she is complaining of bilateral symptoms the cause may result from a lesion of the cervical vertebrae.

89 g. This lady has damaged her ulnar nerve. It runs in the cubital tunnel and may be damaged following injuries to the bones in that area. The symptoms resulting are those mentioned in the case as the ulnar nerve supplies sensation to the medial half of the ring finger and the little finger. It provides motor supply to the intrinsic muscles of the hand and therefore weakness and reduced function may ensue.

90 f. This patient is complaining of pain and burning sensation over the distribution of the lateral cutaneous nerve of the thigh. It passes from the lateral border of psoas major across the iliac fossa to pierce the inguinal ligament. It travels in a fibrous tunnel medial to the anterior superior iliac spine and enters the thigh deep to the fascia lata before continuing distally into the subcutaneous tissues. The nerve can become compressed as it passes under the inguinal ligament resulting in meralgia paraesthetica, provided there are no associated motor signs the treatment of this is conservative.